HEALTHCARE BIOTECHNOLOGY

A Practical Guide

HEALTHCARE BIOTECHNOLOGY

A Practical Guide

DIMITRIS DOGRAMATZIS

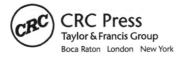

CRC Press
Taylor & Francis Group
Boca Raton London New York

CRC Press is an imprint of the
Taylor & Francis Group, an **informa** business

CRC Press
Taylor & Francis Group
6000 Broken Sound Parkway NW, Suite 300
Boca Raton, FL 33487-2742

© 2011 by Taylor and Francis Group, LLC
CRC Press is an imprint of Taylor & Francis Group, an Informa business

First issued in paperback 2019

No claim to original U.S. Government works

ISBN-13: 978-0-367-45227-8 (pbk)
ISBN-13: 978-1-4398-4746-6 (hbk)

Library of Congress Cataloging-in-Publication Data

Dogramatzis, Dimitris, 1962- , author.
  Healthcare biotechnology : a practical guide / Dimitris Dogramatzis.
    p. ; cm.
  Includes bibliographical references and index.
  Summary: "A first of its kind to focus on the management of health-care related biotechnology, this text is a resourceful practical guide that assists all healthcare related biotech professionals in their day-to-day activities. The book contains chapters on bioeconomy, biolicensing, biofinance, biopartnering, biodrug research, biomarketing planning, biopromotion, product life cycle management, and biobusiness models, among others. Written by a well-established professional and registered pharmacist, this reference is appropriate for graduate students and industry professionals. It contains over 350 tables and figures and end-of-section problems accompany each chapter. There are also extensive references following each chapter to enhance further study"--Provided by publisher.
  ISBN 978-1-4398-4746-6 (hardcover : alkaline paper)
  1. Pharmaceutical biotechnology. 2. Biotechnology. 3. Biotechnology industries. I. Title.
  [DNLM: 1. Biomedical Technology--organization & administration. W 82]

RS380.D64 2011
615'.19--dc22   2010043670

Visit the Taylor & Francis Web site at
http://www.taylorandfrancis.com

and the CRC Press Web site at
http://www.crcpress.com

*To George,
Vasilis, and Maria,
with eternal love.*

Contents

Preface

To encompass modern biotechnology within a book is like rowing across the Atlantic Ocean. However, the book you are currently holding in your hands has a clear vision: To contribute a tiny amount of knowledge but a significant amount of understanding to the modern world of healthcare biotechnology management. In doing so, our mission will be to utilize knowledge available through the biomedical sciences, finance, and marketing so as to understand the process of bringing a healthcare innovation from the laboratory bench to the patient's bedside.

This book is focused on the management of healthcare-related biotech, from its conception stage and throughout the biotech product and company life cycle. More specifically, it aims to become a resourceful practical guide, assisting all healthcare-related biotech professionals in their day-to-day activities, even ruining its pages by lab fluid spillages, executive board meeting coffee accidents, or sales managers' hectic lifestyle habits.

ORGANIZATION

The book is divided into six parts, following the exact journey a biomedical innovation takes through its adventurous life cycle. Part I, "The Healthcare Biotechnology Industry," is devoted to studying the operating environment of healthcare biotechnology. Chapter 1, "Bioeconomy," presents the concept of "red," or healthcare biotechnology within other biotechnology applications, and compares it with its sister pharmaceutical industry. It discusses briefly the commercial progress made to date and the controversy surrounding its business returns. It then goes on to discuss the major players, starting from the companies involved, the products launched, and the participating geographical regions.

Part II, "Intellectual Property," covers the significant topic of intellectual property (IP) protection, a prerequisite to any successful biotechnology commercialization effort. Chapter 2, "Intellectual Property Management," takes us through the various kinds of existing IPs and the issue of the powerful inventions of biotechnology that can be patented around the world. It also focuses on the process of patent application and the significance of strategic IP management, and discusses the consequences that a competitor who attempts to challenge a biopharma's IP portfolio has to go through. Chapter 3, "Biolicensing," focuses on the innovation creation cycle and the arduous steps required to commercialize any biotechnology application. It also focuses on the means to accelerate commercialization and the efforts of every company involved in pursuing the fruits of academic research through the technology transfer process, as well as the licensing of inventions made by other companies in the field. The licensing process is further elaborated upon to include the actual agreement process and the financial objectives involved.

Part III, "Funding," describes how a biopharmaceutical company may support its cash-intensive activities or get involved in partnering with another company in the field. Chapter 4, "Biofinance," focuses on the financing life cycle and the numerous funding alternatives available today. It goes on to discuss the idea of "exiting" by an investor wishing to focus on something new, and the impact of valuation on biotechnology start-ups. Chapter 5, "Biopartnering," discusses why biotechnology firms need each other or a classical pharmaceutical (big pharma) player in order to remain viable through the choppy seas of the commercialization process. In doing so, it also describes the essentials of alliance implementation and management, and how a company can attract and retain the best of biopharmaceutical partners.

Part IV, "New Product," guides us through the challenges involved in biopharmaceutical research and development and biomanufacturing. Chapter 6, "Biodrug Research," takes us through the clinical trial design and the processes mandated by the biggest regulatory agencies in the world. The alternative processes of fast-track approval are also presented, as are the essentials of patient recruitment or collaborating with external partners called contract research organizations. Finally, the idea proposed that there exists a deep innovation gap between resources available and molecules discovered, and various methods proposed to counteract it are presented in detail. Chapter 7, "Biomanufacturing," focuses on the production platforms and processes involved in healthcare biotechnology, as well as the strategies, relevant costs, and timelines involved.

Part V, "Marketing," revolves around the quintessential process of creating and defining a biotechnology product, pricing it appropriately, distributing it to different corners of the world, and promoting it to its diverse audiences, each with its own characteristics and peculiarities. Chapter 8, "Biomarketing Planning," discusses the basic concept of its "four Ps," analyzes the modern healthcare environment, and presents the tools for studying it in detail. It also explains the value of segmenting any market, planning how to launch new products, and thriving in the competitive market. Chapter 9, "Biopromotion," discusses the branding of biopharmaceuticals and promoting them by using any means available, from the traditional sales forces to the emerging social networking sites and beyond. Chapter 10, "Biopricing," discusses the sensitive issues surrounding healthcare costs and government efforts to contain them, and how biopharmaceutical companies choose a product pricing strategy, how they actually price their products before a global launch, and how they attempt to explain the sometimes huge prices to the authorities and consumers alike. Achieving reimbursement is also discussed, as well as the modern trend of innovative deals between biopharmas and insurance providers around the world.

Chapter 11, "Biosupply Chain," takes us through the characteristics of U.S. and European pharmaceutical supply chains and the distribution models existing for biopharmaceuticals today. The concept of special networks setup for specialty pharmaceuticals and the issue of biosupply chain management are also elaborated upon. Chapter 12, "Biobrand Life Cycle Management," covers the distinct life cycle of biopharmaceuticals, from the moment they are commercially launched to patent expiration, product extensions, and market withdrawal, each requiring special resources and tactics to succeed. The strategies and tactics of original medicines against the ever-present generic and bioequivalent biopharmaceuticals are also discussed.

Finally, Part VI, "Running the Business," which consists of Chapter 13, "Biobusiness Models," and Chapter 14, "Biocompany Life Cycle," focuses on the numerous models currently in operation and describes the life period of a biopharmaceutical company itself, through inception, adolescence, maturity, and decline, as well as the steps required along the way to not only remain viable but also to thrive in an extremely competitive world.

SPECIAL FEATURES

This book is not meant to be a complicated research thesis. Instead, it is designed to be a practical guide, allowing the reader to pace his or her reading through the individual chapters, to rethink and redesign the numerous figures and tables as they please, and to transform the appendices into useful tools. There are more than 40 figures, 220 tables, and 180 references. There are also two appendices on the field of healthcare biotechnology management that include a useful list of abbreviations and a biopharmaceutical product business plan outline.

As far as biotechnology management students and educators are concerned, every chapter contains 10 questions and 10 exercises. The questions focus on material contained within the book and the answers can be easily found if you know where to look. The exercises are meant to challenge your curiosity, managerial acumen, and entrepreneurial thinking. Thus, the answers are not provided easily. Instead, they challenge you to take the extra step, to search and discuss, to summarize and present, to defend and object. For example, the exercises frequently ask you to find additional material over the Internet, as per detailed instructions, and then put yourselves in the shoes of healthcare biotechnology entrepreneurs who are in search of their destiny. I can guarantee you this journey is more than exciting. Furthermore, interested educators can get access to a detailed solutions manual by contacting the publisher.

More than two years in the making, this book is now available to students, educators, professionals, consultants, regulators, the media, and to all those who would like to gain a deeper understanding into the world of healthcare biotechnology. In the process, as more questions are solved and new problems arise, I invite the readers to suggest different angles, additional tools and appendices, further needs, or ideas for improvement, all through my e-mail below, as I undertake to include them should a future edition be suggested.

Enjoy reading!

Dimitris Dogramatzis
gamma@otenet.gr

Author

Dr. Dimitris Dogramatzis received a bachelor's diploma in pharmacy from the University of Patras, Patras, Greece. He spent the next seven years at Texas studying and working for the University of Texas System, Austin, Texas. During this period, he completed his PhD in pharmacology and toxicology at the University of Texas Medical Branch at Galveston, Texas. He later went on to complete two successive postdoctoral trainings at the University of Texas Medical Branch at Galveston as well as at the M.D. Anderson Cancer Center at Houston, Texas.

Following his return to his native Greece in 1991, he served a mandatory military service as an army pharmacist with the Greek Army Medical Corps, and after his discharge he joined the pharmaceutical industry. His successful industry career includes field sales, medical affairs marketing, product management, disease management, country management, and regional management positions, with Hoffmann-La Roche, Lundbeck, and Serono. During 2000–2002, he served as the regional vice president of Northern Europe for the Serono International Group, responsible for the U.K., Irish, Dutch, Swedish, Danish, Norwegian, Finnish, and Icelandic markets. He is currently the owner of a retail pharmacy in Athens, a business consultant, and a writer.

He has written extensively in both English and Greek, for either basic research or business publications. His academic publications include congress abstracts, full papers, and review articles, while his business publications include several interviews, full articles, two book chapters, and the book *Pharmaceutical Marketing: A Practical Guide* (CRC Press 2001).

I

The Healthcare Biotechnology Industry

1

The Healthcare Biotechnology Industry

## CHAPTER 1

Bioeconomy

Biotechnology has created more than 200 new therapies and vaccines, including products to treat cancer, diabetes, HIV/AIDS and autoimmune disorders.

Source: Courtesy of Biotechnology Industry Association (BIO), Washington, DC, 2008.

H UMANS HAVE BEEN USING biotechnology to produce food and medicine since prehistoric times. Karl Ereky, a Hungarian engineer, suggested in 1919 the very term "biotechnology." In 1953, James D. Watson and Francis Crick published a paper in *Nature* describing the double helix (1953), eventually receiving the Nobel Prize in Physiology in 1962 (http://nobelprize.org/nobel_prizes/medicine/laureates/1962/). And, in 1976, Robert A. Swanson and Herbert W. Boyer founded Genentech, eventually succeeding in launching the first biosynthetic insulin in 1982, in collaboration with Eli Lilly.

BIOTECHNOLOGY DEFINITIONS

The United Nations' Convention on Biological Diversity (2009; http://www.cbd.int/convention/convention.shtml) defines biotechnology as "any technological application that uses biological systems, living organisms, or derivatives thereof, to make or modify products or processes for specific use." Similarly, the U.S.-based Biotechnology Industry Association (BIO; http://www.bio.org) defines it as "a collection of technologies that capitalize on the attributes of cells, such as their manufacturing capabilities, and put biological molecules, such as DNA and proteins, to work for

TABLE 1.1 Which Are the Most Commonly Used Biotechnologies?

DNA	Proteins	Subcellular Organisms	Cell/Tissue Culture	Processes	Other
Genomics	Sequencing	Gene therapy	Cell culture	Bioreactors	Bioinformatics
Pharmaco-genetics	Glyco-engineering	Gene vectors	Tissue engineering	Fermentation	Nanobio-technologies
Gene probes	Proteomics		Hybridization	Bioprocessing	Advanced materials
DNA sequencing	Hormones		Cellular fusion	Bioremediation	
Genetic engineering	Growth factors		Immuno-stimulation	Biofiltration	
	Cell receptors		Embryo manipulation		

Source: OECD, *Statistical Definition of Biotechnology*, Paris, France, updated in 2005, http://www.oecd.org/document/42/0,3343,en_2649_34537_1933994_1_1_1_37437,00.html (accessed on January 27, 2010). With permission.

us" (2008). Some of these "exotic" biotechnologies have been categorized by the Organization for Economic Cooperation and Development (OECD; http://www.oecd.org) in Table 1.1 (2005). Most of these terms will be further elaborated throughout this book.

WHAT IS HEALTHCARE BIOTECHNOLOGY

Biotechnology is based on a thorough understanding of biological, biochemical, and genetic processes in humans and other species. These processes were greatly elaborated after the description of the double helix, and over the last 50 years have gradually produced a collection of technologies able to describe and, most importantly, influence cellular, molecular, and genetic phenomena. This influence has led to an explosion of scientific and commercial applications across several industrial sectors (see Figure 1.1), geometrically accelerating since the dawn of the twenty-first century, leading many experts to label it as the "biotechnology century."

Red, Green, Blue, and White Biotechnologies

Today, there exist multiple commercial applications of biotechnology (biotech). More specifically, four different commercial sectors exist, each given its own corresponding coding color. In particular, *healthcare biotech is color-coded red* (from the red blood cells) and includes the biosynthetic production of medicines and vaccines, stem-cell research, DNA sequencing, and more. *Agricultural* (*green*) biotech includes biotransformation and biomediation. *Marine* (*blue*) biotech includes species preservation, viral genomics, etc. *Industrial* (*white*) biotech is involved, among other fields, with alternative energy sources. Finally, a fifth, interdisciplinary application, bioinformatics, is involved with sequence analyses, evolutionary biology, etc. For more commercial applications, see Table 1.2.

Healthcare (Red) Biotechnology

Of all the commercial applications mentioned above, healthcare biotechnology has had both a profound significance in saving, extending, and improving human lives, as well as significant commercial returns for the scientists and entrepreneurs involved.

By all accounts, it is the most important commercial stream mentioned above and will, from now on, be the focus of this book. Broadly speaking, healthcare biotech is about diagnosis, prevention, and treatment of disease. For diagnosis of disease, biotech has produced a series of new biomarkers, and the tools to measure them. It has also greatly reduced the

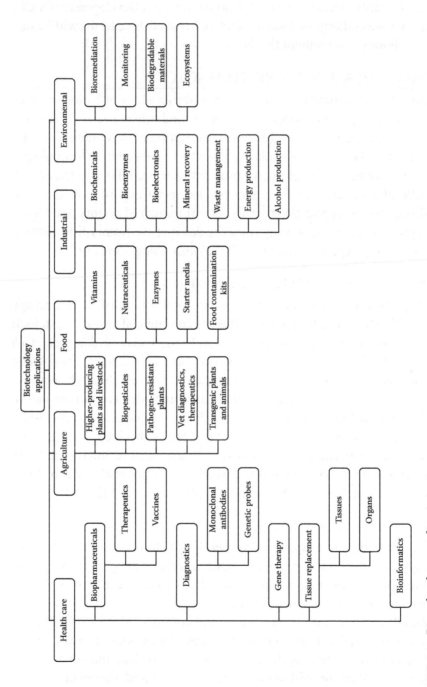

FIGURE 1.1 Biotechnology applications.

TABLE 1.2 Which Are the Commercial Applications of Biotechnology Today?

Health Care (Red)	Agricultural (Green)	Marine (Blue)	Industrial (White)	Bioinformatics
Bionanotechnology	Biomediation	Marine pharmaceuticals	Alternative energy	Genome annotation
Bionics	Bioluminescence	Microbes	Oxidoreductase	Evolutionary biology
Cloning	Biotransformation	Pollutants	Food contamination testing	Protein structures
Cybernetics	New plant varieties	Species preservation	Microbial enzymes	Biodiversity
Diagnostics	Biopesticides	Viral genomics	Organic chemicals	Sequence analysis
DNA sequencing	Pathogen resistant crops		Mineral recovery	Cancer mutations
Enzymes	Improved livestock		Bioelectronics	Combinatorial chemistry
Gene therapy	Biofarming		Waste reduction	Nucleic acid amplification
Genetics	Veterinary therapeutics			
Immune globulins	Veterinary diagnostics			
Molecular energy	Veterinary vaccines			
Monoclonal antibodies				
Pharmacogenomics				
Protein therapeutics				
Stem cells				
Tissue replacement				
Toxins				
Vaccines				

Source: Author's research.

sample volumes required, the diagnostic-related risks, and the waiting periods for results to be known. Furthermore, it has increased diagnostic portability, accuracy, sensitivity, and reproducibility.

For prevention of disease, genomics has led the way of identifying potential disease sufferers and altering their behavior; stem cell technology has led to personalization of treatment regimes, new vaccines have made more humans immune, while immune globulins and growth factors have spearheaded the fight against disease relapse and complications.

Finally, when it comes to treatment, humanity is now at a different level of fighting disease and suffering, the same way that once penicillin gave the world a new hope for survival and life expectancy prolongation. Whether it is recombinant proteins replacing naturally deficient production, or growth hormones boosting the endogenous capabilities, or monoclonal antibodies custom-designed to fight a frightening antigen, or even antibodies against autoimmune attacks, biotech has offered the solutions sought after by philosophers, alchemists, biologists, pharmacologists, and physicians over the ages. Thankfully, we are all standing at the dawn, not the sunset, of this extremely promising scientific endeavor. Healthcare biotechnology will continue to shine the way in offering innovative solutions in diagnosis, prevention, and treatment of disease in the decades to come.

Figure 1.2 shows the relative size of biopharmaceutical sales within the global pharmaceutical market between 1999 and 2009. Over this decade, biopharmaceutical contribution has increased from 6% to 23% of the global pharmaceutical market.

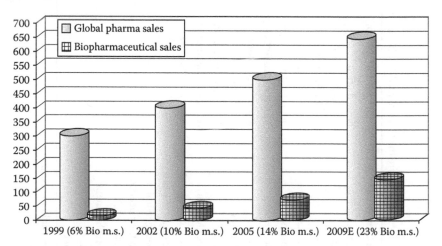

FIGURE 1.2   The global pharmaceutical market (in U.S.$ sales). (Courtesy of IMS Health, Norwalk, CT.)

THE UNFULFILLED PROMISE OF BIOTECH

Bioeconomy

The Organization for Economic Co-operation and Development (OECD; http://www.oecd.org; Paris HQ) defines bioeconomy as "an economy in which the latent value incumbent in biological products and processes is captured through economic, health, environmental and other gains" (OECD, p. 3, 2007). In other words, bioeconomy encompasses all economic activity related to scientific, research, and industrial applications based on the understanding of the generic and molecular processes of human and other species. OECD's Science and Technology ministers convened in 2004 and created a mandate for all their member states to take gradual steps in order to manage the transition to a bioeconomy. Obviously, the expected returns of bioeconomy are of major importance for the economic growth and sustainability of the respective member states in the decades ahead.

In order to better understand the current state, as well as the future prospects of bioeconomy around the world, one has to come into contact with the announcements made or special research conducted by international consulting agencies, life sciences venture capitalists, university biotechnology departments, or the various biotechnology industry associations existing in the major biotechnology nations of the world.

The first group is prominently represented by the likes of Ernst and Young (http://www.ey.com; London HQ), with their annual authoritative "Beyond Borders—Global Biotechnology Report" (2009), as well as Deloitte Recap (http://www.recap.com/; Walnut Creek, California HQ). The second group includes Burrill & Company (http://www.burrillandco.com; San Francisco HQ), a global life sciences–focused group, active in venture capital, private equity, merchant banking and media, and publishers of their own Annual Biotechnology Industry Report (2009). Within the group of academic biotechnology/technology management departments, we distinguish the likes of University of California, Berkeley (http://mot.berkeley.edu/), Cornell University (http://www.biotech.cornell.edu/), Georgetown University (http://biotechnology.georgetown.edu/), Harvard University (http://www.extension.harvard.edu/biotech/), and the University of Cambridge, United Kingdom (http://www.ceb.cam.ac.uk/index.php). Finally, some of the most prominent international biotechnology industry associations include the following: All India Biotechnology Association, AusBiotech, Bio

TABLE 1.3   Global Biotechnology at a Glance in 2008 (U.S.$ Million)

Public Company Data	Global	United States	Europe	Canada	Asia-Pacific
Revenues	89,648	66,127	16,515	2,041	4,965
R&D expense	31,745	25,270	5,171	703	601
Net income (loss)	(1,443)	417	(702)	(1,143)	(14)
Number of employees	200,760	128,200	49,060	7,970	15,530

Source: Courtesy of Ernst & Young, Beyond Borders: Global Biotechnology Report 2009, Boston, MA.

Deutschland, BioIndustry Association (United Kingdom), BioSingapore, BIOTECanada, Biotechnology Industry Organization (BIO; U.S.), EuropaBio, Nederlandse Biotechnologie Associatie, NZBio, Swiss Biotech, and SwedenBIO. Let us now review the global state of the biotechnology industry by the end of 2008. E&Y Global Biotechnology Report 2009 provides us with the top line data, summarized in Table 1.3.

Biotech Proponents

Over the last three decades, healthcare biotechnology companies, starting with Genentech in 1976, have raced to commercially capitalize on the discovery of the double helix (Watson and Crick, 1953), as well as later discoveries on how to manipulate genes by "splitting and splicing" (Professors Richard J. Roberts and Phillip A. Sharp, 1993 Nobel Prize in Physiology or Medicine; http://nobelprize.org/nobel_prizes/medicine).

During this arduous process, countless biotechnology companies have formed in the various bionations (see Major Bionations in this chapter), borrowed huge amounts of money through private or public sources, employed strong scientific minds, and, unfortunately very few have managed to commercially introduce biopharmaceuticals or vaccines into the global marketplace. By the end of 2005, there were 142 biopharmaceuticals already launched, of which 76 had originated in the United States, 21 in Europe, 8 in Japan, 15 in Switzerland, and another 5 in other countries (Australia, South Korea, and India). According to IMS, global prescription sales of biotech drugs increased 12.5% in 2007 to more than $75 billion and 22 biotech products generated sales exceeding $1 billion in 2007 (2008). Of the companies that have commercialized their products, even fewer have managed to reach profitability, thus giving birth to a recent debate on whether biotechnology has capitalized on its promise to patients, employees, and investors alike that it would soon revolutionize medicine, by achieving significant financial returns in the process.

By definition, a debate includes both proponents and critics. We will begin by discussing the views of the biotechnology proponents. As expected, related industry associations, such as the U.S. Biotechnology Industry Association (BIO, http://www.bio.org/; Washington, District of Columbia, HQ), as well as the U.S. Pharmaceutical Research and Manufacturers of America (PhRMA; http://www.phrma.org; Washington, District of Columbia, HQ) argue that biopharmaceuticals: (a) increase life expectancy, (b) decrease disability, and (c) reduce the need for health services. In addition, biopharmaceutical companies employ a significant number of Americans and bolster the U.S. economy. For example, PhRMA reported that during 2006, biopharmas employed 686,442 people, while the sector supported a total of 3.2 million jobs (direct, indirect, and induced). Furthermore, these companies had a net effect on the U.S. economy of $294.6 billion, or 2.2% of the U.S. gross domestic product (as defined by the value of sales generated less the value of raw materials used), had a total sector output of $626.6 billion, while their employees contributed $15 billion in total federal and Social Security taxes (2009).

Fine, but what about industry profitability as a whole? Is this not the epitome of business success and future sustainability? Should not the biotechnology industry, after three decades of innovation and success in therapeutics and disease prevention, be able to turn the corner and offer the promised financial returns to its loyal investors? Well, as this book was being written, two well-known sources were reporting a turn to the positive profitability side. In their 2009 Global Biotechnology Report (http://www.ey.com/Publication), E&Y reported that in 2008 the U.S. biotechnology sector reached aggregate profitability with an aggregate net income of $0.4 billion. This fact, together with Europe's declining net loss, was responsible for the global biotechnology industry profitability in 2008 being reported to have improved by 53% from 2007. The positive U.S. sector profitability was also reported by Burrill & Company, in their "Biotech 2009—Life Sciences: Navigating the Sea Change," 23rd annual report on the biotechnology industry (http://www.burrillandco.com/resources. html), when they mentioned that after 40+ years since the industry began it finally turned a profit in 2008.

The European Commission Joint Research Centre's (JRC) Institute for Prospective Technological Studies (IPTS; http://ipts.jrc.ec.europa.eu/, Seville HQ) is another proponent of the biotechnology contributions. In their "Consequences, Opportunities and Challenges of Modern

Biotechnology for Europe—The Analysis Report—Contributions of modern biotechnology to European policy objectives," published in 2008 (http://ftp.jrc.es/EURdoc/JRC44144.pdf), they reported that modern biotechnology contributes about 5% of the EU pharmaceutical market's gross value-added growth (GVA) and 0.04% to the EU's total GVA, indicating the high value of the comparatively low number of products, and that the European dedicated biotechnology industry directly employs 96,500 people, mostly in small and medium enterprises (SMEs). They also reported that, an analysis of biopharmaceutical turnover during 1996–2005 indicated that their share out of all pharmaceuticals had been constantly growing both in the EU and in the U.S. markets.

EuropaBio, the European Association for Bioindustries (http://www. europabio.org/; Brussels HQ), has 72 corporate and 6 associate members operating worldwide, 4 bioregions and 26 national biotechnology associations representing some 1800 SMEs. They report that the industry in Europe comprises some 1600 companies and represented revenues of approximately €7.8 billion in 2005; biotech companies focusing on healthcare biotech rose from 37 (1996) to 143 (2005); biotech medicines hold a 9% share of the EU pharmaceutical market; and growth rates in biopharmaceuticals are twice as high as non-biotech (2010).

For a biopharma progress towards profitability example see: THROMBOGENICS, Leuven, Belgium, THROMBOGENICS Press Release, 11 September 2009, http://www.thrombogenics.com.

Biotech Critics

Gary P. Pisano is the Harry E. Figgie Jr. Professor of Business Administration at Harvard Business School (http://www.hbs.edu/research/). In his 2006 book entitled *Science Business: The Promise, the Reality, and the Future of Biotech* as well as subsequent writings (2006b), he argues that (a) the combined revenues of all public U.S. biotechs remain close to zero, (b) the combined revenues of all United States combined public and private biotechs remain in the red, (c) R&D spending per new biopharmaceutical launched decreased from $2 billion in 1985 to 1.3 billion in 2004, (d) 30 years since their creation, very few biopharmas have reached profitability, and (e) the biotechnology company business model requires a thorough reevaluation in the face of less-than-impressive financial returns. Paul Nightingale and Paul Martin have also written about the so-called myth of the biotech revolution (2004). They have argued that instead of the "biotech revolution" model of technological change, biotechnology is following a well-established pattern of slow and incremental technology diffusion, and that the translation of this science into new technology is far more difficult, costly, and time-consuming than many proponents advocate.

Nevertheless, the healthcare biotechnology industry has recently started to indicate that better times are yet to come. First, the U.S. industry has reached aggregate profitability in 2008, for the first time ever. Second, R&D productivity is gradually improving, as indicated by the amount of R&D money spent per molecule introduced. Third, the absolute number of profitable biotechnology companies is slowly increasing every year. Fourth, global biopharmaceutical sales have steadily risen from approximately $13 billion in 1998 to 33 billion in 2007. Fifth, biopharmaceuticals are gradually stealing sales away from traditional pharmaceuticals in several therapy areas. Sixth, biopharmaceutical approvals are gradually overtaking chemical medicine approvals. Seventh, the number of annual biopharmaceutical approvals is increasing, compared to the dawn of healthcare biotechnology (first ever approval in 1982). Eighth, the numbers of patients treated, companies formed, employees working, and products and therapy areas involved are steadily and impressively rising. Ninth, the NASDAQ Biotechnology Index (http://dynamic.nasdaq.com/dynamic/nasdaqbiotech_activity.stm) and the AMEX Biotechnology Index (http://www.amex.com/othProd/prodInf/OpPiIndMain.jsp?Product_Symbol=BTK) have significantly outperformed the S&P, DOW JONES, and NASDAQ indices over the 1995–2008 period. Tenth, biotechnology has also outperformed several other newer industries, such as telecommunications, Internet, and the like.

BIOTECHNOLOGY VERSUS BIG PHARMA

The healthcare biotechnology industry performance during 2005 is summarized in Table 1.4. Biotechnology companies (biopharma) have been compared with traditional pharmaceutical companies (big pharma) literally every day over the last three decades.

The comparison has provided different insights used in mutual competitive analyses (see Chapter 8), and also fuelled countless discussions among academic observers, employees, financial analysts, investors, and the media. It has also led to the identification of various similarities and differences that over the years have provided mutual competitive advantages or reasons for imitation, and blurring business models over the same time period. We first focus on the few similarities, and then try to analyze the several differences still in existence today. According to IMS Health, the global

TABLE 1.4   Healthcare Biotechnology Performance, 2005

Share of big pharma sales from biotech products	33%
U.S. public biotechs showing profit in 1 of last 3 years	15%
Biotech share of global Rx revenues	10%

Source: Courtesy of Milne, C.-P., Pharmacogenics: Changing the drug development paradigm Tufts Center for the Study of Drug Development, Boston, MA, BIO IT Coalition, *5th Annual Conference*, George Mason University, May 4–5, 2005.

pharmaceutical sales (pharma + biopharma) reached $773 billion (growing by 4.8% over 2007), and is expected to grow 4%–6% on a constant-dollar basis, exceeding $825 billion in 2010. Global pharmaceutical market value is expected to expand to $975+ billion by 2013 (2009).

Similarities

We start from the similarities. Both industries need a few good scientists, both undertake business risks, both rise and fall on the strength of their R&D, both are after new chemical entities (NCEs), or blockbusters, and both are building powerful fortresses in order to protect their valuable intellectual property armamentaria. Furthermore, human resources, molecules, and financial capital freely flow from one side of the divide to the opposite.

Differences

If that is the case, then why focus on a biotech industry per se? To start with, traditional pharmas have been around for at least four centuries; they have originally started in the old world making vitamins, elixirs, and potions, and have gradually grown to 100,000 employee-plus organizations, with 150 national subsidiaries, or 200 drug-strong portfolios, and over $20 billion in global sales. In contrast, biotechs were born only 30 years ago, most of them have never posted profitability, marketed a commercial product on their own, or even reached the holy grail of FDA (U.S. Food and Drug Administration) approval.

1. *Entrepreneurship*: The author has previously worked for both biotech and big pharma. While the two sides were apparently using the same business model, going after the same therapy areas, and vying for the same prescribers and eventually patients-consumers, the company aspirations were significantly different. For example, big pharma boasted that they were the first, they had the largest number of patients to date, they had launched the "reference" medicine years

back, and that they would continue to thrive in the decades to come using the same old proven business model. The big pharma model was based on large vertical organizations, with thousands of R&D personnel and predictable new product introductions, mainly arising from gradual improvements of existing products. On the opposite side, biopharma was focused on carefully chosen few therapeutic areas; it had a small R&D team with several academic affiliations, and was mainly focused on producing and leveraging its patents toward either commercial affiliations with other companies, or producing new biological entities (NBEs) that would enjoy therapeutic uniqueness over several years.

2. *Academic-like environment*: Once again, let us compare a big pharma with a biotech organization. The first would be sourcing talent from other big pharma competitors, to work within a rigid vertical structure, following detailed standard operating procedures (SOPs) and timelines. In 1999, Jurgen Drews, the former global head of research at Hoffmann-La Roche had written in his book *In Quest of Tomorrow's Medicines* (p. 84, http://www.springer.com) that

the origins of pharmaceutical companies ... are in a 'chemical worldview...' This is an extremely rigorous culture of precision and objectivity, but also of hierarchical dependency, discipline, and subservience... while biotechnology.... stems from a primarily democratic, liberal, indeed libertarian social order, in which formal hierarchies play a much smaller role, while on the other hand, personal development and freedom are more important.

The latter would be going after pharmacology and molecular biology researchers, to work originally in R&D, later in scientific marketing, and eventually in marketing and sales. Moving from subsidiary to corporate or across subsidiaries would also be an option for biopharma, with its adaptive, evolving, and fast-paced mentality. For comparison purposes, let us study two competing organizational structures in the same therapy area, as illustrated in Table 1.5.

3. *R&D focus*: It is common for a big pharma to be active in 15 different therapy areas, some of them affecting large proportions of the general population across the globe, for example, asthma or diabetes. In this case, their approved medicines need to become widely

TABLE 1.5   Big Pharma versus Biopharma Organizational Structures

Level	Big Pharma (15 Levels)	Biotech (4 Levels)
1	Group chief executive officer (CEO)	Chief executive officer (CEO)
2	Pharma CEO	
3	Global head of marketing (senior EVP)	Global head of marketing (senior EVP)
4	European marketing head (EVP)	
5	Northern European marketing head (VP)	
6	Subsidiary managing director (MD)	
7	Subsidiary commercial director	
8	Business unit (BU) A director	
9	BU A commercial director	
10	BU A sales director	
11	Area business unit sales director	Area business manager (ABM)
12	District A sales director	
13	District A sales supervisor	
14	District A senior key account manager	
15	District A key account manager	Key account manager (KAM)

Source: Author's own corporate experience.

known and accepted across national borders within prescribers, other health personnel, health administrators, patients and their families, the media, and the public. For such a gargantuan effort, big pharma is obliged to utilize massive marketing and media campaigns in order to influence its diverse audiences (or stakeholders, see Chapter 8) before their medicines become commercial successes (commonly described as blockbusters, see Chapter 13). The example of PFIZER's Lipitor would fit this focus (http://www.lipitor.com).

In contrast, an emerging biopharma may be focusing on a rare disease, with a limited worldwide number of patients, and an even smaller number of medical experts. For such a targeted effort, it is imperative that the biopharma will focus on its R&D development in an effort to satisfy an unmet medical need, while refraining from mass marketing and media campaigns that would soon exhaust its precious little financial resources before the product is approved, launched, and accepted by the medical and patient community. GENZYME's Cerezyme would be a fitting example here (http://www.cerezyme.com).

4. *Niching*: As mentioned above, a start-up biopharma has limited resources available in order to capitalize on a given scientific discovery, and carry this product through an arduous R&D process,

regulatory approval negotiations, and finally a commercial launch. Be it in the case of asthma, the start-up in question would have to compete throughout this lengthy process with several big pharma competitors, not only for available intellectual property, but also for scientific talent, research facilities and tools, clinical investigator relationships, prescriber attitudes and behaviors, regulatory hurdles, media attention, etc. If, however, the scientific discovery in the bio-pharma's portfolio were to belong to the therapeutic area of infertility, this would immediately lower the number of competitors, the length and cost of the required clinical trials, as well as the eventual marketing budget. The selection of such a targeted therapy area is called "niching," as in the case of a small natural micro-environment (or habitat) existing somewhere on this lovely planet. As far as the infertility niche is concerned, the case of Schering-Plough's (originally Organon's) Puregon (http://www.puregon.com) would be a prominent example.

5. *Risk propensity*: Healthcare biotechnology has been on an uphill competitive pathway since its inception more than 30 years ago. In order for it to succeed, it had to invent a new-to-the-world business model, to convince risk-averse investors, to explain its methods to sceptic regulators, and finally alleviate the fears of traditional prescribers or until-then ignorant consumers. For all these hurdles to be overcome, a significantly higher risk propensity was to become the name of the biotech game. Thus, unproven scientific theories had to be pursued, e.g., producing a biopharmaceutical after a "foreign" gene was inserted into a microorganism host. Research had to start at the earliest, yet untested level of animal model discovery and molecular physicochemical characterization, often bypassed when a well-proven older medicine gives its position to a newer, slight modification. Original clinical investigators had to be adequately educated and convinced about the potential risk-to-benefit ratios of untested biomaterials. Clinical indications had to be selected, often ignored by mainstay therapeutics, e.g., multiple sclerosis. Finally, investors had to be patient enough before they looked for an early and rewarding exit (see Genentech's history at http://www.gene.com/gene/about/corporate/history/). However, biotechnology has overcome these obstacles, finally bringing more than 200 biopharmaceuticals to the marketplace to date. In the process, countless battles were fought and won. Others however

have been lost, leading hundreds of start-ups to an early, unprofitable industry exit, negative industry profitability until today, a severe shortage of R&D funds available to many struggling biopharmas, and the unavoidable financial recessions occurring every few years.

6. *Clinical trials*: Some of the biopharmaceutical clinical trials differ widely from clinical trials for chemically produced medicines. For example, biopharmaceuticals often have smaller clinical indications, fewer clinical trial patient populations, radically different endpoints (e.g., a chronic disease reversal, as opposed to delay of disease progression), different routes of administration, and different diagnostic procedures used. In addition, they more often go against active comparator medicines (the chemical "reference" treatments) instead of placebo, they often require less clinical study times, while the applicable regulatory agencies often agree to approve them expeditiously, due to their revolutionary mechanism of action.

   For example, Imatinib mesylate (Gleevec; Novartis Pharmaceuticals, East Hanover, New Jersey) recently received expedited approval in the United States as an orphan drug for the treatment of chronic myeloid leukaemia. First approved by the FDA in 2001, GLEEVEC (http://www.gleevec.com) is a unique treatment for certain forms of cancer. It works by targeting, and turning off, specific proteins in cancer cells that cause the cancer cells to grow and multiply.

7. *Manufacturing*: Seventh, manufacturing of biotechnology-derived products is fundamentally different from producing their chemical competitors. For example, "biomanufacturing" involves the creation of a "master cell line," the subsequent preparation of a production cell line, tissue culture in specially characterized media, the frequent use of specialized "bioreactors," isolation and purification of the product, and finally characterization and standardization of the resulting bioproduct. This process is more technology- and capital-intensive, requires stricter production conditions, and carries a greater risk of contamination and delays due to its unique process, thus giving the name to the industry phrase "the product is the process!"

8. *Innovation*: Eighth, most biotech introductions to date have been original medications, and even new chemical entities in their purest form. Only recently, biotechs have been involved in biotech me-toos, or even "biosimilars," meaning biotechnology medications

bioequivalent to the original medications that are only surfacing after the patent expirations of the latter. In contrast, big pharma has been involved in countless me-toos, generics, line extensions, and reformulations, strategies we will be discussing deeper into this book. Furthermore, alliances with other biotech firms, university research centers, and pharmaceutical companies are the norm in the industry, providing biotech with faster access to capital and knowledge, enabling companies to react more quickly and flexibly to new developments, and offering better protection of intellectual property rights. Finally, the time line between establishing the company (i.e., initial investment) and return (i.e., product availability in the market) is long. On average, the entire biotech process, from scientific discovery to commercialization, can take up to 15 long and challenging years.

9. *IP dependence*: Ninth, healthcare biotechnology applications are more intellectual property-dependent, and are created or eliminated on strong IP protection. It is common knowledge to the venture capital world that strong IP is the basis for any biotech investment, and that eventual investment returns should commensurate with the IP strength or the R&D risks involved along the way, therefore commanding higher return premiums as compared to big pharma investments.

10. *Patient-friendliness*: Tenth, biotechnology claims to be customer-friendly and safe, but it will still take a long way before establishing itself fully in the minds of the customers, be it the regulators, physicians, patients, their families, or the media. Thus, there is still a battle to be won in the areas of mass-market appeal, patient-friendliness, oral administrations versus injectable, frequency of follow-ups required, or long-term safety, compared to more established (and claiming to be so) traditional pharmaceuticals.

Head-to-Head

Having been through the major similarities and differences between big pharma and biopharma, let us now put them into a head-to-head comparison, as shown in Table 1.6. Every single competitive advantage indicated in Table 1.6 for one side has been contested or imitated by the other side, while the boundaries between the two sides have gradually eroded over the recent years.

TABLE 1.6 How Do Typical Biotechs Compare versus Pharmaceutical Companies?

	Biotech	**Pharmaceuticals**
Balance sheet/cash flow	Burn cash (—)	Strong cash inflow
Capitalization	Small	Big
Dividend	None	Moderate—strong
Financing	Almost all equity	Debt and equity mixed
Globalization	Operates in one site	Operates globally
History	10–30 years old, e.g., Amgen founded in 1980	At least 100 years old, e.g., Roche founded in 1896
Investment risk	Very high	Moderate
Major alliances	1–2 strategic alliances	20–40 strategic alliances
Major cost centers	R&D	R&D, Manufacturing, Marketing
Major investments	80% resources on R&D	20% sales on R&D
Personnel base	Employs 200 people	Employs 50,000 people
Pipeline	Strong	Moderate/Weak
Product sales	No product sales	Annual sales $5 billion+
Profitability	Reports no profits	Reports profits in $ billion

Blurring Pharmaceutical–Biopharmaceutical Boundaries

The higher prices, relative immunity from cost pressure, and lack of follow-on biosimilar or biogenerics in the United States have resulted in pharma push into biologics. Big pharma have undertaken to imitate biotechs in various ways. For example, they are becoming more entrepreneurial by spinning out promising projects, attracting biotech talent, selecting riskier projects, partnering with promising start-ups, eliminating hierarchy levels, and getting closer to their customers (e.g., the CEO becoming the best sales rep to the global medical opinion leaders). The battle continues.

For example, PFIZER (http://www.pfizer.com), the world's foremost pharmaceutical company, is claiming in its corporate R&D page that (a) with the integration of Pfizer and Wyeth, they continue to build the world's premier biopharmaceutical R&D organization, (b) they now have broader and deeper disease area knowledge in their research units, and increased modality and technology capabilities in their biotech units, and that (c) their biotechnology units, namely the Center for Integrated Biology & Biotherapeutics; CovX; Indications Discovery; Regenerative Medicine; Rinat; and RTC/Coley possess the deep scientific excellence and skills associated with delivering large molecule medicines and vaccines, while remaining modality agnostic.

At GlaxoSmithKline (GSK), a specialized R&D business unit is driving growth in external drug discovery to complement the late-stage GSK pipeline. The Center of Excellence for External Drug Discovery (CEEDD; http://www.ceedd.com/) builds and personally manages unique risk/reward-sharing drug discovery alliances with world-class biotech companies. Another example of big pharma internalizing biotech is obviously Roche (http://www.roche.com). Headquartered in Basel, Switzerland, Roche is one of the world's leading research-focused healthcare groups in the fields of pharmaceuticals and diagnostics. They proclaim that, as the world's biggest biotech company and an innovator of products and services for the early detection, prevention, diagnosis, and treatment of diseases, the Group contributes on a broad range of fronts to improve people's health and quality of life.

Big Pharma Example: NOVARTIS

Mission: We want to discover, develop, and successfully market innovative products to prevent and cure diseases, to ease suffering, and to enhance the quality of life.

Businesses: Novartis offers a wide range of healthcare products through our Pharmaceuticals, Vaccines and Diagnostics, Sandoz and Consumer Health Divisions.

Locations: We operate in 140 countries, with our global headquarters in Basel, Switzerland.

Company history: Novartis was created in 1996 through the merger of Ciba-Geigy and Sandoz. 2008 Net Sales: USD 41.459 billion; 2008 Operating Income: USD 8.964 billion Number of associates: 98,200.

Source: Courtesy of NOVARTIS, Basel, Switzerland, http://www.novartis.com

BIOPHARMACEUTICAL COMPANIES

The distinctions between biopharmaceuticals and drugs carry over to the organizations, usually companies, involved in the discovery, development, and marketing of these products. Compared with firms with drug products, biopharmaceutical companies generally have staff with different training and expertise, higher costs of goods, greater investment in different types of manufacturing facilities, and more product-dedicated marketing/sales organizations.

TABLE 1.7   Top 20 Companies by Biologic Sales during 2007 (U.S.$ Billion)

1	Amgen	15,964	11	BiogenIdec	1,773
2	Roche/Genentech	15,469	12	Bayer	1,714
3	Johnson & Johnson	6,285	13	Merck	1,360
4	Novo Nordisk	5,890	14	Pfizer	0.849
5	Eli Lilly	3,931	15	AstraZeneca	0.825
6	SanofiAventis	3,201	16	Genzyme	0.726
7	Abbott	3,145	17	Imclone	0.686
8	MerckSerono	2,734	18	GlaxoSmithKline	0.654
9	Schering-Plough	2,577	19	Baxter Intl.	0.616
10	Wyeth	2,254	20	Novartis	0.521

Source: Courtesy of IMS Health, Norwalk, CT.

IMS Health (http://www.imshealth.com/portal/site/imshealth) is among the world's leading providers of market intelligence to the pharmaceutical and healthcare industries, collecting and analyzing data from drug manufacturers, wholesalers, retail pharmacies, hospitals, long-term care facilities, and healthcare professionals in more than 100 countries. In 2008, they reported the top 20 companies by biologic sales during 2007, as shown in Table 1.7.

According to the Genetic Engineering and Biotechnology News (Napodano, 2009) of the 225 publically traded biotechnology firms in their database, only 10 traded with a market capitalization over $2 billion, according to the Zacks database. Only 18 traded with a market capitalization over $1 billion. In June 2009, there were only five large-cap firms, or those that have a market capitalization over $10 billion, namely, Amgen, Genzyme, Gilead Sciences, Biogen Idec, and Celgene.

Biopharma Stellar Examples: Amgen and Genentech
As Burrill & Company (2009a) reported, the top two biotechnology companies in the world remained at their respective spots during 2008, ending the year up 24% and 23%, respectively. Amgen's increase in share price came largely from expectations over its future blockbuster sales potential with the osteoporosis drug denosumab. Genentech gained on strong sales and continued potential for its key blockbuster cancer drug Avastin. Total biopharmaceutical revenues were $14.3 billion (up 3%) and 9.4 billion (up 24%), respectively. For more detailed information on the world's two foremost biotechnology companies during 2008, take a look at Table 1.8 (Contract Pharma, 2009).

TABLE 1.8   Amgen versus Genentech during 2008

Amgen (http://www.amgen.com)	Genentech (http://www.gene.com)
Headcount: 17,000	Headcount: 11,000
Year established: 1980	Year established: 1976
Biopharma sales: $14,687 + 3%	Biopharma sales: $10,531 + 12%
Royalty revenues: $316 + 4%	Royalty revenues: $2,539 + 28%
Total revenues: $15,003 + 2%	Total revenues: $13,418 + 14%
Net income: $4,196 + 33%	Net income: $3,427 + 24%
R&D budget: $3,003 − 7%	R&D budget: $2,800 + 14%
2008 Top selling drugs—Drug indication sales (±%)	2008 Top selling drugs—Drug indication sales (±%)
Enbrel rheumatoid arthritis, psoriatic arthritis: $3,598 + 11%	Avastin colorectal cancer: $2,686 + 17%
Neulasta chemotherapy-induced neutropenia: $3,318 + 11%	Rituxan lymphoma, rheumatoid arthritis: $2,587 + 13%
Aranesp chemotherapy-induced anemia: $3,137 − 13%	Herceptin breast cancer: $1,382 + 7%
Epogen anemia: $2,456 − 1%	Lucentis wet AMD: $875 + 7%
Neupogen chemotherapy-induced neutropenia: $1,341 + 5%	Xolair asthma: $517 + 10%
Sensipar renal disease complications: $597 + 29%	Tarceva lung cancer: $457 + 10%
	Nutropin/Protropin HGH deficiency: $358 − 4%
Account for 98% of total pharma sales, same as in 2007.	Account for 84% of total pharma sales, same as in 2007.

Source: CONTRACT PHARMA, Top 10 Biopharmaceutical Companies Report, July/August 2009. With permission.

BIOPHARMACEUTICAL THERAPY AREAS

According to IMS Health, oncologics was the therapy area showing the largest global combined biopharmaceutical/pharmaceutical sales, among both the top therapeutic classes (Table 1.9) and the top specialty classes (Table 1.10) during 2008. Specialty pharmacy is defined as the service created to manage the handling and service requirements of specialty pharmaceuticals, including dispensing, distribution, reimbursement, case management, and other services specific to patients with rare and/or chronic diseases, and will be further discussed in Chapter 11.

Looking into biopharmaceuticals per se, the La Merie Business Intelligence firm has previously reported that tumor necrosis factor inhibitors (anti-TNF antibodies) were the best selling class of biologics in 2008 with total sales of $16.4 billion. Erythropoetins fell down to position 4 with 2008 sales of $10 billion, superseded by the class of anticancer antibodies ($15.6 billion) and insulin products ($10.9 billion) due to the continuing success of insulin analogs. Overall, the 13 major classes of biologics

TABLE 1.9   Top 10 Therapeutic Classes by Worldwide Sales, 2008

Rank	Audited World Therapy Class	2008 Sales (U.S.$ Billion)	% Sales	% Growth over 2007 (Constant U.S.$)
1	Oncologics	48.2	6.7	11.3
2	Lipid regulators	33.8	4.7	−2.3
3	Respiratory agents	31.3	4.3	5.7
4	Antidiabetics	27.3	3.8	9.6
5	Acid pump inhibitors	26.5	3.7	0.6
6	Angiotensin-II antagonists	22.9	3.2	12.6
7	Antipsychotics	22.9	3.2	8.0
8	Antidepressants	20.3	2.8	0.6
9	Anti-epileptics	16.9	2.3	9.7
10	Autoimmune agents	15.9	2.2	16.9
	Top 10 therapy classes	266.0	36.7	6.6

Source: Courtesy of IMS Health, MIDAS, Norwalk, CT, December 2008, http:// www.imshealthcanada.com. © 2009 IMS Health Canada. All rights reserved.

TABLE 1.10   Top 10 Specialty Therapeutic Sales by Worldwide Sales, 2008

Specialty Pharmaceuticals	Examples	% Market Share 100.0	% Growth U.S.$ 8.8	% CAGR, 03-07 13.9
Oncologics	Avastin, Herceptin, Sutent	35.7	11.4	18.1
HIV antivirals	Kaletra, Truvada	9.1	11.9	12.5
Immunosuppressants	Cellcept, Prograf	9.1	17.9	13.8
Erythropoetins	Procrit, Aranesp	8.5	−14.0	4.5
Specific antirheumatics	Humira, Enbrel, Kineret	8.2	18.2	35.5
Immunostimulants	Neupogen, Neulasta	6.6	6.0	14.2
Interferons	Avonex, Betaseron	4.2	8.1	7.6
Immunoglobulins	Octagam, Gamunex	3.7	11.5	12.0
Blood coagulation	Helixate FS	3.0	8.6	11.7
Antivirals (Hepatitis)	Copegus, Rebetol	2.9	6.2	5.1
Total others		9.0	9.8	11.4

Source: Courtesy of IMS Health, MIDAS, Norwalk, CT, December 2008, http://www. imshealthcanada.com. All rights reserved.

together posted 2008 sales of $80.6 billion of which 43.4% originated from antibody sales. The second cluster of successful classes of biologics consisted of interferon beta ($5.4 billion), G-CSF ($5.2 billion), and recombinant coagulation factors ($4.9 billion) (La Merie, HQ: Barcelona, http://www.lamerie.com/, 2009. With permission.)

For a biologic agent example, see the American College of Rheumatology Factsheet on Rheumatoid Arthritis, http://www.rheumatology.org/public/factsheets/ra.asp

BIOPHARMACEUTICAL PRODUCTS VERSUS CHEMICAL MEDICINES

Biopharmaceutical products are inherently different from chemically synthesized pharmaceuticals. Nearly all aspects of a biopharmaceutical's life cycle, i.e., from inception, patenting, clinical testing, manufacturing, approval, marketing, to life after patent expiration are fundamentally different from the respective phases of a chemical medicine. We review their comparison from the start.

Small Molecules

Chemically synthesized medicines are small molecules—hence the name—composed of a limited number of atoms, with well-known physicochemical properties, and a high degree of purity. They have a guaranteed manufacturing reproducibility, and are physicochemically- and bio-equivalent to their generic counterparts that are introduced following the expiration of the original patent. The top five pharmaceutical products by global sales during 2008 are shown in Table 1.11, with PFIZER's Lipitor (atorvastatin calcium; a cholesterol- and triglyceride-lowering medication) reaching annual global sales of $13.7 billion.

TABLE 1.11   Top Five Pharmaceutical Products by Global Sales, 2008

Rank	Product	Sales (U.S.$ Million)	% Growth 2008 (Local Currencies)
1	Lipitor	13,655	−0.9
2	Plavix	8,634	16.9
3	Nexium	7,842	7.8
4	Seretide	7,703	7.0
5	Enbrel	5,703	5.6

Source: Courtesy of IMS Health, Norwalk, CT, http://www.imshealth. com. © 2009 IMS Health. All rights reserved.

Biopharmaceuticals

IMS defines biologics as a class of medicines under four key principles— "Molecular Structure," as biologic molecules are complex macromolecules, typically with some form of polymer structure; "Molecular Identification," as biologic molecules must be clearly identified; "Active Substance," as biologic molecules must be, or are intended to be, clearly defined active therapeutic ingredients in a product; and "Regulatory," as biologic molecules must have undergone or are undergoing a regulatory human clinical trial program under the auspices of a national or regional regulatory authority (2009). Table 1.12 lists the top five biopharmaceutical products by global sales during 2008.

Biopharmaceuticals are significantly more complex than their chemical counterparts. Instead of a few atoms, they comprise of thousands of molecular subunits, for example, various amino acids and nucleotides that have two direct implications. First, their combined molecular weight is several orders of magnitude larger than that of the average small molecule pharmaceuticals. Second, the presence of such a complex structure is exacerbated by the fact that several of their subunits form, often with the help of only naturally encountered enzymes, three-dimensional bridges and ligands, the slight alteration of which may lead to physicochemistry and bioequivalence modifications that render the new molecule significantly different than its original copy. Figure 1.3 describes a representative matrix of protein types, which have been commercially launched as biopharmaceuticals. For example, Rituximab (Rituxan; http://www.rituxan.com), a chimeric murine/human monoclonal antibody, approved in the United States for the treatment of refractory or relapsed B-cell lymphomas, is composed of two heavy chains of 451 amino acids and two light chains of 213 amino acids with a molecular weight of 145 kDa. Several molecular weight examples of chemical versus biological medicines are shown in Table 1.13.

TABLE 1.12   Top Five Biopharmaceutical Products by Global Sales, 2008

Rank	Product	Sales (U.S.$ Million)	% Growth over 2007 (Local Currencies)
1	Enbrel	5703	5.6
2	Remicade	4935	14.0
3	Mabthera	4435	8.9
4	Humira	4075	39.5
5	Avastin	4016	37.4

Source: Courtesy of IMS Health, Norwalk, CT, http://www. imshealth.com. © 2009 IMS Health. All rights reserved.

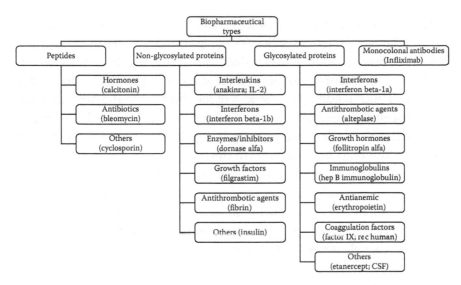

FIGURE 1.3 Matrix of protein types. (From Bhattycharyya, L. et al., *AAPS J.*, 7(4): E786, 2005, United States Pharmacopeia. With permission.)

TABLE 1.13 Molecular Weight Examples of Chemical versus Biological Medicines

Chemical	Molecular Weight (Da)	Biological	Molecular Weight (Da)
Glucophage	166	Neupogen	18,800
Prozac	346	Intron-A	19,625
Zantac	351	Humatrope	22,125
Paxil	375	Avonex	22,500
Claritin	383	Epogen	30,400
Zocor	419	Pulmozyme	37,000
Augmentin	420	ReoPro	47,615
Crixivan	712	Enbrel	755,000
Taxol	854	Zenapax	144,000
		Rituxan	145,000

Source: EuropaBio, *Biological and Biosimilar Medicines*. EuropaBio, Brussels, Belgium, January 2005, http://www.europabio.org/. With permission.

Complexity

As mentioned above, biopharmaceuticals are inherently bigger and more complex molecules than their small molecule counterparts. These differences are not only theoretical subjects for a chemistry class, but actually play a role in influencing the therapeutic efficacy and safety of the biopharmaceuticals under question. For example, slight modifications between biopharmaceutical molecules lead to completely different efficacy profiles mandating different recommended dosages and frequencies of administration, as is the case between interferons beta one- alpha and beta. Furthermore, the absence or presence of multidimensional bridges among the biopharmaceutical molecule's subunits may lead to the alteration of significant molecular positions ("loci"), leading to the loss of identical "lock-and-key" similarities between the molecule and its biological ligand, eventually leading to the recipient's body developing antibodies against the biopharmaceutical in question, thus reducing its long-term efficacy and safety.

The two problems originating from the biopharmaceutical products' complexity just mentioned form the fiercely debated principle of therapeutic reproducibility of an original biopharmaceutical by its generic equivalent (often called biogeneric, biosimilar, or follow-on biological), which will be further elaborated in Chapter 14.

Intellectual Property

It is often said that the essence of a thriving biopharmaceutical industry is a strong intellectual property system, a subject that will be thoroughly discussed in Chapter 2. However, for comparison purposes between chemical and biopharmaceutical medicines, we need to emphasize the fundamental differences in the content of intellectual property protection between them. For example, in the case of small molecules, a patent may be based around a chemical manufacturing process, an enzyme molecule, a precursor molecule, or the chemical combination of an inactive with an active ingredient, leading to the final molecule. What happens though, when all these processes and precursors are abundant in nature? For example, could and should a biopharmaceutical manufacturer patent the way the human hypophysis regulates the biosynthesis of insulin in our bodies? This dilemma is at the heart of the biotechnology patentability issue that will be presented in Chapter 2 (for an important decision on the subject, see the U.S. Supreme Court decision on DIAMOND v. CHAKRABARTY, 1980).

For the time being, it suffices to describe that international patenting organizations have accepted that instead of what happens in the human or other species' bodies, manufacturers may patent the way they have inserted a human gene into another host organism, for example, Chinese hamster ovary (CHO) cells, and directed it to produce a human hormone, or the structure of the gene inserted, or the cell lines developed for this purpose, and the purification methods for the hormone's eventual isolation and purification. Furthermore, all these processes may be covered by other forms of intellectual property, for example, a trade secret—not patented—which prohibits a biopharmaceutical manufacturer's employee to take this secret to a competitor.

Manufacturing

The differences between small molecules and biopharmaceuticals are nowhere more apparent than in their respective manufacturing processes. On the one hand, small molecules comprise of a limited number of atoms (carbon, nitrogen, oxygen, calcium, etc.), which can be mixed in various concentrations and under various chemical reaction conditions leading to the formation of a more complex chemical structure, the small molecule in question. Obviously, the purity of all these prime materials can be precisely characterized, while the bulk manufacturer is not a critical issue for the final product (apart from price competitiveness).

In the case of biopharmaceuticals, the process is essentially different. There is no such thing as a well-characterized, generic, no-name bulk molecular antibody, ready to be used for further biosynthesis of the final biopharmaceutical. Why? Because, our precious therapeutic monoclonal antibody can either be synthesized by only living organisms, hence the need for a carrier host organism specifically designed and created for this purpose following years of sophisticated development. Furthermore, the antibody may not even occur in nature, but may be a biosynthetic construct, a combination of existing subfragments, or a "chimeric" construct (comprised of parts of different species origin), also synthetically biomanufactured under the strictest conditions. Finally, because both complex molecules are to be produced by obliging host cells, for example, a bacterium called *Escherichia coli*, special care needs to be devoted to the eventual isolation and purification of the active ingredient, free of any contaminants of biological nature, before administration into human patients. The issue of complex biomanufacturing processes and procedures will be further discussed in Chapter 7.

For a chemical and biopharmaceutical company expertise example, see the corporate profile of MerckSerono at: http://www.merckserono.com/en/merck_serono/what_we_do/what_ we_do.html

Head-to-Head

We have previously analyzed various differences between small molecules and biopharmaceuticals. Now it is time to put them both into a head-to-head comparison. We attempt to encompass all different aspects of their respective life cycles. Let us study Table 1.14 and compare.

TABLE 1.14 How Are Biopharmaceuticals Different from Small Molecules?

Characteristic	Small Molecules	Large Molecules
Antigenicity	Nonantigenic, unpredictable antigenicity	Usually antigenic
Body distribution	Any combination of organs/tissues	Usually limited to plasma and/or extracellular fluids
Conditions treated	Treats a chronic or an acute condition	Treats a difficult, often terminal condition
Frequency of administration		Biologics have a long half-life in the human body. Patients do not need to take biologics as often as LMW medicines
Inorganic and/or organic compounds	Organic and inorganic compounds. Examples include antibiotics and statins	Organic. Monoclonal antibodies, cytokines, enzymes, immunomodulators, growth factors
Marketing and sales	Needs a big sales force with DTC advertising	Needs a small sales force, rarely DTC advertising
Metabolism	Metabolized to non-active and active metabolites	Catabolized to endogenous amino acids
Molecular stability	Generally stable and not extremely sensitive to heat	Both heat and shear sensitive (aggregation)
Molecular structure	Do not exist in small molecules	Mostly glycoprotein that forms 3D structures—secondary, tertiary, quaternary
Molecular weight	Typically <500 Da	Typically >5000 Da (5 kDa)
Origin	Small molecule organic compounds obtained by screening large libraries of natural or synthetic compounds. Produced by chemical or semisynthetic synthesis	Purified from natural sources or, more commonly, produced by recombinant methods
Patients	Targets big populations like acne and high blood pressure	Targets smaller populations like HIV and specific cancer types
Physicochemical properties	Mostly well defined	Complex (e.g., tertiary structure, extent, and type of glycosylation)
Prescriber	Prescribed in primary care by a GP	Prescribed in a hospital by a consultant
Pricing	Relatively low priced	Relatively high-priced, even for $100,000 a year or more

Purity	Single entity, high chemical purity, purity standards well established	Often heterogeneous mixture, broad specifications which may change during development, difficult to standardize
Quality assurance	Usually one bioanalytical method (mostly LC/MS) for pharmacokinetic studies needed	Several bioanalytical assays (mass assay, bioassay, antibody assays) (mostly ligand binding assay) necessary for pharmacokinetic studies
Regulation	Regulated by FDA Center for Drug Evaluation and Research (CDER)	Regulated by FDA Center for Drug Evaluation and Research (CDER) Other biologics: Vaccines, antitoxins, antivenins, blood components, cellular products—Regulated by FDA Center for Biologic Evaluation and Research (CBER)
Route of administration	Oral administration often possible	Usually administered parenterally
Safety		Being proteins are degraded exactly the same way as other proteins in the body. As a result, patients taking biologics drugs tend to have fewer side effects than with synthesized chemical drugs
Selectivity		More selective than traditional low-molecular-weight (LMW) drugs. They usually only "attack" their disease target and do not affect healthy tissues or cells
Synthesis	Chemically synthesized	Biotechnologically produced by host cell lines
Systemic absorption	Rapidly enter systemic circulation through blood capillaries	Larger molecules (>15–20 kDa) primarily reach circulation via lymphatic system, subject to proteolysis during interstitial and lymphatic transit
Targets	Intracellular and nuclear proteins	Cell surface receptors, soluble or circulating proteins
Therapeutic aim	Aims to either cure the patient or effectively cure with chronic administration	Aims to extend survival, or improve QoL, after diagnosis
Toxicity	Often specific toxicity (toxicological is dissociated from primary pharmacological effect)	Mostly receptor-mediated toxicity, including both exaggerated pharmacodynamic responses and biological toxicity

HEALTHCARE BIOTECHNOLOGY IN NUMBERS

There are various, publicly available information tools for a biotechnology reader to study and analyze the evolution of the biotechnology industry over the years. As previously mentioned, major biotechnology information sources are global biotechnology consultants' public releases (e.g., IMS Health, Ernst & Young, Burrill & Company, and Bioworld). In addition, several stock exchanges measure and publicly announce the evolution of specific biotechnology indices, such as those belonging to AMEX, NASDAQ, and Burrill & Company. We briefly study some of their recent observations on the state of the global biotechnology industry.

The global market for biotechnology or biologics medicines was strong in 2008 with double-digit growth and was over $125 billion. There were over 40 biologic brands with sales of over $1 billion in 2008. The total sales of these 40 brands were $115 billion and the additional $10 billion was from brands with sales exceeding $100 million. (MEDPEDIA, 2009).

In March 2010, Burrill & Company reported that biotech maintained its positive climb in February in lockstep with the general markets, which despite a few bumps in the road, also continued to strengthen. The Burrill Biotech Select Index posted an almost 3% jump in value in February buoyed by Affymetrix, whose shares surged and closed the month up 38% after reporting an unexpected profit in the fourth quarter. In addition, most of the companies in the group posted modest single-digit percentage gains in their share values.

Biotech Industry Statistics (compiled by the Burrill Report):

The industry closed the month with a collective market cap of $362.42 billion (up 1.6 percent for the month and 3.9 percent for the year)

56 companies (18.5 percent) have market caps greater than $1B (there were 49 companies at the beginning of 2008)

Top five biotech companies are Amgen ($56.3B, unchanged YTD), Gilead Sciences ($42.8B, up 10 percent YTD), Celgene ($27.4B, up 6.8 percent YTD), Genzyme ($15.2B, up 16 percent YTD), and Biogen ($14.8B, up 2.7 percent YTD).

Source: Courtesy of Burrill & Company, San Francisco, CA, Press Release, March 2, 2010, http://www.burrillandco.com

MAJOR BIONATIONS

According to OECD, between January 1989 and January 2009, 138 bio-therapies received marketing approval in one or more national jurisdictions in the world (see Table 1.15). These consisted of 2 experimental therapies, 10 in vivo diagnostics, 11 bio-vaccines and 115 therapeutics. A review of the ownership and development records for all 138 approved bio-therapies identified the firm that originally developed the bio-therapy and the current owner of the bio-therapy. For 56 (40.6%) of the 138 bio-therapies, the firm that originally developed the molecule differs from the current owner. For most of these cases, the developer was a small dedicated biotechnology firm that was later purchased by a large pharmaceutical firm. In total, only 21 (15.2%) of the 138 bio-therapies were originally developed by one of the major pharmaceutical firms. Bio-therapies that were jointly developed by two firms were assigned a value of 0.5 to the head office country of each firm.

One or more approved bio-therapies were developed by firms based in 12 OECD and 3 non-OECD countries (China, Cuba, and Israel). Firms based in the United States developed 91.5 (66.3%) of the 138 bio-therapies that received marketing approval between January 1989 and January 2009. European firms developed 21.5 (15.6%) and Japanese firms developed 10.5 (7.6%) of the approved

TABLE 1.15 Nationality of the Developer Firm for 138 Approved Bio-Therapies, January 1989–2009

United States	91.5	Cuba	3.0
Japan	10.5	Israel	2.0
Switzerland	7.5	Canada	2.2
United Kingdom	5.0	Netherlands	1.0
Germany	3.5	Ireland	1.0
France	3.5	Denmark	1.0
Korea	3.0	Australia	0.5
China	3.0		

Source: van Beuzekom, B. and Arundel, A., *OECD, Biotechnology Statistics* 2009. Paris, France, OECD, May 25, 2009, http://www.oecd.org/dataoecd/4/23/42833898.pdf. With permission.

Note: Six biopharmaceuticals that were jointly developed by two firms in two different countries were assigned a share of 0.5 to each country.

TABLE 1.16 Number of Dedicated Biotechnology Firms, 2006

	Dedicated Biotechnology Firms	Dedicated Biotechnology R&D Firms		Dedicated Biotechnology Firms	Dedicated Biotechnology R&D Firms
United States	2075	2744	Austria	111	86
EU average			Switzerland		77
Canada	532		Finland		75
Germany	496		Italy		72
France		461	Ireland		
Australia	384		Brazil	71	
Korea		265	Czech Republic		52
Netherlands		221	South Africa	38	
Spain	211		Portugal		20
Sweden	148		Philippines		13
Belgium	122		Slovak Republic		6
New Zealand	120		Poland		3

Source: van Beuzekom, B. and Arundel, A., *OECD Biotechnology Statistics 2009*, OECD, Paris, France, May 25, 2009, http://www.oecd.org/dataoecd/4/23/42833898.pdf. With permission.

Definitions: Dedicated biotechnology firm: a biotechnology firm whose predominant activity involves the application of biotechnology techniques to produce goods or services and/or to perform biotechnology R&D. These firms are captured by biotechnology firm surveys. Dedicated biotechnology R&D firms devote 75% or more of their total R&D to biotechnology R&D. These firms are captured by R&D surveys.

TABLE 1.17   Top Pharmaceutical Markets Worldwide, 2008

Rank		Sales (Billions, U.S.$)	% Growth over 2007
1	North America	311.9	1.3
2	Europe	237.4	5.4
3	Asia, Africa, Australia	72.3	15.7
4	Japan	68.6	2.6
5	Latin America	34.3	12.9
	Top 10 pharma markets	564.0	3.1

bio-therapies. In the last five years (since January 2004), the share of approved bio-therapies developed by US firms declined slightly to 63.2% (24 of 38 bio-therapies). The number of approved bio-therapies per million inhabitants in 2000 of the head office country of the developer firm ranges from 1.040 bio-therapies per million in Switzerland to 0.002 bio-therapies per million in China. Other leading countries include Israel (0.342 per million) and the United States (0.324 per million).

Source: van Beuzekom, B. and Arundel, A., *OECD Biotechnology Statistics 2009*, OECD, Paris, France, http://www.oecd.org/dataoecd/4/23/42833898.pdf, 2009. With permission.

Table 1.16 shows the number of dedicated biotechnology firms existing in major bionations at the end of 2006. The leading bioregions were the United States and Europe.

As far as the size of the pharmaceutical market is concerned, IMS Health data on Table 1.17 describe its size by continent, during 2008.

QUESTIONS

1. Which are the most commonly used biotechnologies?
2. Which are the main commercial applications of red, green, blue, and white biotechnology to date?
3. How does the North American Industry Classification System (NAICS) classify healthcare biotechnology?
4. What are the proponents and critics of healthcare biotechnology saying about its performance to date?

5. What are the main similarities and differences between pharmaceutical (big pharma) and biopharmaceutical (biotech) companies to date?
6. Is big pharma converging with modern biopharmaceutical companies and in what way?
7. Which were the top 10 therapeutic classes and the top 10 specialty therapeutic classes by worldwide sales in 2008?
8. What are the main similarities and differences between small molecule pharmaceuticals and biopharmaceuticals?
9. What was the performance of global healthcare biotechnology during 2008, and which are the main sources of information for these rankings?
10. What are the major global bionations, and what are the most commonly used parameters in their ranking?

EXERCISES

1. Figure 1.1 lists some of the most common biotechnology applications today. Name two examples for each application.
2. Choose your standing among healthcare biotechnology's proponents or critics. Identify 10 arguments supporting your side, as well as specific arguments negating your opponents' views. Present them in a debate.
3. Identify 10 big pharmas that have launched biopharmaceuticals as well as 10 biopharmaceutical companies that are developing small molecules. Provide details.
4. Describe the size of the global pharmaceutical markets in diabetes, rheumatoid arthritis, psoriasis, and multiple sclerosis. Start with epidemiological data, and proceed into major biological treatments, their annual sales, their patent expirations, and their planned successors under development.
5. What are some of the metrics used to define a biopharmaceutical enterprise's innovation? Use several metrics to compare Amgen, Genentech, and Genzyme between them.
6. Monoclonal antibodies are one of the most important biopharmaceutical R&D platforms. Name the major molecules launched and their applications, as well as additional molecules under development.
7. How are biologicals regulated by the U.S. FDA? Describe the relevant procedures for the regulation of their R&D, manufacturing, advertising, and pharmaco-vigilance.

8. What are the predictions of major healthcare biotechnology analysts and consultants for the industry evolution over the next few years? What are the major drivers for growth or potential downsides anticipated during the present decade?

9. Using publicly available stock exchange data, describe the standing of the healthcare biotechnology sector, as well as its most important global companies? How was the sector affected by the global financial crisis of 2008–2009?

10. How can you rate the top five global bionations? What is their respective healthcare biotechnology productivity, and what national/state initiatives are they respectively using to boost it?

REFERENCES

American College of Rheumatology Factsheet on Rheumatoid Arthritis, Atlanta, GA, http://www.rheumatology.org/practice/clinical/patients/medications/biologics.asp

Bhattycharyya, L., Dabbah, R., Hauck, W., Sheinin, E., Yeoman, L., and Williams, R., 2005. Equivalence studies for complex active ingredients and dosage forms. *AAPS Journal* 7(4): E786–E812.

Biotechnology Industry Organization, 2008. *Guide to Biotechnology 2008*. BIO: Washington, DC, 2008. Posted at: http://www.bio.org/speeches/pubs/er/BiotechGuide2008.pdf

Burrill & Company, 2009a. *Biotech 2009—Life Sciences: Navigating the Sea of Change*. San Francisco, CA: Burrill & Co.

Burrill & Company, 2009b. Biotech holds up well in the face of financial crisis and market turmoil, Press Release, January 2, 2009.

Burrill & Company, San Francisco, CA, Press Release, March 2, 2010, http://www.burrillandco.com

CONTRACT PHARMA, 2009. Top 10 biopharmaceutical companies report, July/August 2009.

Drews, J., 1999. *In Quest of Tomorrow's Medicines*. New York: Springer-Verlag.

Ernst & Young. 2009. Beyond borders: The global biotechnology report 2009. Boston, MA: E&Y.

EuropaBio, 2005. *Biological and Biosimilar Medicines*. Brussels, Belgium: EuropaBio.

EuropaBio, 2009. Healthcare biotech facts & figures, http://www.europabio.org/Healthcare/HC_facts.htm (accessed on January 30, 2010).

European Commission Joint Research Centre's (JRC) Institute for Prospective Technological Studies, 2008. Consequences, opportunities and challenges of modern biotechnology for Europe—The analysis report—Contributions of modern biotechnology to European policy objectives, http://ftp.jrc.es/EURdoc/JRC44144.pdf

IMS Health, December 2008. MIDAS, Norwalk, CT, http://www.imshealthcanada.com

IMS Health, 2008. IMS health reports global biotech sales grew 12.5 percent in 2007, exceeding $75 billion, Press Release, June 17, 2008.

IMS Health, 2009a. IMS forecasts global pharmaceutical market growth of 4%–6% in 2010; predicts 4%–7% expansion through 2013, Press Release, October 7, 2009.

IMS Health, 2009b. IMS launches MIDAS global biologics, delivering new market insights for enhanced portfolio planning, Press Release, October 14, 2009.

La Merie, 2009. Top 20 biologics 2008, Press Release, March 9, 2009.

MEDPEDIA, 2009. Biotechnology industry performance in 2008, http://wiki.medpedia.com/Biotechnology_Industry_Performance_in_2008 (accessed on January 30, 2010).

Merck Serono, Geneva, Switzerland, http://www.merckserono.com/en/merck_serono/what_we_do/what_we_do.html

Milne, C.-P., 2005. Pharmacogenics: Changing the drug development paradigm. Tufts Center for the Study of Drug Development, Boston, MA, BIO IT Coalition, *5th Annual Conference*, George Mason University, May 4–5, 2005.

Napodano, J., 2009. Biotech companies face the key question—Deal or no deal? Genetic Engineering & Biotechnology News Special Reports, June 5, 2009. Posted at: http://www.genengnews.com/analysis-and-insight/biotech-companies-face-the-key-question-deal-or-no-deal/55682893

Nightingale, P. and Martin, P., 2004. The myth of the biotech revolution. *Trends in Biotechnology* 22(11): 564–569.

NOVARTIS, Basel, Switszerland, http://www.novartis.com

OECD, 2007. Health biotechnology to 2030, Report to the Third Meeting of the Steering Group, OECD International Futures Project, on The Bioeconomy to 2030: Designing a Policy Agenda. Paris, France: OECD.

Organization for Economic Co-Operation and Development (OECD). *Statistical Definition of Biotechnology*, Paris, France, updated in 2005, http://www.oecd.org/document/42/0,3343,en_2649_34537_1933994_1_1_1_37437,00.html (accessed on January 27, 2010).

Pharmaceutical Research and Manufacturers of America, 2009. Pharmaceutical industry profile 2009. Washington, DC: PhRMA.

Pisano, G.P., 2006a. *Science Business: The Promise, the Reality and the Future of Biotech*. Boston, MA: Harvard Business School Press.

Pisano, G.P., 2006b. Can science be a business? Lessons from biotech. *Harvard Business Review* 84(10): 114–124.

ThromboGenics Press Release, Leuven, Belgium, http://www.thrombogenics.com

United Nations Environment Program, Text of the convention on biological diversity, updated on 11–8–2009, http://www.cbd.int/convention/convention.shtml (accessed on January 27, 2010).

U.S. Supreme Court DIAMOND v. CHAKRABARTY, 1980. 447 U.S. 303 (1980)—447 U.S. 303—No. 79-136. Argued March 17, 1980. Decided June 16, 1980.

van Beuzekom, B. and Arundel, A., 2009. *OECD Biotechnology Statistics 2009.* Paris, France: OECD, May 25, 2009, http://www.oecd.org/dataoecd/4/23/42833898.pdf

Watson, J.D. and Crick, F.H.C., 1953. Molecular structure of nucleic acids—A structure for deoxyribose nucleic acid. *Nature* 171: 737–738.

II

Intellectual Property

## CHAPTER 2

Intellectual Property Management

During 2008, there were 2983 patents granted by the USPTO within the U.S. Patent Classification System Class #514 (Drug, Bio-Affecting and Body Treating Compositions).

Source: Courtesy of United States Patent and Trademark Office (USPTO), Alexandria, VA.

B EFORE ANY ANALYSIS OF the healthcare biotechnology management process is to be undertaken, the role of intellectual property (IP) rights in this process needs to be elaborated. IP rights have evolved over the last 150 years, with one intention in mind: to offer protection of someone's ideas from imitation, by conferring a period of exclusivity. There are two main themes of creativity of the human mind. These are its artistic or commercial ideas. The first may come in the form of a poetry, or literature, music, painting, sculpture, or software. The second may come in the form of a new device, an industrial process, a tool, a chemical reaction, etc. Either of these two forms may be protected by various forms of IP rights, for example, patents, trademarks, or copyrights. In this book, we focus on the commercial IP rights, especially those relevant to the healthcare biotechnology industry.

Three conditions are mandatory for a commercial idea to be protected: Newness, usefulness, and nonobviousness. In plain words, it would be impossible in 2010 to protect the invention of trousers (not new), styling one's hair with his bare hands (too obvious), and finally staring at a rainbow (not so useful). As far as the types of protection available are concerned, there are various kinds, for example, patents—a new, nonobvious, and useful method of producing a commercial product (e.g., a new medicine) or trademarks (a specially created sign that is not only indicative, but also distinctive). In addition, a trade secret may describe the not-publicly known method or "recipe" of doing things, or an industrial design, for example, a wristwatch or a vacuum cleaner. The IP protection system that has gradually been evolving over more than a century is based on a set of mutual incentives, for either the idea creator–inventor, or the society as a whole. On the other hand, despite its countless incremental evolutions that have taken place to date, it is still not free of criticism. But let's start from those incentives.

INTELLECTUAL PROPERTY INCENTIVES

As described above, an inventor is enticed by society to come up with a commercially applicable idea, that is new and nonobvious, and come forward with an application to protect it, in order to be awarded a regional monopoly (be it national or international). Society's intention is twofold: first, to provide incentives for a new technology to be widely implemented and second, to stimulate economic growth. It really makes no sense to the society to utilize its natural resources in order to offer a better education, health care, and long-term sustainability to its citizens, while disregarding the creations of their mind that could potentially supplement the natural resources with intangible resources, i.e., their inventions.

On the other hand, the inventor is asked to prove that his or her idea is new, nonobvious, and has a useful application, while making a detailed description of such an invention. The invention is awarded a financial monopoly that lasts a certain period of years (usually 20 years from filling the application, during which the inventor may commercially exploit it himself or herself, or decide to license it to a manufacturer for a given fee or proportion of future commercialization profits—"royalties"). At the end of the given period, the invention loses its monopoly, and fellow society members may utilize the invention or even improve it, and successfully patent their improvement, and so on.

INTELLECTUAL PROPERTY CRITICISM

There have been various criticisms against the IP system expressed over the years. Some of them may belong to the philosophical domain, while others may hold huge consequences for mankind. The practical guide you are holding in your hands would soon exhaust its pages in discussing the pros and cons of all such criticisms. Instead, it will only briefly mention some of them, leaving the interested reader of monopoly rights to further his or her knowledge by visiting the Web sites of either the proponents of the global IP system in existence (such as the international patent organizations), or some of the global not-for-profit organizations (NGOs) that have campaigned in favor of a freer IP environment.

First, IP rights usually cover items that are called non-rival, that is, goods that may be used by many individuals at a time, for example medicines. Non-Rival goods would be those that can only be used by one individual (in other words, what good would a patent be for a medicine that would be so personal, it could only be used by a single individual due to his or her genetic predisposition?). If that's the case, don't medicines that could save mankind from a global, deadly pandemic belong to mankind as a whole?

Second, inventions may have not been invented, if there were a complete vacuum of IP protection in the form of a commercial monopoly. In other words, why would an inventor of earlier years devote an entire lifetime, countless man-hours, incalculable expenses, and even his own life (think of a researcher self-injecting himself with a new vaccine), if there were no incentives to commercialize it? And even if royalties were not his lifelong aim, what if recognition went to an early imitator who had no fear of a monopoly surrounding the invention? OK, fine, fame or fortune would be a sufficient incentive for innovation. But what if the original inventor charged an exorbitant amount to potential recipients of this vaccine injection? How would the society prosper by the researcher becoming super-rich while the masses remained unprotected from the antigen?

Third, how long should the monopolistic period be for a given healthcare invention? Logic would suggest a sufficient period for the inventor to recuperate the invention's research and development costs, and a nominal profit. Here the danger lies in how much were the total R&D costs (not easily accountable for), or how much should the additional profit be in the face of healthcare inequalities. In other words, if societies cannot afford paying for rising healthcare costs (not only medicine-related), while healthcare manufacturers thrive against all expectations, why shouldn't the monopoly protection period be shortened?

Fourth, except for the monopoly protection period, should we be concerned with what "goods" can be protected? In plain words, it is fine to

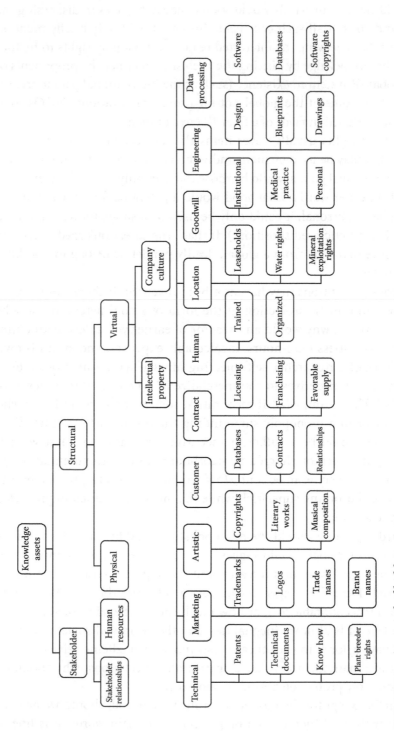

FIGURE 2.1   A myriad of hidden assets.

TABLE 2.1   Which Are the Main Types of Intellectual Property Protection?

Type	Covers	Rights	Terms	Examples
Patent	Device, process, composition of matter	Inventor	20 years	Biopharmaceutical
Copyright	Material form of composition	Author, creator	Author's life + 50 years	Books, software, music
Trademark	Identifiable mark		15 years (renewable)	Logo, slogan
Plant breeder rights	Variety of plant	Breeder	18 years	Quantum Canola
Industrial design	Aesthetic design of product	Designer	10 years	Rug, robot design/ shape
Trade secrets	Anything	n/a	Indefinite	Secret sauce, soft-drink recipe

protect a biopharmaceutical or a medical device with IP protection. What about more "natural," or more "ethereal" goods? Let's be provocative for a minute (it's called writing anyway). How about patenting a genetically modified microorganism? Or a plant and an animal? Should we patent a human being (for example, he could have a genetically modified super-strong muscular system—a "eugenic" clone)? How about the "theory of relativity"—someday it was new, nonobvious, and remains commercially immensely useful. Finally, what about an alien virus arriving to Earth on a meteorite? Or the color of nuclear fusion?

The list keeps on enlarging. For us, it's time to become pragmatists again. We now focus on the role of IP in biotechnology innovation and diffusion. Before we further study the main forms of IP relevant to health-care biotechnology, let's take a look at the various forms of IP protection available today, as shown in Figure 2.1 and Table 2.1.

INTELLECTUAL PROPERTY TYPES

There currently exists a myriad of hidden IP assets, as indicated in Figure 2.1. These assets cover domains belonging from the technical and engineering worlds, to the more artistic and even goodwill environments. As far as the main types of IP protection are concerned, Table 2.1 summarizes what some of these cover, and their respective rights and terms.

Patents

Like every other form of IP, a patent is an exclusive right to a creation of the mind—an invention—surrounding a product or a process. In the case of healthcare biotechnology, a patent may cover a biopharmaceutical product, for example with a unique ability to stimulate the production of neutrophils thus enhancing the body's immune system (see http://www.neupogen.com), or a biotechnology process, such as the one involved in the genetic engineering of a monoclonal antibody, based on the discovery of N.K. Jerne, G.J.F. Kohler, and C. Milstein who received the Nobel Prize in medicine in 1984 (see http://nobelprize.org/nobel_prizes/medicine/laureates/1984/index.html). As previously described, a patent provides a commercial exclusivity to the patent holder, which in the case of pharmaceuticals lasts for 20 years from the day the patent application was filed.

The exclusive rights arising from a patent are awarded to the inventor, who becomes the patent holder. He or she can then decide to capitalize on this invention by self-commercializing it, a case not applicable to the biopharmaceutical industry due to the huge resources required to bring a new medicine to the market place. Instead, the patent holder may decide to license the rights to the invention to an organization or multiple organizations for that purpose. The new patent right holder may then relicense those exclusivity rights to others, for example on a regional basis. Finally, when the patent protection period expires, the rights to the invention become public and everyone can use them for their own purposes.

Patent Privileges and Obligations

As previously described, patents offer the inventor a limited monopoly protection period during which he or she may commercially capitalize on the invention. Following the expiration of this period, anyone may use this invention for either personal or commercial purposes, without any obligations to the original inventor. However, how would the monopoly end, unless the inventor was obliged to reveal the ins and outs of his or her invention? That's exactly what the current patent protection system mandates. In order for someone to protect an invention, he or she has to make a patent application and describe how it works. In other words, if you don't describe it, you fail to protect it, and someone else may claim rights to it. For more information, visit the Web sites of the U.S. Patent and Trademark Office (under the Department of Commerce; http://www.uspto.gov/) or the European Patent Office (created on the basis of the 1973 European Patent Convention—EPC; http://www.epo.org/).

The patent holder's obligation is meant to increase the technological knowledge of the society as a whole, and upon patent expiration, to be disseminated among all society members who may then study it, rework it, improve it, and hopefully patent-protect the improvement. The end result is a regulated, incremental increase of public knowledge that remains at the heart of rewarding the commercial applications of all inventions, in the era of biotechnology.

Inventor versus Patent Holder

The international patent system awards patents to the original inventor, which in the case of healthcare biotechnology is usually a scientist. Obviously, this scientist either works for an academic institution or a company, who are then given rights to this invention, as the inventor's employers who provided him or her with the funds, the facilities, the chemical reagents, the apparatuses, as well as the benefits of working with a team complementing each other's abilities. For example, think of the history-making discoveries of DNA fingerprinting (1984 by molecular biologist Alec Jeffreys; Jeffreys et al. 1985), the polymerase chain reaction (1985 by biochemist Kary Mullis; Saiki et al. 1985), and the genetic sequencing of the human genome (2001, http://www.ornl.gov/sci/techresources/Human_Genome/home.shtml, by both private and government teams). The individual inventor who patented his or her idea on their own, or the respective employer of the biotechnology scientist mentioned above, may then decide to transfer the rights to their invention, to someone who is willing and capable of commercially capitalizing on this invention, for either a one-time fee, or an initially smaller fee plus a proportion of all future profits under patent, the later called a royalty.

All regional patent systems, such as the ones named above, are supervised by Courts who make decisions in times of patent disputes. Therefore, patents can be challenged, they can be found invalid, and they can be annulled. As far as the holders and challengers are concerned, the patents need to be protected, monitored, licensed, sold, further protected with additional patents, researched, reworked around, challenged, limited, invalidated, negotiated, and constantly cared for by a dedicated team of IP specialists.

Patent Function

We have previously described how the patent system makes a compromise between the individual inventor's rights to a limited monopoly, and the society's rights to collectively learn and be improved by the invention. In the process, the patents play several important roles simultaneously. Let's study some of them.

First, they provide an *incentive*. The incentive is in the form of monetary reward for the inventor during a period of exclusivity. Without it, there would be no race to invent it, protect it, and commercially launch a related product. Second, there would be no incremental knowledge added to the world's heritage if it weren't for the individual inventor describing his or her invention in order for a patent to be issued, thus the patent system encourages the *disclosure* of this specialized knowledge by the individual to the society. Third, patents enjoy a limited *monopoly*, which in the case of biopharmaceuticals lasts for 20 years from the patent application filing. With careful analysis, experienced sales and marketing experts may forecast the future potential earning of this biopharmaceutical during its patent protection period (usually 10 years after all required clinical testing and approval procedures are completed and the product is launched under monopoly). Thus, a patent immediately confers a *commercial value* to the invention, and patent holders may negotiate these rights should they decide to license them. Fourth, a biopharmaceutical company's patent family (usually called a *portfolio*) is a dependable and valuable asset, although an intangible asset liable to patent challenges. In most cases, that's what the biopharma industry thrives on, and that's what leads potential investors and employees alike to follow it to the horizon. In other words, patents indicate value, and value is a strong beacon of future financial success and stability. Fifth, patents are a prerequisite for commercial success, thus attracting profits, which are then reinvested into R&D, thus leading to future patents, and so-on. It is this *positive spiral* of research and discovery that has been driving our societies at a faster pace of development over the last 100 years, compared with countless centuries before them. Sixth, patents are a prerequisite to the existence of *free enterprise* societies, as opposed to totalitarian state monopolies where originality and invention are discouraged. The future will prove the retrospective value of the patent system in not only technological, but also general society evolution over the years.

Despite the positive patent functions just mentioned, the patent system is not devoid of criticisms, some of which have been mentioned at the beginning of this chapter. For a shining example of a patent portfolio, see some of Genentech's holdings below (Table 2.2).

Patent Holder Example: Genentech

TABLE 2.2   Selected Genentech Patents

Product	Latest-to-Expire Product-Specific U.S. Patent(s)	Year of Expiration
Avastin	6,884,879	2017
	7,169,901	2019
Rituxan	5,677,180	2014
	5,736,137	2015
	7,381,560	2016
Herceptin	6,339,142	2019
	6,407,213	2019
	7,074,404	2019

Source: Courtesy of GENENTECH 2008 Form 10-K with Exhibits 23.1, 31.1, 31.2, and 32.1, San Francisco, CA, http://www.gene.com

Trademarks

We have previously described how an inventor comes up with an idea, which is finally patented, and licensed to an organization which takes it through a rigorous R&D process until it is approved by the relevant regulatory authorities (in the case of biopharmaceuticals) and is ready for launch. Before doing so, however, the company's marketers must create a thoroughly enticing, distinctive, and memorable visual identity that is to surround the already approved product name in all its future uses, either on the product's packaging, or in promotional materials, Web sites, TV advertisements (where allowed), and so on. Such a visual identity needs to be legally protected, in this case in the form of a trademark, by the relevant trademark approval authorities around the world.

The duration of trademark protection is variable, but can be renewed indefinitely by the holders, provided they pay the required renewal fees. Eventually, through well-designed and persistent efforts by the manufacturer, it becomes globally recognizable and sought-after, enhancing and protecting the product's value from unauthorized copying or counterfeiting, an issue of immense proportion in the field of biopharmaceuticals. Trademarks apply to products or services, an example for the latter being the home-care services that usually accompany the administration of a specialty biopharmaceutical (see Chapter 11).

Now, what does a trademark cover? It covers words (Neuron), names (Roche), letters (TCA Cellular Therapy), numerals (454 Life Sciences), drawings (Lunesta), symbols (Efexor XR), colors (Viagra), signs (Avastin), and even music and sounds when promoting these medicines to healthcare professionals or to the public (only some countries allow—see Chapter 9). For reviewing some of the world's best known medicinal trademarks, see the Physicians' Desk Reference (http://www.pdr.net), or google-search for a trademark's image.

Before we review a famous pharmaceutical trademark holder's example, let's briefly mention the availability of trademarks not belonging to private organizations, but instead to international associations that play a role in biopharma development. For example, a biopharmaceutical company may be given the right to advertise a service quality qualification with the use of a global, well-recognized quality trademark (such as ISO 9000), or the stamp of approval by a regulatory agency (such as FDA-approved manufacturing facilities), or even a patient association's recommendation (visit the International Alliance of Patients' Associations; http://www.patientsorganizations.org/).

For several trademark examples see: GENENTECH's Trademarks, GENENTECH 2008 Form 10-K with Exhibits 23.1, 31.1, 31.2 and 32.1, San Francisco, CA, http://www.gene.com

Trade Secrets

According to the U.S. Patent and Trademark Office (http://www.uspto.gov/ip/global/patents/ir_pat_tradesecret.jsp), trade secrets consist of information and can include a formula, pattern, compilation, program, device, method, technique, or process. As a member of the World Trade Organization (WTO) and a party to the Agreement on Trade Related Aspects of Intellectual-Property Rights (TRIPS), the United States is obligated to provide trade secret protection. Article 39 paragraph 2 requires member nations to provide a means for protecting information that is secret, commercially valuable because it is secret, and subject to reasonable steps to keep it secret. The United States fulfils its obligation by offering trade secret protection under state laws, which are mostly based on the Uniform Trade Secrets Act (http://www.law.upenn.edu/bll/archives/ulc/fnact99/1980s/utsa85.htm). Courts can protect trade secrets by enjoining misappropriation, ordering parties that have misappropriated a trade secret to take steps to maintain its secrecy, as well as ordering payment of a royalty to the owner.

Trade secrets are an alternative to patents. Whether a biopharma company decides to protect its discoveries with one or the other depends on the nature of the secrets to be protected. For example, a patent offers a monopoly protection for a given period of time, while trade secrets are indefinite. A patent requires the secret to be described, and later become publicly known, while trade secrets never divulge this sensitive information. On the other hand, if the trade secret owner does not take proper steps to guard it, or another entity accidentally discovers the same thing, then protection is lost forever. Also, a patent is a guaranteed protection over 20 years, and provided it's not challenged, nothing can legally break it. A trade secret needs to be constantly guarded from prying eyes of vying competitors or malicious employees, but if it is properly guarded it can last for centuries and beyond. In other words, a patent is more predictable, while a trade secret is more hopeful but lasting.

As previously mentioned, in 1982, the collaboration between the biopharmaceutical start-up Genentech with the pharmaceutical powerhouse Eli Lilly resulted in bringing the first biopharmaceutical insulin into the marketplace. Later in 1987, Genentech sued the very same Eli Lilly for stealing its trade secrets over recombinant DNA technology, in creating non-insulin products. Eventually, Eli Lilly managed to have its growth hormone Humatrope approved as an orphan drug (for more on orphan drugs, see Chapter 13).

Trade Secret Protection
As far as trade secret protection is concerned, biopharmas are not only protecting themselves from competition but they are even required by law to protect them, in order for these processes, formulas, or recipes to enjoy a trade secret status in the beginning. In other words, a biopharma publishing its confidential research procedure in an internal R&D department newsletter cannot possibly protect it later by saying it had taken all necessary steps to protect it.

What constitutes trade secret protection practices anyway? Biopharmaceutical researchers are extensively trained in learning and upholding these practices in whatever they do in the laboratory or elsewhere. These may range from keeping detailed, hardcover, bound laboratory notebooks with accompanying dates and signatures of the researchers on each process described in the laboratory notebook; making the employees sign confidentially and non-compete agreements; using laboratory computers with only network hard drives that monitor any suspicious copying;

implementing strict employee web surfing policies; and utilizing the latest software and hardware firewalls. As previously described, trade secrets will remain secret if only well protected indefinitely.

Comparison with Patents

In most cases, biopharmas file for patents and start enjoying the respective monopoly period on their respective discoveries. During this period, the biopharma scientists may come up with invaluable improvements, be it in the form of new subprocesses, better yields, newer tools, alternative raw materials, and so on. The additional improvements immediately become a trade secret and must be protected accordingly. What happens though when the biopharma decides to license its original patent to another company? Obviously, the licensee will require the licensor to reveal any such improvements and modifications they have not protected until then. On the other hand, the licensor will not be able to come up with another patent in the future, unless the improvements had been previously protected as trade secrets. In addition, if the licensor wanted to share a trade secret of its own in exchange for another company's secrets, any such communication should be based on exchanging the appropriate nondisclosure agreements first. For an excellent overview of biotechnology IP issues, see Spruson and Ferguson (2001).

Freedom to Operate

Let's take a simple example. An aspiring biochemist enjoys mixing and matching reagents at his home garage during the weekends. He has previously stocked various sophisticated reagents, some still under patent, from a well-known laboratory supplier. During Thanksgiving holiday he comes up with a mixture recipe, which, when tried on home-lab-grown bacteria, makes them secrete a brownish excretion, proven to be a powerful new antibiotic. Should he rush to the patent office on Monday morning? He'd better not.

The same example applies to most biopharmaceutical upstarts. They have a core team of bright scientists who continuously labor for the next "best thing." In the process, they come up will all kinds of inventions, potentially useful in human therapeutics. Are they free to patent them as their own? Only, if they have not used any other patented products, processes, or tools in the process. If all this applies, then we can declare that they possess "freedom to operate."

What Is Meant by "Freedom to Operate"?

Freedom to operate is the ability to capitalize on an invention, without challenges from any other parties, private or companies. It also means that throughout one invention's creation period, the inventor took extra care in ensuring that he or she has not used any other products or processes that have been previously patented by others. Freedom to operate is therefore a right to commercially capitalize on your biotechnological invention and is not interchangeable with the patent, that is, you may hold a patent but not the freedom to operate. In order to avoid such a serious obstacle, you need to ensure freedom to operate preferably in advance of acquiring the patent.

Ensuring Your Freedom to Operate

In the case of biopharmaceutical inventions, it usually takes more than a decade to bring a new invention to the marketplace. Over this time- and resource-consuming process (see Chapter 6), a plethora of raw materials, tools, chemical reactions, techniques, and processes are used by countless R&D professionals. In order for any biopharma to ensure that it eventually has the freedom to operate, it will take two complementary steps: First, to collect and record every single material, tool, process etc. required for coming up with the invention, and, second, to identify and study any potentially existing exclusivity claims on each and every ingredient used along the way to the invention. Let's review these two steps in detail.

Biopharmaceutical research and development is a sequential process, comprising of seven major steps, namely, (1) discovery and technology, (2) identification of candidate molecules, (3) manufacturing, (4) selection of indications and dosages, (5) validation of target product profile, (6) compilation of the regulatory dossier, and (7) regulatory submission. Step 1 entails the use of in vitro and in vivo disease models, and the application of dedicated process, discovery, and manufacturing technologies. Step 2 includes the lead identification and preclinical development. Step 3 includes the selection of a host system, isolation, and purification of the active substance, improving the production yield, scaling up, and full-scale production.

Every single process during these three significant R&D steps needs to be fully described. In other words, every biopharma needs to record who did what, how, with the help of what, and where. This process will reveal thousands of steps, each with respective inputs, processes, and outputs. All the inputs, processes, and outputs are then taken through an IP screening, for example, who has patent claims, what do these include, where are they valid, and for how long? The search is conducted by experienced IP professionals, over free or proprietary (with high fees) databases. When this step is completed, patent attorneys undertake the task of ascertaining which one of the biopharma thousand R&D steps infringes on someone's patents. Finally, getting the freedom to operate is the decisive step, before the biopharma may proceed with its own commercial applications of the patent.

Getting the Freedom to Operate

There are four main methods for a biopharma to get the required freedom to operate before it takes a new biopharmaceutical candidate through its rigorous clinical trial process. It can pay for the freedom to operate, or it can exchange one of its technologies with somebody else's technology rights. It can also bypass a licensed obstacle by "inventing around" it, or create a "patent pool" with other interested biopharmaceutical or pharmaceutical companies. We study each of these options in detail.

Paying for It   A biopharma in need of an important patent it does not already own can request the patent holder to either sell the patent outright, or license it. For the licensee, it's a go-ahead with its own development plan, which will hopefully repay the costs of acquiring a patent from the outside. For the licensor, it may not be a priority patent, or letting someone else also use it for a different product gives them additional revenue over the patent life. The price of such license or sale is commensurate with the rarity of the patent in question, or the anticipated sales potential of the new product based on the licensed patent.

Exchanging a Technology   Two biopharmas holding large patent portfolios on their own may decide to exchange patent rights on some of their portfolio holdings that will give them access to much needed new expertise and future sales potentials. For example, one company may hold a patent on fast-screening thousands of candidate molecules, each a chemical modification of an archetype, while the other may hold rights on an animal disease model, for example, rat-type II collagen arthritis, an animal model useful for the study of rheumatoid arthritis. Once again, terms and conditions are based on future valuations of the technologies involved (see Chapter 4).

Inventing Around   A biopharma has managed to sequence the gene responsible for interferon alpha, naturally occurring in the body, and later succeeded in inserting the gene into a host system, eventually producing the recombinant molecule with a given yield (see Chapter 7). Later into development, the use of a patented chromatography column has led to a 50-fold increase in the yield. Before licensing the expensive rights to the proprietary column used, the internal development department comes up with a similar column, using a different absorbent material which not only is patent-free, but may revolutionize the interferon biomanufacturing in the future. The discovery eventually leads to their own chromatography patent, as well as a means to "invent around" the manufacturing technique.

Patent Sharing   Three academic institutions, active in the fields of gene sequencing, come up with complementary ideas for enhancing and accelerating the process of gene sequencing on the way to sequencing the first-ever mammalian species' complete genome. Instead of laboring individually for years, in the race to the genome characterization, they come together by forming a patent-sharing pool, each allowing the others to share, use, and improve upon the respective patents, with all eventual improvements to be shared among the three. In the end, their pooled patents attract the interest of a major biopharmaceutical company, which licenses the pool from the three academic parties. In retrospect, if it weren't for the patent pool, no individual parties would have progressed enough in the sequencing, neither would they have access to any significant royalties, nor would the biopharma ever capitalize on the genome knowledge to produce its own therapeutic interventions.

For a freedom to operate example see: Molecular Partners Press Release, Zurich, Switzerland, http://www.molecularpartners.com

Biotechnology Patentability
General Patentability Qualifications
At the beginning of this chapter, we mentioned the three basic requirements for an invention's patentability, namely, novelty, usefulness, and nonobviousness. The same requirements also apply for any biotechnology patent, although these characteristics are sometimes debatable, for example, the future usefulness of a first-to-the-world genetic manipulation can hardly be described.

The three requirements needed are evaluated by the relevant patent office on the basis of how the inventor describes his or her invention in the patent application documents, where he or she is obliged to make certain "claims" on the invention. When it comes to these claims, there is a "tug-of-war" between claiming narrow claims, for example, "our technique can precisely cleave aptamer XYZ of chromosome 17XY," or for that matter broader claims, for example, "our techniques can split and splice every aptamer belonging to the human genome." The difference in these claims is obviously enormous, and has even wider commercial ramifications in the future. A rule of thumb is that it makes more practical sense to make as wider the claims as the patent office will allow.

When it comes to biotechnology patentability, there exist significant differences between the biggest patent offices (United States, Europe, and Japan) in the world. We attempt to review some of the applicable differences below.

U.S. Patent Example Covering ENBREL (U.S. Patent 5712155)

Title: DNA encoding tumor necrosis factor-α and -β receptors

Inventors: Smith, Craig A. (Seattle, WA), Goodwin, Raymond G. (Seattle, WA), Beckmann, Patricia M. (Poulsbo, WA). Claims: What is claimed is:

1. An isolated DNA sequence selected from the group consisting of: (a) a DNA sequence that encodes a polypeptide having the amino acid sequence selected from the group consisting of amino acids 1 to X of FIG. 2A and amino acids 1 to 233 of FIG. 3A, wherein X is an amino acid from 163 to 235; and (b) a DNA sequence capable of hybridization to the complement of the DNA sequence of (a) under moderately stringent conditions (50°C., 2× SSC) and which encodes a polypeptide that is capable of binding to TNF and which is at least 88% identical to a polypeptide encoded by the DNA of (a).

2. An isolated DNA sequence selected from the group consisting of: (a) a DNA sequence that encodes a polypeptide having the amino acid sequence selected from the group consisting of amino acids 1 to X of FIG. 2A and amino acids 1 to 233 of FIG. 3A, wherein X is an amino acid from 163 to 235; and (b) a DNA sequence capable of hybridization to the complement of the DNA sequence of (a) under moderately stringent conditions (50°C., 2× SSC) and which encodes TNF-R protein that is capable of binding greater than 0.1 nmoles TNF per nmole

TNF-R and which is at least 88% identical to a polypeptide encoded by the DNA of (a).

3. An isolated DNA sequence selected from the group consisting of: (a) a DNA sequence that encodes a polypeptide having the amino acid sequence selected from the group consisting of amino acids 1 to X of FIG. 2A and amino acids 1 to 233 of FIG. 3A, wherein X is an amino acid from 163 to 235; and (b) a DNA sequence capable of hybridization to the complement of the DNA sequence of (a) under moderately stringent conditions (50°C., 2× SSC) and which encodes TNF-R protein that is capable of binding greater than 0.5 nmoles TNF per nmole TNF-R and which is at least 88% identical to a polypeptide encoded by the DNA of (a).

4. A recombinant expression vector comprising the DNA sequence according to claim 1.

5. A recombinant expression vector comprising the DNA sequence according to claim 2.

6. A recombinant expression vector comprising the DNA sequence according to claim 3.

7. A host cell transformed or transfected with the vector according to claim 4.

8. A host cell transformed or transfected with the vector according to claim 5.

9. A host cell transformed or transfected with the vector according to claim 6.

10. An isolated DNA sequence selected from the group consisting of (a) a DNA sequence that encodes a polypeptide having the amino acid sequence selected from the group consisting of amino acids 1 to X of FIG. 2A and amino adds 1 to 233 of FIG. 3A, wherein X is an amino acid from 163 to 235; and (b) a DNA sequence that encodes a polypeptide identical to the polypeptide encoded by the DNA of (a) except for modification(s) to the amino acid sequence selected from the group consisting of: (i) inactivated N-linked glycosylation sites; (ii) altered KEX2 protease cleavage sites; (iii) conservative amino acid substitutions; (iv) substitution or deletion of cysteine residues; and (iv) combinations of modifications (i)-(iv); wherein such polypeptide is capable of binding TNF.

11. An isolated DNA sequence selected from the group consisting of: (a) a DNA sequence that encodes a polypeptide having the amino acid sequence selected from the group consisting of amino acids 1 to X of FIG. 2A and amino acids 1 to 233 of FIG. 3A, wherein X is an amino acid from 163 to 235; and (b) a DNA sequence that encodes a polypeptide identical to the polypeptide encoded by the DNA of (a) except for modification(s) to the amino acid sequence selected from the group consisting of (i) inactivated N-linked glycosylation sites; (ii) altered KEX2 protease cleavage sites; (ii) conservative amino acid substitutions; (iv) substitution or deletion of cysteine residues; and (v) combinations of modifications (i)-(iv); which encoded polypeptide is capable of binding greater than 0.1 moles TNF per nmole of such polypeptide.

12. An isolated DNA sequence selected from the group consisting of (a) a DNA sequence that encodes a polypeptide having the amino acid sequence selected from the group consisting of amino acids 1 to X of FIG. 2A and amino acids 1 to 233 of FIG. 3A, wherein X is an amino acid from 163 to 235; and (b) a DNA sequence that encodes a polypeptide identical to the polypeptide encoded by the DNA of (a) except for modification(s) to the amino acid sequence selected from the group consisting of (i) inactivated N-linked glycosylation sites; (ii) altered KEX2 protease cleavage sites; (ii) conservative amino acid substitutions; (iv) substitution or deletion of cysteine residues; and (v) combinations of modifications (i)-(iv); which encoded polypeptide is capable of binding greater than 0.5 moles TNF per nmole of such polypeptide.

13. A recombinant expression vector comprising the DNA according to any of claims 10, 11 or 12.

14. A host cell transformed or transfected with the vector according to claim 13.

15. A DNA sequence that encodes a polypeptide having the amino acid sequence selected from the group consisting of (a) amino acids 1-235 of FIG. 2A; and (b) a DNA sequence capable of hybridization to the DNA sequence of (a) under moderately stringent conditions (50°C., 2× SSC) and which encodes a polypeptide that is capable of binding to TNF and which is at least 88% identical to a polypeptide encoded by the DNA of (a).

16. A recombinant expression vector comprising the DNA sequence according to claim 15.
17. A host cell transformed or transfected with the vector according to claim 16.

Source: Courtesy of freepatentsonline, Miami Beach, FL, http://www.freepatentsonline.com/5712155.html

United States For a thorough review of biotechnology patentability by the U.S. Patent and Trademark Office (USPTO), see the *Manual of Patent Examining Procedure (MPEP)*, 2008.

We begin our overview by referring to a historic decision by the U.S. Supreme Court in 1980, in *Diamond vs. Chakrabarty*, 447 U.S. 303 (U.S. Supreme Court, 1980) 447 U.S. 303—Argued March 17, 1980—Decided June 16, 1980. Title 35 U.S.C. 101 provides for the issuance of a patent to a person who invents or discovers "any" new and useful "manufacture" or "composition of matter."

The respondent filed a patent application relating to his invention of a human-made, genetically engineered bacterium capable of breaking down crude oil, a property which is possessed by no naturally occurring bacteria. A patent examiner's rejection of the patent application's claims for the new bacteria was affirmed by the Patent Office Board of Appeals on the ground that living things are not patentable subject matter under 101. The Court of Customs and Patent Appeals reversed, concluding that the fact that microorganisms are alive is without legal significance for purposes of the patent law. Held:

A live, human-made microorganism is patentable subject matter under 101. Respondent's microorganism constitutes a "manufacture" or "composition of matter" within that statute (pp. 308–318).

(a) In choosing such expansive terms as "manufacture" and "composition of matter," modified by the comprehensive "any," Congress contemplated that the patent laws should be given wide scope, and the relevant legislative history also supports a broad construction. While laws of nature, physical phenomena, and abstract ideas are not patentable, respondent's claim is not to a hitherto unknown natural phenomenon, but to a nonnaturally occurring manufacture or composition of matter—a product of human ingenuity "having a distinctive name, character [and] use." Hartranft vs. Wiegmann, 121 U.S. 609, 615. Funk Brothers Seed Co. vs. Kalo Inoculant Co., 333 U.S. 127, distinguished (pp. 308–310).

(b) The passage of the 1930 Plant Patent Act, which afforded patent protection to certain asexually reproduced plants, and the 1970 Plant Variety Protection Act, which authorized protection for certain sexually reproduced plants but excluded bacteria from its protection, does not evidence congressional understanding that the terms "manufacture" or "composition of matter" in 101 do not include living things (pp. 310–314). [447 U.S. 303, 304]. (c) Nor does the fact that genetic technology was unforeseen when Congress enacted 101 require the conclusion that micro-organisms cannot qualify as patentable subject matter until Congress expressly authorizes such protection. The unambiguous language of 101 fairly embraces respondent's invention. Arguments against patentability under 101, based on potential hazards that may be generated by genetic research, should be addressed to the Congress and the Executive, not to the Judiciary (pp. 314–318, decision posted at http://caselaw.lp.findlaw.com/scripts/getcase.pl?court=us&vol=447&invol=303).

In reviewing the U.S. Supreme Court decision, USPTO's MPEP-Chapter 2100 clearly states that "The tests set forth by the Court are:

(A) 'The laws of nature, physical phenomena and abstract ideas' are not patentable subject matter.

(B) A 'non-naturally occurring manufacture or composition of matter—a product of human ingenuity—having a distinctive name, character, [and] use' is patentable subject matter.

(C) '[A] new mineral discovered in the earth or a new plant found in the wild is not patentable subject matter. Likewise, Einstein could not patent his celebrated $E = mc^2$; nor could Newton have patented the law of gravity. Such discoveries are "manifestations of… nature, free to all men and reserved exclusively to none."'

(D) '[T]he production of articles for use from raw materials prepared by giving to these materials new forms, qualities, properties, or combinations whether by hand labor or by machinery' [emphasis added] is a 'manufacture' under 35 U.S. 101."

Source: U.S. Patent and Trademark Office (USPTO), 2008. *The Manual of Patent Examining Procedure (MPEP)*, Chapter 2100 on Patentability. 8th edn., Alexandria, VA, August 2001, Latest Revision July 2008, p. 2105. Posted at: http://www.uspto.gov/web/offices/pac/mpep/mpep_e8r6_2100.pdf

Leaving the legalese behind us, natural products can NOT be patented, while recombinant products CAN be patented. In addition, the USPTO

TABLE 2.3   Patents in Biotech: Key Hurdles in Protecting IP

Subject Matter	In What Category Does the Invention Fit?
Utility	How can it be used? Does it have proven value to humans?
Novelty	Is it different from the "prior art"?
	Is the invention known or previously published in the art?
Obviousness	Did the inventor simply take "the next obvious step"?
Disclosure	Is there sufficient information disclosed to allow one skilled in the art to repeat the invention?

may award biotechnology-related patents for a novel method of manufacturing a naturally occurring protein (manufacturing patents), a device used for its administration into humans (device patents), as well as the use of that protein in treating a disease (use patents), but not all diseases. Irrespective of the type of patent sought, all biotechnology-related patents must clear the hurdles summarized in Table 2.3.

Examples of Patentable Organisms in the United States   The U.S. Biotechnology Industry Organization (BIO) gives an excellent review of patentable organisms in the United States in its *Guide to Biotechnology 2008* (Guilford-Blake and Strickland, 2008. With permission). For example:

Natural compounds: A human protein is natural, but not living. It can be isolated, sequenced, its encoding gene encoded in a host system, and reproduced in the laboratory. For this process, the protein can be patented, although it's natural.

Genes: The human genome was fully sequenced in 2003 (see http://www.ornl.gov/sci/techresources/Human_Genome/home.shtml). It has been found to contain approximately 25,000 genes, some of them previously characterized and used in the biosynthetic engineering of therapeutic proteins. The manipulations that led to the protein production were patented, since they did not occur in nature. Such patents were, once again, based on novelty, usefulness, and non-obviousness. In contrast, the human genome, or a single gene within it cannot be patented, since they are obvious and NOT useful for anything specific.

Microbes: The history-making case of Chakrabarty's invention of a new bacterium genetically engineered to degrade crude oil was mentioned above. In 1980, the U.S. Supreme Court clearly stated that new micro-organisms not found in nature were patentable, and Chakrabarty received a patent in 1981 (U.S. Pat. No. 4,259,444).

Plants: In 1930, the U.S. Congress passed the Plant Patent Act, which specifically provided patent protection for newly invented plants that are asexually reproduced. In 1970, Congress provided similar protection for newly invented sexually reproduced plants.

Animals: In 1988, P. Leder and T. Stewart were granted a patent on transgenic nonhuman mammals (U.S. Pat. No. 4,736,866; http://www.freepatentsonline.com/4736866.html) that covered the so-called Harvard mouse, a genetically engineered model for the study of cancer. For more information on transgenics, see Chapter 7.

Source: Molecular Partners Raises 18.5 Mio CHF in Series A Financing, Zurich–Schlieren, Switzerland, August 14, 2007.

Europe   The European Patent Office (EPO; http://www.epo.org) is part of the European Patent Organization that currently has 36 member states. EPO awards biotechnology patents based on the same principles of novelty, usefulness, and nonobviousness, while there are also special considerations made for special biotechnology fields, for example, living organisms, genes, etc. that are discussed below. EPO has reported that during 2008, there were 7597 patent applications filed and 2858 patents granted in the field of biotechnology (EPO, 2009).

The European Biotech Patent Directive
Following a multiyear debate among member states, the EU Directive 98/44/EC on the legal protection of biotechnological inventions—the Biotech Patent Directive—was adopted on July 6, 1998. This was later incorporated into the Implementing Regulations to the European Patent Conference (EPC) as secondary legislation (European Patent Convention, 2007). According to the Directive, biotechnological inventions are basically patentable:

- Isolated biological material is patentable even if it has occurred previously in nature (Rule 27 (a) EPC).

- Plants or animals are patentable if the technical feasibility of the invention (e.g., a genetic modification) is not confined to a particular plant or animal variety (Rule 27 (b) EPC).

- An invention relating to gene sequences can be patented as long as the industrial application of the sequence is disclosed in the application and all other patentability criteria are fulfilled (Rule 29 (3) EPC).

However, according to the EPC, no European patent can be granted for the following:

- Any invention whose commercial exploitation would be contrary to public order or morality (Art. 53 (a) EPC).

- Plant and animal varieties (Art. 53 (b) EPC).

- Essentially biological processes for the production of plants and animals (Art. 53 (b) EPC), e.g., classical breeding, crossing, and selection.

- Methods for treatment of the human or animal body by surgery or therapy, and diagnostic methods practiced on the human or animal body (Art. 53 (c) EPC).

- Discoveries (e.g., the discovery of natural substances, such as the sequence or partial sequence of a gene) are not patentable because, without a description of the technical problem they are intended to solve and a technical teaching, they are not regarded as inventions (Art. 52 (2) (a) EPC).

- The entire human body in all its developmental phases (Rule 29 (1) EPC). The same applies to processes for cloning human beings, processes for modifying the germ-line genetic identity of human beings, and the use of human embryos for industrial or commercial purposes. Also excluded from patentability are processes for modifying the genetic identity of animals which are likely to cause them suffering without any substantial medical benefit to man or animal, and animals resulting from such processes. This catalog of exceptions to patentability is not exhaustive (Rule 28 EPC).

Table 2.4 describes some of the major U.S.–Europe biotechnology patentability differences.

EPO Patent Example: Genentech/Roche
REGISTER ENTRY FOR GB2079291. Form 1 Application No GB8120279.8 filing date 01.07.1981.

TABLE 2.4   U.S.–Europe Biotechnology Patentability Differences

	United States	**EPO**
Methods of treatment or therapy	Patentable	Not patentable
Inventions from collaborative research	Not patentable	Patentable

Title INTERFERONS AND PROCESS FOR THEIR PREPARATION
Applicants/Proprietors
  GENENTECH INC., 460 Point San Bruno Boulevard, South San Francisco, California, United States of America   [ADP No. 00467670001]
  F HOFFMANN-LA ROCHE & CO AKTIENGESELLSCHAFT, Incorporated in Switzerland, 124–184 Grenzacherstrasse, CH-4002 Basle, Switzerland   [ADP No. 00854356001]
Inventors
  SIDNEY PESTKA, 82 Brookside Terrace, North Caldwell, New Jersey, United States of America   [ADP No. 02192631001]
  DAVID VAN NORMAN GOEDDEL, 1449 Benito Avenue, Burlingame, California, United States of America   [ADP No. 02554897001]
Publication No GB2079291 dated 20.01.1982. Examination requested 09.02.1982
Patent Granted with effect from 13.06.1984 (Section 25(1)) with title INTERFERONS AND PROCESS FOR THEIR PREPARATION

Source: Courtesy of http://www.espacenet.com/index.en.htm

Australia   IP Australia (Phillip ACT HQ; http://www.ipaustralia.gov.au/) administers Australia's IP rights system, specifically patents, trademarks, designs, and plant breeder's rights. According to the Australian Patents Act 1990 (prepared on March 27, 2007, taking into account amendments up to Act No. 106 of 2006; http://www.comlaw.gov.au), patentable inventions for the purposes of a standard patent are

(1) Subject to subsection (2), an invention is a patentable invention for the purposes of a standard patent if the invention, so far as claimed in any claim:

  (a) Is a manner of manufacture within the meaning of Section 6 of the Statute of Monopolies.

  (b) When compared with the prior art base as it existed before the priority date of that claim:

    (i) Is novel

    (ii) Involves an inventive step

  (c) Is useful

  (d) Was not secretly used in the patent area before the priority date of that claim by, or on behalf of, or with the authority of, the patentee or nominated person or the patentee's or nominated person's predecessor in title to the invention.

Patentable inventions for the purposes of an innovation patent

(1A) Subject to subsections (2) and (3), an invention is a patentable invention for the purposes of an innovation patent if the invention, so far as claimed in any claim:

(a) Is a manner of manufacture within the meaning of Section 6 of the Statute of Monopolies

(b) When compared with the prior art base as it existed before the priority date of that claim:

(i) Is novel

(ii) Involves an innovative step

(c) Is useful

(d) Was not secretly used in the patent area before the priority date of that claim by, or on behalf of, or with the authority of, the patentee or nominated person or the patentee's or nominated person's predecessor in title to the invention.

(2) Human beings, and the biological processes for their generation, are not patentable inventions. Certain inventions are not patentable inventions for the purposes of an innovation patent.

(3) For the purposes of an innovation patent, plants and animals, and the biological processes for the generation of plants and animals, are not patentable inventions.

(4) Subsection (3) does not apply if the invention is a microbiological process or a product of such a process.

Japan and China   For an excellent review of the practice of the United States, the European Union, Japan, and China for the protection of biotechnology inventions, see Xinqi and Tanaka (2006) posted at the Japan Patent Office Web site (http://www.jpo.go.jp).

Biotechnology Patentability Controversies
As previously discussed, the Chakrabarty bacterium (U.S. Patent. No. 4,259,444) and the Harvard onco-mouse (EU Patent No. 0 169 672) have provided ample material for a huge biotechnology patentability controversy across the two sides of the Atlantic. This discussion continues unabated to date, with both sides of the controversy fiercely protecting their interests. Some of the currently controversial issues are stem cell cultures, which promise to revolutionize therapeutics, but their isolation from human embryos is seen by many as immoral; the application of transgenic

crops into commercial agriculture for reasons of disease resistance and enhanced productivity is also opposed by proponents of the planet's biodiversity as well as food-chain contamination fears; transgenic animals are not devoid of the accusation of immoral and creation-interfering artificial life forms; hybrid human/animals pose the question of what lies ahead, for example the controversial theory of eugenics; animal cloning is another hotly contested issue; and finally natural (un-programmed) mutations of transgenics in the future pose further questions about the soundness of the underlying science meant for the service of all mankind.

Patent Application

In order for any given patent office to award a patent, a proper patent application needs to be filed first, following set rules concerning its contents. In general, such patent application is comprised of three parts, namely (1) a written document entitled the specification and containing the description and claims, (2) a drawing, if needed, and (3) appropriate fees for filing, searching, and examination.

Let's focus on the patent specification part, as it pertains to a biotechnology patent. It starts with (1) an abstract and (2) a title. It then moves into the invention specification, namely, (3) the relevant technical field, and (4) a description of the invention background, called "prior art." It then focuses on (5) the object of the invention, and then (6) a full disclosure of the invention. Such a disclosure should be in a clear language and sufficient detail so that a person knowledgeable in the field should be able to reproduce it. The invention description is usually followed by (7) a short description of the attached drawings, and (8) a short description of the proposed method of reproducing the invention. In addition, because inventions pertaining to genetic material need to be accompanied by proper specimens, the patent application also contains (9) a description of the microorganism deposits, or (10) a sequence listing of any DNA, RNA, and/or protein sequences involved. In addition, the application contains (11) a description of the industrial applicability of the invention, (12) the previously described patent claims that the patent seeks to uphold, and (13) all relevant drawings.

Essential Patent Conditions

The essential patent conditions that need to be satisfied before any patent is awarded are (1) novelty, namely, that the invention has added an inventive step over the preexisting knowledge in the field, usually referred to as "prior art," (2) usefulness, namely, that the invention is commercially useful and

TABLE 2.5   How Does One Decide to Patent a Biopharmaceutical Invention?

Have the prospects of obtaining a valid patent been assessed?

Has a novelty search been conducted?

Has the extent of possible protection been assessed?

Could infringement of the patent be easily detected?

Is there relevant competitor activity?

Has the relationship of the patent with other intellectual property been assessed?

Does the commercial potential or return justify the cost of enforcement if necessary?

Have countries where patent protection may be required been identified?

Does the organization have the capability and intention to commercialize the invention itself?

If not, do possible licensing opportunities exist?

Has the invention been published?

Has the invention been used commercially?

Source: Adapted from, Biotechnology Intellectual Property Manual, Biotechnology Australia, Canberra, Australian Capital Territory, Australia, 2001.

may lead to a practical application; and (3) nonobviousness, namely, that a superficial reading of prior art would not have led any given person to come up with the said invention. In addition, biotechnology patents need to pass a fourth hurdle, namely that of being patentable, since their immense implications for life and disease among several species cannot extend the boundaries that a civilized society would allow, for example, for reasons that contradict the society's ethics, religious beliefs, the protection of the human as well as other species, the necessity to protect individualism over a species cloning, etc. As previously described, biotechnology patentability varies across the world's most influential patent offices.

The special conditions that need to be fulfilled mentioned above require the careful screening of any potential patent application by trained IP specialists, in advance of the patent application. Such a screening may include, but is not limited to the questions posed in Table 2.5, as summarized by Biotechnology Australia.

Patenting Procedures

We have previously mentioned some of the foremost patent offices in the world of biotechnology, namely, the U.S., European, and Japanese offices. Furthermore, the World Intellectual Property Organization (WIPO; Geneva HQ; http://www.wipo.org) is a United Nations agency dedicated to developing a balanced and accessible international IP system.

There are three potential avenues for a biopharma company considering filing a patent application. First, it may file an application with a national patent office, such as the USPTO. Second, it may file an application with a regional patent office, such as the EPO or the African Regional Industrial Property Organization (ARIPO, Harare HQ, http://www.aripo.org), or the Eurasian Patent Office (EAPO, Moscow HQ, http://www.eapo.org/eng/ea/). For a thorough international directory of national and regional Patent Offices visit the WIPO's web page at http://www.wipo.int/directory/en/urls.jsp).

Third, the biopharma may also apply to the WIPO and seek patent protection for an invention simultaneously in each of a large number of countries by filing an "international" patent application, which is thus subjected to an "international search" the report of which is communicated to the applicant who may decide to withdraw the application if the report makes the granting of license unlikely. According to WIPO, the procedure under the PCT has great advantages for the applicant, the patent offices, and the general public, such as

(i)   the applicant has up to 18 months more than he has in a procedure outside the PCT to reflect on the desirability of seeking protection in foreign countries, to appoint local patent agents in each foreign country, to prepare the necessary translations and to pay the national fees; he is assured that, if his international application is in the form prescribed by the PCT, it cannot be rejected on formal grounds by any designated Office during the national phase of the processing of the application; on the basis of the international search report or the written opinion, he can evaluate with reasonable probability the chances of his invention being patented; and the applicant has the possibility during the international preliminary examination to amend the international application to put it in order before processing by the designated Offices;

(ii) the search and examination work of patent offices can be considerably reduced or virtually eliminated thanks to the international search report, the written opinion and, where applicable, the international preliminary examination report that accompany the international application;

(iii) since each international application is published together with an international search report, third parties are in a better position to formulate a well-founded opinion about the patentability of the claimed invention.

Source: Courtesy of WIPO, Geneva, Switzerland, http://www.wipo. int/pct/en/treaty/about.htm

Filing U.S. Applications   The U.S. Patent and Trademark Office (USPTO) gives a brief outline of the patents process in its web pages (http://www. uspto.gov/patents/process/index.jsp). Basically, acquiring a U.S. patent can be broken down into five simple steps:

1. Search the Patent Full-Text and Image Database (PatFT) to see if an idea has already been patented.

2. View Fee Schedule for current fees and information related to the patent process.

3. Apply for a patent using the Electronic Filing System (EFS-Web) as a registered eFiler or unregistered eFiler.

4. Check Status of a current patent application or any published application using the Patent Application Information Retrieval (PAIR) system.

5. Maintain a patent by paying maintenance fees using the Revenue Accounting and Management (RAM) system.

There are additional optional steps that you may encounter in the patent process: (a) Appeal the decisions made on your patent application with the Board of Patent Appeals and Interferences (BPAI), and (b) Assign Ownership of a patent using the Electronic Patent Assignment System (EPAS).

Filing European Applications   The European Patent Office (EPO) explains in its web pages the procedure for filing a European patent application (http://www.epo.org/patents/One-Stop-Page.html). We review an excerpt of these instructions below:

> The European Patent Office accepts applications under the European Patent Convention (EPC) and the Patent Cooperation Treaty (PCT). If you are seeking protection in only a few countries, it may be best to apply direct for a national patent to each of the national offices. A European patent application consists of: a) a request for grant, b) a description of the invention, c) claims, d) drawings (if any), and an abstract. Applications can be filed at the EPO in any language. However, the official languages of the EPO are English, French and German. If the application is not filed in one of these languages, a translation has to be submitted.

Filing and formalities examination:

The first step in the European patent granting procedure is the examination on filing. This involves checking whether all the necessary information and documentation has been provided, so that the application can be accorded a filing date. The following are required: a) an indication that a European patent is sought, b) particulars identifying the applicant, c) a description of the invention or d) a reference to a previously filed application. If no claims are filed, they need to be submitted within two months. This is followed by a formalities examination relating to certain formal aspects of the application, including the form and content of the request for grant, drawings and abstract, the designation of the inventor, the appointment of a professional representative, the necessary translations and the fees due.

Search: While the formalities examination is being carried out, a European search report is drawn up, listing all the documents available to the Office that may be relevant to assessing novelty and inventive step. The search report is based on the patent claims but also takes into account the description and any drawings. Immediately after it has been drawn up, the search report is sent to the applicant together with a copy of any cited documents and an initial opinion as to whether the claimed invention and the application meet the requirements of the European Patent Convention.

Publication of the application:

The application is published—normally together with the search report—18 months after the date of filing or, if priority was claimed, the priority date. Applicants then have six months to decide whether or not to pursue their application by requesting substantive examination. Alternatively, an applicant who has requested examination already will be invited to confirm whether the application should proceed. Within the same time limit the applicant must decide in which states protection is needed and confirm this by paying the appropriate designation fees and, if applicable, the extension fees. From the date of publication, a European patent application confers provisional protection on the invention in the states designated in the application. However, depending on the relevant national law, it may be necessary to file a translation of the claims with the patent office in question and have this translation published.

Substantive examination: After the request for examination has been made, the European Patent Office examines whether the European patent application and the invention meet the requirements of the European Patent Convention and whether a patent can be granted. An examining division normally consists of three examiners, one of whom maintains contact with the applicant or representative. The decision on the application is taken by the examining division as a whole in order to ensure maximum objectivity.

The grant of a patent:
If the examining division decides that a patent can be granted, it issues a decision to that effect. A mention of the grant is published in the European Patent Bulletin once the translations of the claims have been filed and the fees for grant and printing have been paid. The decision to grant takes effect on the date of publication. The granted European patent is a "bundle" of individual national patents.

Validation: Once the mention of the grant is published, the patent has to be validated in each of the designated states within a specific time limit to retain its protective effect and be enforceable against infringers. In a number of contracting states, the patent owner may have to file a translation of the specification in an official language of the national patent office. Depending on the relevant national law, the applicant may also have to pay fees by a certain date.

Opposition: After the European patent has been granted, it may be opposed by third parties—usually the applicant's competitors—if they believe that it should not have been granted. This could be on the grounds, for example, that the invention lacks novelty or does not involve an inventive step. Notice of opposition can only be filed within nine months of the grant being mentioned in the European Patent Bulletin. Oppositions are dealt with by opposition divisions, which are normally made up of three examiners.

Limitation/revocation: This stage may also consist of revocation or limitation proceedings initiated by the patent proprietor himself. At any time after the grant of the patent the patent proprietor may request the revocation or limitation of his patent. The decision to limit or to revoke the European patent takes effect on the date on which it is published in the European Patent Bulletin and applies ab initio to all contracting states in respect of which the patent was granted.

Appeal: Decisions of the European Patent Office—refusing an application or in opposition cases, for example—are open to appeal. Decisions on appeals are taken by the independent boards of appeal. In certain cases it may be possible to file a petition for review by the Enlarged Board of Appeal.

Filing Japanese Applications   Similarly to the other patent offices, the Japan Patent Office (JPO) describes in its own web pages (http://www.jpo.go.jp/cgi/linke.cgi?url=/tetuzuki_e/t_gaiyo_e/pa_right.htm) the procedures for obtaining a patent right, as excerpted below:

(1) Application: No matter how good an invention may be, a patent right naturally cannot be obtained unless it is applied for. An application requires that one fills out the forms prescribed in the relevant ordinances and submit them to the JPO. Japan has adopted the first-to-file system, i.e. the principle that where two parties apply for a patent for the same invention, the first party to file will be granted the patent. Accordingly, it is advisable to file as soon as possible after the invention. It is also advisable not to make the invention public before filing a patent application.

(2) Formality Examination: An application document submitted to the JPO will be checked to see whether it fulfils the necessary procedural and formal requirements. An invitation to correct will be made where necessary documents are missing or required sections have not been filled in.

(3) Publication of Unexamined Application: The JPO will publish the content of an application in the Official Gazette after 18 months have elapsed from the date of filing.

(4) Request for Examination: Patent applications are not necessarily examined. An examination will be carried out only for the application for which the applicant or a third party has filed a request for examination and paid the examination fees.

(5) Deemed Withdrawal (No Request for Examination). Any application for which a request for examination has not been filed

within a period of *three years from filing date will automatically be regarded as withdrawal and cannot be patented thereafter.

(6) Substantive Examination: An examination will be carried out by an examiner of the JPO, who will decide whether or not the claimed invention should be patented. The examiner firstly checks whether the application fulfils requirements prescribed by law, i.e., whether or not there are any reasons for refusal.

(7) Notification of Reasons for Refusal: If the examiner finds reasons for refusal, a notification to this result will be sent to the applicant.

(8) Written Argument/Amendment: An applicant who has received the notification of reasons for refusal shall be given an opportunity to submit either a written argument claiming that the invention differs from the prior art to which the notification of reasons for refusal refers, or an amendment of the claims in the case that this would nullify the reasons for refusal.

(9) Decision to Grant a Patent: As a result of the examination, the examiner will make a decision to grant a patent as the final assessment of the examination stage if no reasons for refusal have been found. The examiner will also make the same decision if the reasons for refusal have been eliminated by an argument or amendment.

(10) Decision of Refusal: On the other hand, if the examiner judges that the reasons for refusal have not been eliminated, a decision of refusal (the final assessment of the examination stage) will be made.

(11) Appeal against Decision of Refusal: When dissatisfaction is in the decision of refusal of the examiner, the applicant may appeal against the decision of refusal.

(12) Appeal Examination (against Decision of Refusal): The appeal examination against the decision of refusal is performed by a collegial body of three or five appeal examiners. Decision of the appeal examiners is called an appeal decision. When it is judged as a result of appeal examination that the reasons for refusal was solved, an appeal decision to grant a patent is performed, and when the appeal examiners judge that the reasons cannot be cancelled and the patent cannot be registered, an appeal decision of refusal is performed.

(13) Registration (Patent Fee Payment): Provided that the applicant pays the patent fee, once the decision to grant a patent has been

made the patent right will come into effect as it is entered in the Patent Register. At the same time, the invention acquires a patent number. After a patent is registered, a certificate of patent will be sent to the applicant.

(14) Publication of Patent Gazette: The contents of the patent right entered in the Register will be published in the Patent Gazette.

(15) Appeal for Invalidation: Even after a patent is registered, any person may appeal for invalidation of the patent if it has a flaw.

(16) Appeal Examination (Invalidation): An appeal examination of invalidation is carried out by a collegial body of three or five appeal examiners. If the appeal examiners judge that there is no flaw in the decision to grant a patent, they will make a decision to maintain the patent. If however they judge that the decision to grant was flawed, they will make a decision to invalid the patent right.

(17) Intellectual Property High Court: An applicant who is dissatisfied with an appeal decision of refusal of an appeal against decision of refusal, and an interested party who is dissatisfied with an appeal decision of invalidation or maintenance, may appeal to the Intellectual Property High Court.

Patent Life

As previously described, a patent for a biopharmaceutical lasts for 20 years from the day of the patent application filing. Obviously, following the application and while the patent is still pending, the manufacturer undertakes a series of preclinical tests in a race against time in order to submit an application to the U.S. Food and Drug Administration (FDA, Washington, DC HQ, http://www.fda.gov) for subsequent clinical tests, and after several years hopefully files for a marketing authorization before launching the product into the marketplace (see Chapter 6).

Based on the fact that preclinical, clinical, and regulatory approval times collectively add upto approximately 10 years, the biopharmaceutical product has a limited time to recuperate the large R&D costs before patent expiration, namely, the remaining 10 years, a period often called the patent's "effective life." Should the biopharma manufacturer achieve a more expeditious approval, more time will obviously be left for the patent's effective life. Another means of lengthening the effective life is to file for a patent following a series of preliminary preclinical tests performed under secrecy, so that patent filing is closer to clinical testing and eventually the product's marketing approval.

A Biopharmaceutical Patent before Regulatory Approval or Vice Versa?
If the effective patent date is practically limited to 10 years, then why should a biopharma not file for a patent following the drug's FDA approval and enjoy the maximum patent protection of 20 years? There are multiple reasons for inhibiting this option.

First, it is practically easier to get a patent than a marketing approval. While both organizations require the satisfaction of safety standards, those set by the PTO are only "sufficient probability of safety" based on preclinical information, while FDA requires extensive clinical studies spanning several phases, multiple years, dozens of research centers, and thousands of treated patients. Second, it is practically impossible to conduct the clinical testing phase of the magnitude just mentioned while keeping a biopharmaceutical invention secret or even a competitor from rushing to file a patent before the inventing biopharma manages to do so. Third, a prerequisite for filing a patent application is that the invention has been kept secret or has been disclosed only within the prior year before filing, otherwise the invention enters the public domain forever. Fourth, FDA approval is accelerated for patented biopharmaceutical compounds.

Fifth, conducting clinical trials requires significant amounts of money, the majority of which is usually provided by external investors. These investors will obviously demand for patent protection, before they commit significant amounts in any investigation of the drug. Sixth, before clinical trials can be conducted, the biopharma needs to submit to the FDA an Investigational New Drug (IND) application (see Chapter 6), containing the following parts: (1) animal pharmacology and toxicology studies, (2) manufacturing information, and (3) clinical protocols and investigator information. Obviously, by doing so, it jeopardizes the product's secrecy and also the 1 year patent filing deadline. Seventh, instead of going for a marketing approval first and then a patent for an effective patent life of 20 years, a biopharma avoids risking it all (e.g., losing the patent right all together) and opts for a shorter effective life, but the opportunity to prolong the product's commercial life cycle (see Chapter 12) past the patent expiration date through intensive product branding and marketing, that can theoretically prolong the product's revenue stream for even beyond 100 years—think of reference medicines such as aspirin (since 1897) and penicillin (since 1945).

Patent Life Importance Example: European Biopharmaceutical Enterprises

ONE IN FIVE OF EUROPE'S SMALL BIOPHARMACEUTICAL COMPANIES FACING FINANCIAL DIFFICULTY—EBE CALLS FOR URGENT ACTION

Brussels, 16th March 2009—One of Europe's most innovative sectors is facing potential catastrophe in the current financial crisis, as many small European biopharmaceutical companies face increasing difficulties to access the funding they need to keep afloat. A new study by French research group Alcimed, on behalf of the European Biopharmaceutical Enterprises, paints a grim picture of the impact of the crisis on the sector. The problem is particularly acute in healthcare biotechnology because product development can take up to 12 years of research before companies have a viable, marketable product. This means many companies are dependent on external funding for liquidity—a resource that almost disappeared as the financial crisis continues to bite.

The new study confirms that the healthcare biotechnology sector is already looking at a major funding shortfall, putting 20% of Europe's small biopharmaceutical companies at risk of bankruptcy by the end of 2009. This could mean the loss of 20,000 high-skill, high-value jobs and a permanent damage to Europe's research. The figures underline the fact that the majority of these small companies only have enough funding to cover 18 months of operation or less. For many, the clock on those 18 months has been ticking ominously for some time. The crisis could deepen further in 2010 if the current situation persists. This unprecedented state of affairs means that over 50% of small biopharmaceutical companies already feel under threat. Whilst the immediate impact would be highly damaging, the long-term ramifications would be much greater. In the medium to long term, it could spell a major setback to Europe's future competitiveness. Bankruptcies on any scale could mean that the benefits of health research already undertaken by biotech SMEs may be lost. For medicinal products under development, which already have a limited patent life, this will further reduce their appeal to potential investors...

Source: Courtesy of European Biopharmaceutical Enterprises (EBE) Press Release, Brussels, Belgium, March 16, 2009, http://www.ebe-biopharma.org

Biopharmaceutical Patents versus Market Exclusivities

The U.S. FDA provides a useful comparison between patents and exclusivity at its Web site (http://www.fda.gov/Drugs/DevelopmentApprovalProcess/ ucm079031.htm). Let's compare these two similar—but not identical— meanings below.

Patents are granted by the patent and trademark office anywhere along the development lifeline of a drug (expired before drug approval, or issued after drug approval, and anywhere in between). Patent information is required to be submitted with all new drug applications at the time of submission of the NDA. If appropriate, the patent information is published at the time of approval of the NDA. For patents issued after approval of the NDA, the applicant holder has 30 days in which to file the patent to have it considered as a timely filed patent. Patents may still be submitted beyond the 30 day timeframe but the patent is not considered a timely filed patent.

Exclusivity is exclusive marketing rights granted by the FDA upon approval of a drug if the statutory requirements are met, and can run concurrently with a patent or not (see 21 C.F.R. 314.108). Exclusivity was designed to promote a balance between new drug innovation and generic drug competition. Some drugs have both patent and exclusivity protection while others has just one or none. Patents and exclusivity may or may not run concurrently and may or may not encompass the same claims. Exclusivity is not added to the patent life. How long is exclusivity granted for? It depends on what type of exclusivity is granted: Orphan Drug (ODE)—7 years; New Chemical (NCE)—5 years; "Other" Exclusivity—3 years for a "change" if criteria are met; Paediatric Exclusivity (PED)—6 months added to existing Patents/Exclusivity; and Patent Challenge (PC)—180 days (this exclusivity is for ANDAs only).

In the United States, the Hatch–Waxman Act (1984) allows for two components: the extension of patent term for brand name companies who have lost term during FDA approval, and protection for generic manufacturers. The Act allows patent holders to seek extension of period lost during FDA approval. It allows for ANDA applications, and it allows for ANDA suitability positions where you can have variations from the drug components. Incentives for the brand name companies include patent term extension and non-patent market exclusivity. For a new chemical, irrespective of patents, you can have up to 5 years of market exclusivity because the FDA will not approve a drug of that same chemical entity.

Applications for new variations of other drugs that require new clinical investigations can get a 3 year extension. There is also 180 day exclusivity for the first generic to successfully challenge a listed drug's patent.

In order to obtain patent term extension under Hatch–Waxman Act, the following criteria must be met: (1) the patent must not have expired; (2) the term must never have been extended; (3) the application must be submitted by the record owner, not a licensee; (4) the product must have been subject to a regulatory review period before market approval; and (5) it must be the first permitted commercial marketing or use of the product. The application must be made within 60 days of market approval.

Supplementary Protection Certificates in the European Union
Since 1992 (find the original EU Regulation No. 1768/92 at http://eur-lex. europa.eu/LexUriServ/LexUriServ.do?uri=CELEX:31992R1768:EN:H TML), the European Union has taken steps to allow for a pharmaceutical drug patent protection extension, due to the very long time it takes for such a product under patent protection to receive regulatory approval. This is allowed in the form of supplementary protection certificates (SPCs) that come into force after the corresponding patent expires, and may last for up to five additional years. According to EU regulation, the total combined duration of market exclusivity of a patent and an SPC cannot exceed 15 years. In fact, there is a special formula that estimates the duration of any SPC as follows:

$$\text{SPC Term} = ([\text{date of first marketing authorization within EU}] - [\text{Date of corresponding patent filing}]) - 5 \text{ years}$$

In 2006 (find the original EU Regulation No. 1901/2006 at http://www. ema.europa.eu), the SPC term was further given an additional 6 months extension if the new marketing authorization application contained data from trials conducted according to an agreed Paediatric Investigation Plan (PIP). The issue of clinical trial exclusivity which refers to the protection of such data from being submitted to a regulatory agency to prove safety and efficacy of a generic drug by a generic pharmaceutical manufacturer will be discussed in detail in Chapter 12.

STRATEGIC MANAGEMENT OF IP

The U.S. Biotechnology Industry Organization (BIO) states in its Web site: "The biotechnology industry as we know it did not exist prior to the landmark U.S. Supreme Court decision of *Diamond vs. Chakrabarty* of 1980.

TABLE 2.6   Which Are the Five Elements of Managing Intellectual Property?

Element	IP Recognition	IP Extraction	IP Portfolio Management	IP Creation	Strategic Alignment
Metric	Outcome from IP	Output from IP	In-process handling of IP	In-process handling of IP	Overall
Driver	Start with the end in mind	Know what drives value	Organizing assets	Building assets	Know what business you are in
Examples	Stock price increase	Freedom to operate	Inventory segment	Invention	Vision
	Access to investors	Freedom to exclude	Assess	Innovation	Mission
	Standards impact	License	Values	Develop	Values
	Customer alignment	Sell	Manage	Joint develop	Strategies
	Recruiting tool	Barter		License-in	Tactics
				Purchase	

The court held that anything made by the hand of man was eligible for patenting. Since this decision, the biotechnology industry has flourished and continues to grow" (http://bio.org/ip/).

We have previously mentioned that young biopharmaceutical enterprises rise and fall on the basis of their IP portfolio strength and that going after additional IP is the basis of business success and sustainability. Under this environment, it is not sufficient to acquire and protect IP, but instead it is mandatory for survival to manage all IP under a strategic, proactive, and long-term plan. The implementation of such a plan by every biopharma is also mandatory due to the fact that intangible assets almost always surpass the value of all tangible assets of most biopharmas, begging the common logic that it is vain to try to accumulate and protect tools, devices, and buildings, while on the other hand countless patents and other forms of IP remain hidden and unproductive in the company's vault. Table 2.6 lists the five elements of managing IP. Before we progress into the essentials of a strategic IP management, let's first review the various ways of patent use by biopharmas.

Patent Use by Biopharmas
Offensive Use   A fictitious biopharma named INNOVACON may come up with a patent surrounding a laboratory technique for isolation and

characterization of a gene sequence encoding a protein with human biological activity, for example the stimulation of insulin production. Since such a protein may play an important role in diabetes management, INNOVACON races to the applicable patent office for such a process patent, lasting 20 years from filing. If, during this period, a second company named DIABECON attempts to launch a biopharmaceutical based on that same technique, INNOVACON may decide to launch an IP offensive against DIABECON, bringing a lawsuit to the applicable court. Should the relevant court decide on the validity of INNOVACON's claims, it may prohibit DIABECON from ever using the said patent, and force it to pay damages, or royalties of any future proceeds to INNOVACON throughout the patent period.

Such an offensive may thus be extremely damaging to the unauthorized imitator and reinforces the importance of strong IP for every biopharma. As discussed above, it is thus recommended that DIABECON undertakes a thorough evaluation of its "freedom-to-operate" status, preferably for all future inventions and their applications. In case the search identifies a missing link in their "freedom to operate," the legal owners of that IP right should be sought and identified, contacted, and further asked to provide DIABECON with the much-needed license, for a mutually agreed fee and/ or future royalties.

Defensive Use   A defensive IP use refers to the common practice among knowledge-intensive biopharmaceutical companies of building a fortress surrounding their most precious inventions, for the following reasons: (1) making it more difficult for competitors to follow in their scientific discovery path to commercialization, (2) allowing them to protect a fundamental process, so that additional products may be pursued in the future when the required funds will be secured, (3) holding a bargaining chip when forced to ask another competitor for a missing license to operate, and (4) creating a network of companies sharing certain fundamental patents in a so-called patent pool, where each contributing company is entitled to a share of the profits from any use of the patent pool by newcomers.

One effective patent strategy in the biotech sector involves acquiring secondary patents or rights to mundane or very basic research discovery that would otherwise block or lessen the value of core technology. The secondary patent may block out others and the owner of the primary patent from applying techniques that enhance the value of the primary patent. The secondary patent may also provide incentive to the owner of the primary patent and competitors to share technologies by cross-licensing.

Intellectual Property Management Example: ALNYLAM

Alnylam Grants New InterfeRx(TM) Intellectual Property License to Calando for Development and Commercialization of RNAi Therapeutics—New Target-Specific License Provides Non-Exclusive Access to Alnylam Intellectual Property for an RNAi Therapeutic Product. CAMBRIDGE, Massachusetts and PASADENA, California—July 21, 2008 Alnylam Pharmaceuticals Inc. (NYSE: ALNY), a biopharmaceutical company, engages in the development and commercialization of therapeutic products based on RNA interference (RNAi) in the United States. "We are pleased to be granting Calando a new InterfeRx license, providing them access to Alnylam intellectual property, which we believe is critical for the development and commercialization of all RNAi therapeutic products," said Jason Rhodes, Vice President, Business Development of Alnylam Pharmaceuticals. "Calando has demonstrated exciting progress with the only clinical stage RNAi therapeutic oncology program, currently in Phase I trials, and we are encouraged by the potential for similar success with this new target. Calando exemplifies the progress in our InterfeRx program, an important part of our overall strategy to create value today by leveraging our intellectual property portfolio for the development of RNAi therapeutics."

Source: Courtesy of ALNYLAM Press Release, Cambridge, MA, July 21, 2008, http://www.alnylam.com

QUESTIONS

1. What are the pros and cons of the IP system?
2. Which are the main types of IP protection?
3. How does an inventor compare with a patent holder under the modern IP protection system?
4. What are the main functions a patent plays in modern society?
5. What can a modern biopharmaceutical trademark cover? Describe a detailed example.
6. How does a trade secret compare with a patent?

7. What are the major methods of obtaining a biotechnology "freedom-to-operate"?
8. What was the essence of the verdict in the famous U.S. Supreme Court decision in DIAMOND vs. CHAKRABARTY, 447 U.S. 303 (1980).
9. Which are the potential filing application avenues for a biopharma company considering filing a patent application?
10. How do biopharmaceutical patents compare with market exclusivities for these products?

EXERCISES

1. Choose your standing among IP protection system proponents or critics. Identify 10 arguments supporting your side, as well as specific arguments negating your opponents' views. Present them in a debate.
2. Identify one of the top-selling biopharmaceuticals in 2009. Then, using publicly available databases identify some of the patents protecting it, challenges they may have faced along their lifecycle, as well as their expiration dates.
3. Identify three of the top selling biopharmaceuticals in 2009. Then, by using free, international patent office resources, describe their respective trademarks and what these cover.
4. By using publicly available web resources, identify a biopharmaceutical-related trade secret and describe its nature, its potential use by the legal holders, as well as legal challenges that it may have faced over the years. What was the legal outcome of any disputes?
5. Name five examples of start-up biopharmaceutical companies owning or vying to acquire freedom to operate on a significant biotechnological invention. What did it take to finally secure such a right?
6. What role have the so-called Chakrabarty bacteria and the Harvard onco-mouse played in modern healthcare biotechnology? Describe a brief history of both cases and their eventual consequences on the field.
7. A biopharmaceutical start-up is asking for your help in guiding them through the maze of international patenting processes. Visit the web pages of the U.S., European, and Japanese Patent offices, and identify the major steps, fees, and timelines involved for the start-up's research project to be patented.
8. Name some examples of patentable organisms in the United States, Europe, and Australia, and identify some prominent differences between these jurisdictions.

9. Why is it better to patent a biopharmaceutical molecule before entering clinical trials? What are the potential rewards and risks in speeding-up or postponing its patent application until a later stage?

10. Choose two major global biopharmaceutical enterprises. Then, using publicly available web resources compare them as far as their strategic IP management processes are concerned. How do they align or differ? Defend either side in a debate.

REFERENCES

ALNYLAM Press Release, July 21, 2008, Cambridge, MA, http://www.alnylam.com

Biotechnology Australia, 2001. *Biotechnology Intellectual Property Manual*, Canberra, Australian Capital Territory, Australia.

European Biopharmaceutical Enterprises (EBE) Press Release, Brussels, Belgium, March 16, 2009, http://www.ebe-biopharma.org

European Patent Convention, 2007. 13th edn. EPO: Brussels, Belgium. Posted at: http://www.epo.org/about-us/publications/procedure/epc-2000.html

European Patent Office (EPO), 2009. *Patents on Life? European Law and Practice for Patenting Biotechnological Inventions*. EPO: Munich, Germany.

freepatentsonline, Miami Beach, FL, http://www.freepatentsonline.com/5712155.html

GENENTECH 2008 Form 10-K with Exhibits 23.1, 31.1, 31.2 and 32.1, San Francisco, CA, http://www.gene.com

GOEDDEL DAVID VAN NORMAN; PESTKA SIDNEY (Inventors). HOFFMANN LA ROCHE; GENENTECH INC (Applicants). INTERFERONS AND PROCESS FOR THEIR PREPARATION, Patent number: MY71187 (A), Publication date: 1987-12-31. European Classification: C07K14/56; C12N15/10; C12N15/71. Posted at: http://v3.espacenet.com/publicationDetails/biblio?DB=EPODOC&adjacent=true&locale=en_gb&FT=D&date=19871231&CC=MY&NR=71187A&KC=A.

Guilford-Blake, R. and Strickland, D. (Eds.), 2008. *Guide to Biotechnology*. Biotechnology Industry Organization: Washington, DC (http://bio.org/speeches/pubs/er/BiotechGuide2008.pdf).

Jeffreys, A.J., Wilson, V., and Thein, S.L., 1985. Hypervariable 'minisatellite' regions in human DNA. *Nature* 314: 67–73 (Abstract).

Molecular Partners Press Release, Zurich, Switzerland, http://www.molecularpartners.com

Saiki, R., Scharf, S., Faloona, F., Mullis, K., Horn, G., and Erlich, H., 1985. Enzymatic amplification of beta-globin sequences and restriction site analysis for diagnosis of sickle cell anemia. *Science* 230: 1350.

U.S. Patent and Trademark Office (USPTO), 2008. *The Manual of Patent Examining Procedure (MPEP)*, Chapter 2100 on Patentability. 8th edn., Alexandria, VA. August 2001, Latest Revision July 2008, p. 2105. Posted at: http://www.uspto.gov/web/offices/pac/mpep/mpep_e8r6_2100.pdf

U.S. Supreme Court DIAMOND vs. CHAKRABARTY, 1980. 447 U.S. 303 (1980)—
447 U.S. 303 —No. 79-136. Argued March 17, 1980. Decided June 16, 1980.

WIPO, Geneva, Switzerland, http://www.wipo.int/pct/en/treaty/about.htm

Xinqi, Y. and Tanaka, Y., 2006. Final report: The challenge of patent related practitioners from the rapid development of biotechnology—a comparison of the practice of the United States, the European Community, Japan and China for the protection of biotechnology inventions. Graduate School, Tokyo Institute of Technology (JPO Long Term Fellowship Program of October 11, 2005 to March 31, 2006): Tokyo, March 2006.

## CHAPTER 3

Biolicensing

The total value of M&A transactions involving US biotechs was more than US$28.5 billion—a record high not counting megadeals in prior years, such as the 2007 acquisition of MedImmune by AstraZeneca. In Europe, M&A transactions totalled US$5.0 billion (€3.4 billion).

Source: Ernst & Young, Beyond borders: The global biotechnology report 2009, E&Y, Boston, MA, 2009.

INTELLECTUAL PROPERTY (IP) HAS immense importance for healthcare biotechnology companies. Therefore, possessing the freedom to operate is a must for any biopharma that plans to introduce a new biotechnology application into the marketplace. When this is not the case, biopharmas are obliged to enter into a licensing agreement with the entity that holds such right, whereas such entity "licenses out" the invention and is called the "licensor," and the company receiving the right is "licensing-in" and is called the licensee. Biolicensing describes the practice of biopharmaceutical companies to exchange licenses for biotechnological inventions, where the licensor receives an outright fee, or an initial down payment plus a proportion of future profits from the invention, called a royalty. On the other hand, the licensee agrees to pay such terms in order to obtain the necessary freedom to operate, and either receives an exclusive right to the invention, or a nonexclusive one, over the patented life span of the invention (permanent) or a time-limited permission to use it (for example, in case the licensee is in the process of completing its own in-house-developed process).

In most of biolicensing cases, a biopharma wishes to in-license an invention not from another company, but instead from a research-focused academic institution, and take it through the essential technology transfer and commercialization process, both of which are further discussed below.

INNOVATION CREATION AND MANAGEMENT

Innovation Creation

The Random House Dictionary defines invention as "an act or instance of creating or producing by exercise of the imagination" (http://dictionary.reference.com/browse) and innovation as "the introduction of new things or methods." Focusing on innovation, its main goal is introducing something useful to the society, something that could potentially bring positive change. When it comes to healthcare biotechnology, a new biopharmaceutical therapeutic or a prophylactic vaccine and a revolutionizing disease diagnostic are some of the invaluable contributions to the society made in the last 25 years.

Innovation Diffusion

Following an innovation's creation, this innovation can be adapted by other members of the society, ultimately leading to positive change as we have just mentioned. This process has been previously called the diffusion of innovations, attracting the interest of sociologists and anthropologists trying to study this process. Everett M. Rogers, in his book *Diffusion of Innovations* (1995), defined diffusion as "the process by which an innovation is communicated through certain channels over time among the members of a social system" (p. 35).

According to Rogers, the diffusion of innovations follows a diffusion curve, shaped in the form of an S-curve. This is based on the fact that each new innovation follows a five-step process before being adopted by an individual, namely, (1) knowledge, (2) persuasion, (3) decision, (4) implementation, and (5) confirmation. Furthermore, the rate of the innovation's adoption varies amongst individuals, making them characterizable by one of five proposed categories, namely, (1) innovators, (2) early adopters, (3) early majority, (4) late majority, and (5) laggards. As far as the S-curve shape is concerned, the adoption of a biopharmaceutical innovation can be mapped by the gradually increasing number of prescribers, or the patients using it, or the product's revenue growing through an initial slow uptake phase, a subsequent faster rate of growth, a stabilizing "plateau" phase, and an eventual phase of decline with the introduction of competitive and improved innovations. This process lends a product and even a company "life-cycle" entity, which will be further discussed in Chapters 12 and 14, respectively. It further becomes apparent that, since all products will eventually go through the rise and fall predicted by the S-curve, it becomes essential for these products to be constantly researched, improved, supported, and even replaced by newer and better introductions, thus leading to a long-term sustainability of the biotechnology company's commercial life. The phrase "innovate or die" may now sound like a cliché, but new product development (NPD) has become the essence of modern biotechnology.

There are multiple reasons for NPD's importance, namely, (1) satisfaction of changing customer needs, (2) creation of competitive advantage, (3) replacement of out-of-patent products, (4) perpetual regeneration of new products, bringing new revenue, funding new research, bringing new products, (5) sustainability of revenue streams, (6) ability to innovate into new therapy areas or other businesses all together, and (7) an overall superiority in biotechnology research, development, and commercial long-term growth.

Innovation Models

Biotechnology companies across the world rise and fall on the strength of their internally created innovations. These innovations may arise through a variety of innovation models, some of them gradual, others vying for the largest invention of its kind ever. Whatever the model is, the outcomes can be quantified in terms of patents produced, innovations approved, products launched, or revenues created. Let us take a brief look at some of the innovation models used by biotechnology companies today, some of them borrowed from other high-tech industries, and others showing off their advanced age by now.

If following the introduction of a certain biopharmaceutical, prescribers and patients ask for a longer half-life resulting in less frequent drug administrations into the body, then the manufacturer may attempt to slightly modify the product's molecule by adding a slowly degradable chemical side chain, giving the molecule a depot form. The innovation model just mentioned is an "incremental approach." If a biomanufacturer (see Chapter 7) is faced with high production costs, he will look for new innovations improving the yield of the manufacturing process. Because it is not financially feasible to build a new facility in order to test each new innovation, it might be useful to apply all these innovative process changes in a small, experimental scale. This model of innovation is called "piloting."

The lengthy biopharmaceutical R&D process is described in detail in Chapter 6. If all preclinical and clinical phases are divided in stages, and the crossing between stages is decided by a set of criteria at a so-called stage gate, then the resulting innovation model is called the "stage-gate" model. Small biotechnology start-ups often are forced to compete with industry giants. In doing so, they have to invent around preexisting technologies by taking a huge leap in innovation. This model of innovation far surpasses in boldness the previous three, but often is the only available means of progressing and competing in biotechnology. This model is humorously called the "big, hairy, audacious goal" or BHAG, in short for a feat not easily attempted and challenging.

A different model of innovation is the one avoiding the vertically integrated R&D expertise setup at various industry R&D centers, but instead focusing on the "centers-for-excellence" model. For example, instead of a North American center responsible for discovery-to-commercialization of neurology-related innovations, a company can set up a European "center-of-excellence" focusing on early discovery and lead identification for neurology, autoimmune, and diabetes, as well as an Indian center of excellence focused on animal studies on all three therapy areas.

In the previous model, R&D focused away from therapy areas to centers of excellence. Another variant model of innovation is the one focusing instead on disease targets, in other words, structural cellular elements or functional proteins that play a role in a range of physiological mechanisms and may participate in diverse disease pathogenesis. The "molecular target" model may lead to diverse applications from the manipulation of an endogenous protein or the invention of a monoclonal antibody capable of binding on a specific receptor.

Another process of innovation in biotechnology is based on a model first created by the aerospace industry in need of top secrecy. Under such a model, all required expertise for a given project is isolated from everyday contact with their company colleagues and housed in a dedicated unit, where daily brain-storming and close interaction may eventually need to accelerated discovery processes. This model is called "skunk works," a term borrowed from the now-famous Lockheed unit. There are even innovation models that seem to be in complete opposition to the secrecy at the basis of the previous model. For example, a biotechnology organization may decide to completely outsource all critical activities, even the essential R&D process, and focus on a small in-house core team of experienced industry professionals with diversified background. Such an organization may then subcontract preclinical development to a specialized vendor and clinical development to another vendor, eventually bringing these activities together under a "virtual R&D model."

An innovation model with even greater openness is the "open model," where a group of companies agree to participate in a patent pool, sharing their discoveries with each other, and agreeing to individually capitalize on them possibly in a different therapy area each. Such a model eliminates the need for vertical R&D organizations spanning the whole spectrum of discovery and research, eliminating costly infrastructure duplications and saving significant funds. A variant of the open model above is the knowledge-sharing "experts' exchange portal" now emerging in diverse fields, including biotechnology. Under such a model, a biotechnology organization lacking the in-house know-how posts an R&D problem on the portal, offering a monetary award to any scientist expert in the field to think about, research, and hopefully post an answer for the biotechnology company to first test and later even patent and use commercially. The whole process is a major example of the emerging Web 2.0 or even Web 3.0 applications, and will be further discussed in Chapter 9.

Process, Product, Service, and Business Model Innovation

Innovation in the field of healthcare biotechnology is not synonymous to only new product introductions. Instead, it can invariably focus on product, service, process, competitive position, pricing, and business model. First, product innovation may involve the introduction of a new biological entity that treats human disease. Second, service innovation may include the bundling of a biopharmaceutical with a revolutionary diagnostic kit that allows for better disease prognosis and treatment along the disease progression map. Third, process innovation may focus on an improved technique to isolate and characterize a manufacturing extract. Fourth, competitive position innovation may indicate the move of a biopharmaceutical company into imitating big pharma, e.g., through the use of DTC advertising, or conversely, taking an ultra-niche market position (see Chapters 9 and 13, respectively).

Pricing innovation (see Chapter 10) may involve the adaptation of a biopharma facing the rising approvability and reimbursement scrutiny by major pharmaceutical market governments. For example, instead of selling its products at a consistently high price, offering a varying pricing scale based on clinical outcomes, i.e., reduced payments for limited efficacy following a certain observation period. Finally, a business model

TABLE 3.1   What Are the Four Types of Innovation?

1. Product innovation	2. Process innovation
New biological entity	New manufacturing process
New molecular target	New research and development process
New biopharmaceutical or diagnostic	New supply chain management process
New disease monitoring testing	New human resource management process
New long-acting formulation	New company financing processes
New therapeutic modality, e.g., hyperthermia	New knowledge management process
3. Marketing innovation	4. Management innovation
New promotional tactics	New R&D models, e.g., centers-of-excellence
Web and social marketing	New business models, e.g., virtualization
Efficacy-based product pricing	New work environment, e.g., open, sharing, academic, informal
New tamper-proof packaging	New cross-functional collaboration
New supply chain tools, e.g., RFID	New decision-making process
New marketing system, e.g., B2B	New global organizational structure, e.g., identical area business units (ABMs)
New patient adherence services and tools	

innovation may involve the diversification of a product company into a platform company (Chapter 13), for example, out-licensing its platform technologies, e.g., DNA microchips, to any interested product companies. Table 3.1 provides additional examples of various types of innovations.

Biopharmaceutical Innovations

We have previously mentioned several different innovation models. Table 3.2 attempts to summarize some of them, according to their degree of innovativeness.

TABLE 3.2   Innovation Matrix

Disruptive

Existing target		New target
New pathway or disease state targeted (creates new category), e.g., Enbrel		New indication or application, e.g., Serostim
Same indication with new patient benefits—second generation—e.g., Neulasta		New target along an old pathway (creates a new category), e.g., Simponi

Incremental

TABLE 3.3   Breakthrough Innovations from the Biopharmaceutical Industry

Activity	Description	Name	Year
Insulin	First recombinant protein drug	Humulin®	1982
Anti-CD20	First anticancer monoclonal antibody	Rituximab	1997
Anti-CD33+ enediyne antibiotic	First antibody-targeted cancer chemotherapy	Gemtuzumab ozogamicin	2000
IgE blocker	First anti-asthma antibody therapy	Omalizumab	2003
Anti-EGFR	First anti-EGFR antibody	Cetuximab	2003
Anti-VEGF	First angiogenesis inhibitor	Bevacizumab	2004

Source: Betz, U.A.K., *DDT*, 10(15), 1057, August 2005. With permission.

Healthcare biotechnology includes several stellar breakthrough innovations, dating back to the introduction of the first biosynthetic pharmaceutical, namely, insulin in 1982. A brief collection of such innovations is contained in Table 3.3.

For an excellent innovation example see: The Birth of Healthcare Biotechnology at Genentech, GENENTECH, San Francisco, CA, http://www.gene.com/gene/about/corporate/history/

COMMERCIALIZATION PROCESS

Commercialization is the process of introducing a new product into the marketplace. In the case of a biopharmaceutical product, the process consists of an initial discovery taken through a very rigorous research and development program that culminates into clinical testing in humans, and hopefully regulatory approval before launch (see Chapter 6). In this chapter, we focus on the process of identifying a promising invention, usually in the academic setting, and taking this invention through the technology transfer process until it is licensed out to a biopharma company for eventual testing, approval, and commercialization.

Start-Up versus Ongoing Commercialization

The process of commercialization within the healthcare biotechnology industry can be distinguished between two different situations, namely, (1) start-up commercialization and (2) commercialization as a part of business operation. In the first case, a fledging biopharma start-up undergoes a prohibitively difficult early discovery and preclinical development program before it seeks significant funding from either private or public sources (see Chapter 4) so that it can proceed through an intensive clinical trial and regulatory approval program. Biopharmaceutical companies such as Exelixis (http://www.exelixis.com) and Cyclacel (http://www.cyclacel.com) are representative examples of biotechnology start-up commercialization.

In the second case, one of the very few biopharmaceutical companies with several products already launched in the marketplace seeks to identify as many promising new molecular targets as possible, before it takes them through a predefined and well-trodden path of in-house discovery and development, aided by the significant revenue streams already in existence. Fully integrated biopharmaceutical companies (FIBCOs) such as Amgen (http://www.amgen.com) and Genentech (http://www.gene.com) are shining examples of companies undergoing continuous product commercialization as a part of business operation.

When, Where, Whom, and How

According to Professor Philip Kotler (http://www.kellogg.northwestern.edu/faculty/bio/Kotler.htm), any given company planning to enter its product commercialization phase needs to address four fundamental questions, namely, (1) when, (2) where, (3) to whom, and (4) how. Let us review these four issues, as they relate to biopharmaceutical commercialization.

First, a biopharma needs to decide when, for example, how soon will they complete the preclinical and clinical testing, how long will it take for the product to be approved and reimbursed by the proper authorities, when should they start preparing for commercial launch, which of their own products will be affected by the new launch, what reference and other competitive products will they compete against when they launch, and whether the product will be sufficiently ready to satisfy an unmet customer need.

Second, the biopharma will have to decide where to launch, for example, a small subnational area, a larger national area, a supernational regional area, or even the international arena. The most important considerations here have to do with the availability of sales and marketing resources, be it in the form of finances, professionals, organizational structures, subsidiaries, intermediaries, distribution or promotional partners, prescriber-proponents, etc. In the case of biopharmaceutical start-ups, they had initially started by out-licensing their products to big pharma, they later progressed in launching in their home market while out-licensing the foreign markets, a little later they had created their first subsidiaries in the major markets (e.g., United States, Japan, Germany, United Kingdom,

France, Spain, Italy), and lately the larger of them pride of having their own structures present in dozens of markets.

Third, a biopharma needs to decide to who the product should be launched, for example, which therapeutic area (e.g., neurology), which indication (e.g., Alzheimer's disease), which prescribers (e.g., neurology specialists versus gerontologists versus family physicians), which scientific association to be presented first at (e.g., European Neurological Society; http://www.ensinfo.com), which scientific congress (e.g., the Annual Meeting of the American Neurological Association), which patient association (e.g., U.S.'s Alzheimer's Association; http://www.alz.org/index. asp), which state or private insurance funds (e.g., Medicare; http://www. medicare.gov), or which reimbursement agencies (e.g., U.K.'s NICE; http:// www.nice.org.uk).

Fourth, a biopharma ready to enter the marketplace needs to be concerned with how the product is going to be commercialized, for example, which brand name, which promotional messages, what promotional media, what budgets, what kind of advertising, direct-to-consumer or not, an internal sales force and with what specialization, what media and public relations, what web tactics, and so on (see Chapters 8 and 9).

The four basic commercialization questions will be further discussed in subsequent book chapters. Figure 3.1 describes the decision factors of commercialization, according to Kotler.

Main Phases of Commercialization Process

As described above, the biopharmaceutical commercialization process can be envisaged to get under way the moment a new invention is identified, usually in the academic setting, and later follows a product through its preclinical and clinical testing, through regulatory approval and launch. Therefore, the commercialization process runs in parallel with the new product development process, but is not identical to it. Instead, it precedes and outlasts NPD, and usually is in effect until the said product reaches the plateau phase of its market diffusion phase. At that point, the biopharmas usually switch focus on the product's improved replacements and start switching away focus, personnel, and resources into the new products (see Chapter 12). As far as commercialization and budgeting are concerned, these typically fall into gear at the end of preclinical testing, and maximize their intensity at least 2 years before commercial launching, since a series of important launching activities need to programmed, prioritized, and budgeted before approval.

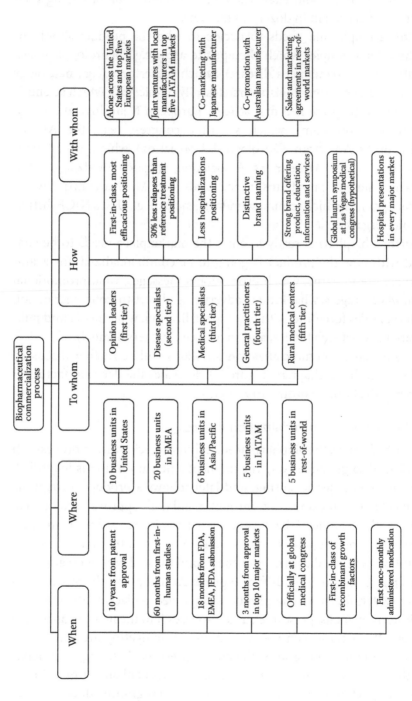

FIGURE 3.1 The decision factors of commercialization. (Modified from Kotler, P., *Marketing Management: Analysis, Planning, Implementation, and Control*, Prentice Hall: New York, 1994.)

Biopharmaceutical Commercialization Is Sequential

We have previously described how a biopharmaceutical company identifies an invention in the academic domain, and having secured a license for it, takes it through the rigorous path of preclinical and clinical research, until finally, it is submitted for regulatory approval, and if approved is launched into the marketplace. The commercialization process we have just described is linear and sequential.

Let us review this process in more detail. The whole process starts with a promising invention, coming either from an academic institution, or a team of scientists at a company's R&D department. Having secured a patent, either side evaluates the commercial opportunity of the invention (opportunity identification phase), and comes up with a potential therapy area, a distinct indication, a desirable molecule, and possibly a target product profile (TPP; see Chapter 12).

Having secured a patent of its own or a license for the academic invention, the biopharma then enters the preclinical development phase, which resembles the design phase seen in the commercialization of consumer goods. During this phase, the company sets up an in vitro test (cells or tissues extracted from an organism and now living in an artificial medium, e.g., tissue culture) to screen the efficacy and safety of the original test compound and countless modifications. These modifications lead to carefully selected lead compounds, which are then taken into animal studies, for the determination of the optimal lead, its dosage spectrum, and its pharmacodynamic (what happens to it when it enters the animal body) and pharmacokinetic profile (the speed of tissue absorption, metabolism, and elimination).

When this preclinical phase is complete, the company submits an application to the applicable regulatory agencies for testing the lead compounds into humans (testing phase). During the clinical trial phases, the compound is tested first in volunteers, then in a limited patient population, and later in a much wider population where all potential effects of the study drug are tested, recorded, and analyzed.

Having been found efficacious and safe, the drug candidate is taken through a meticulous approval phase, where all available documentation is reviewed by experts who recommend the approvability or not of the said compound. When all drug characteristics are beneficial, while potential side effects are within an acceptable scale, the drug is approved and is ready for commercial launch.

Before launching, the approved drug is taken through the when, where, whom, and how questions we have just discussed, while the biopharma prepares a thorough launch plan for its introduction into the marketplace. During its commercial launch phase, the product is supported by a series of sales and marketing activities with the use of carefully selected messages, aimed at select prescriber, regulator, patient and media groups, following the adoption S-curve.

Very often, the biopharma start-up is unable to fully commercialize its product in the target markets and may decide to out-license the rights of its approved drug to a larger, financially stronger, and commercially mature and capable pharmaceutical or biopharmaceutical partner. Once again, the issue of biolicensing takes the primary stage, this time for the exclusive or nonexclusive, global or geographically limited product commercialization rights across the world. Several important aspects of the biolicensing process are presented in the following sections.

For a commercialization example see: Yale's Office of Cooperative Research (OCR), New Haven, CT, http://innovators.yale.edu/commercializing.asp

INTELLECTUAL PROPERTY LICENSING

The Cambridge Advanced Learner's Dictionary (http://dictionary.cambridge.org/dictionary/british/licence# licence_3) defines license as "an official document which gives you permission to own, do or use something, usually after you have paid money and/or taken a test." In the field of healthcare biotechnology, it often covers the rights to use a patented invention, to promote and sell it, to distribute it, to co-promote or co-market it (see Chapter 5), to use its brand name or trademark, etc.

The licensing of biotechnology innovations among biopharmaceutical and pharmaceutical companies has been constantly expanding in the last three decades. Some of the reasons responsible for this rise are the (1) increasing costs of R&D, (2) decreased R&D productivity, (3) increasing demands of investors, (4) increasing competition, (5) strengthening patent protection, (6) increased emphasis on IP, (7) better partnering infrastructure, (8) globalization, (9) more outsourcing, (10) virtualization of biotechnology, and (11) maturation of the industry.

Licensing Advantages

We have just discussed some of the reasons for biolicensing rising. Not all of the reasons mentioned come from within the biopharmaceutical industry involved, as some have to do with society's role (in investing or consuming). What about the industry itself? Are there specific advantages or even disadvantages to be considered?

We will start from the multiple advantages of biolicensing, especially those concerning the licensor.

1. It may lack the financial resources, the R&D infrastructure, the regulatory agency contacts, the insurance company contracts, the sales and marketing skills, the customer relationships, the therapeutic area experience, and the foreign market presence.

2. It may have other molecule priorities, different therapeutic areas in the portfolio, or specific market priorities that leave room for out-licensing the non-core assets.

3. Out-licensing an IP asset may generate a revenue stream that will in turn allow internal R&D and commercialization of a different asset.

4. A licensor, especially in its start-up phase or when faced with an enormous project, may decide to limit its risks, by taking a molecule until the end of phase I clinical trials (limited funds required), and out-licensing it for the remaining phases II and III, and the regulatory approval.

5. Having secured an out-licensing deal, a small licensor will have immediate access to much-needed funds to complete its part of the deal, sales and marketing information, opinion leader recommendations, and efficient decision-making coming from a bigger licensee (such as in the case of a small biopharma out-licensing to big pharma).

Looking at biolicensing advantages with the eyes of a licensee, first, the commercialization costs are limited if an IP asset is acquired at a progressed state of development. Second, the long R&D time requirements are shortened when a compound is in-licensed. Third, it might have been impossible for the licensee to develop something in-house if a basic expertise, assay, tool, or whole facility was missing. Fourth, a licensee might have succeeded to bringing its own injectable biopharmaceutical into the marketplace, but its in-house-developed multi-injector device (e.g., insulin injector pen) might have been inferior to the competition's, suggesting the need for an in-licensed competitive advantage. Fifth, the licensee may have developed its own Parkinson's biomedicine, but it would only make sense to complement its marketed neurology portfolio with in-licensed compounds in Alzheimer's, or the multiple

TABLE 3.4 Which Are the Main Reasons for Biopharmaceutical Licensing?

1 Sharing risk	8 Reducing costs
2 Generating revenue	9 Saving time
3 Increasing market penetration	10 Accessing expertise
4 Accessing funds to complete a project phase	11 Obtaining competitive advantage
5 Accessing sales and marketing information	12 Supplementing a product portfolio
6 Acquiring opinion leader input	13 Acquiring a foothold in a new indication
7 Getting help in decision-making	14 Mutually exchanging licenses

sclerosis indications. Sixth, if its own discovery is long before launch, it might make sense to in-license and launch immediately another noncompetitive medicine in the same indication so as to acquire a prescriber and patient base in anticipation of its own future launch. Seventh, exchanging a license with the licensor may allow both organizations to proceed faster in the respective indications. The multiple advantages of biolicensing for either the licensor or licensee are summarized in Table 3.4.

For an excellent IP licensing example, namely the Cohen-Boyer patents, see the review by Bills, K., A guide to licensing biotechnology, *LES les Nouvelles*, 86–94, June 2004.

Licensing Disadvantages

Apart from advantages, there are also several potential disadvantages to a biotechnology licensing agreement. Let us review some of them, starting from the licensor's perspective.

First, an exclusive out-licensing limits the future rights of the licensor to commercialize its own IP and obviously derive a larger stream of revenue as compared to in-house development and commercialization. Second, out-licensing a technology for any R&D process will obviously increase the internal know-how of the licensee, over and above the commercialization of the agreed compound, giving them a future boost in more of their own R&D efforts (a common thorny issue in out-licensing a technology to an emerging market manufacturer). Third, out-licensing a technology to the highest bidder may hinder the licensor possibilities for more cooperative or open innovation, and eventually slower but larger revenue returns. Fourth, out-licensing may often mean the loss of focus from an invented discovery, which may be associated with essential personnel turnover, loss of opinion leader contacts, or even damages to the remaining licensor brands.

Fifth, if the licensee is a small biopharma, the invention may never reach its full commercialization potential, or the company may go under before returning the royalties expected by the licensor. On the other hand, if the licensee is big pharma, the promised royalties may only represent a tiny fraction of real sales, underestimating the invention's potential. Additionally, a big pharma licensee may be overpowering and intimidating to a small licensor. Sixth, biolicensing does not come easily. It is time- and resource-consuming; it requires constant research, monitoring, and management, and may distract a licensor from its other priorities. Seventh, a licensor may be faced with a devastating abandonment of its out-licensed invention by a big pharma partner, due to lack of efficacy or other unexpected priorities of the licensee, leaving it without the much-needed returns, as well as lost patent time in the race for commercialization.

On the other hand, a biotechnology invention licensee is often faced with its own disadvantages, for example: First, in-licensing a technology may require vast amounts of down payment or future royalties, making the future profitability of the potential compounds limited. Second, the IP under negotiation may be weak, that is not comprehensive and prohibitive one for other imitators to copy or invent-around, thus rendering it of limited value for the licensee. Third, the IP may be challengeable in the applicable courts, and may even run the risk of being found invalid, thus useless for the licensee. Fourth, the licensing rights offered may be nonexclusive, thus allowing another competitor to beat the licensee in the race to commercialize the patented invention. Fifth, the licensor may not be willing to divulge essential trade secrets that are required for the full exploitation of the patented invention, or certain patent aspects may necessitate the hiring of the original inventing scientist, which however may not be feasible. Sixth, in-licensing any technology will certainly inhibit the licensee from any attempt to invent around, or possibly acquire the know-how slower but with multiple benefits for its future growth. Finally, seventh, in-licensing an unproven technology will certainly impose new risks and strains to internal R&D efforts, thus making the licensing investment seem questionable for a long period of time before finally proving commercially exploited and proving successful.

Whatever the advantages and disadvantages of biolicensing are, they have to be constantly compared with those offered by in-house development, or other forms of partnering (see Chapter 5), such as mergers, acquisitions, co-development agreements, and others. Forming a capable team of business development professionals that have a close interaction with all other in-house functions (finance, legal, R&D, marketing, medical affairs) will make the biolicensing process less risky and more rewarding in the long run.

TECHNOLOGY TRANSFER

According to *The Random House Dictionary* (http://dictionary.reference. com/browse/technology), technology is "the branch of knowledge that deals with the creation and use of technical means and their interrelation with life, society, and the environment, drawing upon such subjects as industrial arts, engineering, applied science, and pure science." As far as technology transfer is concerned, the Association of University Technology Managers (AUTM; http://www.autm.net) defines it as follows:

> Technology transfer is the process of transferring scientific findings from one organization to another for the purpose of further development and commercialization. The process typically includes: 1) Identifying new technologies, 2) Protecting technologies through patents and copyrights, and 3) Forming development and commercialization strategies such as marketing and licensing to existing private sector companies or creating new start-up companies based on the technology.

For more information on the significance and the processes involved in technology transfer, visit the web pages of the U.S. National Institutes of Health (NIH) Office of Technology Transfer (OTT) (http://ott.od.nih.gov/ index.aspx) and those of the Licensing Executives Society International (http://www.lesi.org/Article/Home.html).

Technology Transfer Methods

The reasons for technology transfer are multiple, for example, scientific recognition of the institution, prior obligation for government research grants received, attraction of new national or regional financial incentives, attraction of corporate funds, attraction of new faculty and undergraduate/graduate students, local economic development, future royalties from licensed inventions that provide significant long-term income for the institution, media and public recognition, creation of combined academia-industry educational, or research programs and more.

There are various methods of technology transfer. The determining factor is mostly the degree of involvement and therefore risk undertaking of the licensor. For example, in a typical out-licensing agreement, the licensor agrees to transfer exclusive or nonexclusive rights for an invention to a designated licensee, in exchange for a down payment and royalties on future profits. Here the licensor involvement and risk are minimized, both responsibilities undertaken by the licensee who expects to get return on the investment through future sales of the commercialized invention. Occasionally, the transfer of licensing rights is accompanied by the setup of a new organizational entity, called a spin-out, which may be funded by scientists investing their own funds, or external investors, either in the form of venture capital (VC) or public markets (see Chapter 4).

In other technology transfer deals, both the licensor and licensee maintain involvement and future risk, by entering other types of partnering, such as a joint venture or a merger/acquisition agreement. The licensee may also be a virtual company, i.e., one maintaining a very small core team and project-managing the outsourcing of all R&D, manufacturing, and even marketing efforts. In other occasions, the licensee may be an investment fund that acts by managing large investments of individuals, insurance funds, or banks through in-licensing product rights, expediting the commercialization efforts, and quickly exiting the venture through a public offering (IPO). Most of these activities are presented in Chapter 4.

Technology Transfer Process Steps

The technology transfer process for a biopharmaceutical invention made by an academic scientist typically follows the following six steps: (1) invention disclosure, (2) technology assessment, (3) patenting, (4) licensing, (5) preclinical and clinical testing, regulatory approval, and finally, (6) commercial launching and marketing. We study the first four steps in the following paragraphs, while step #5 is presented in Chapter 6, and step # 6 is discussed in Chapters 8 and 9.

At the beginning of the process, the inventor needs to disclose her/his invention to the academic institution's technology transfer office (TTO). The disclosure involves a special form where the invention is described in detail, together with the supporting science, as well the inventor's prior announcements in the form of scientific congress abstracts, full research papers, interviews, or web postings, as well as prior patents. In addition, the inventor provides information about competitive work either coming from the scientific research literature or other patent listings. Finally, the TTO may ask the inventor to give an indication of future commercial applications of the invention, an initial gross valuation, and potentially interested parties, such as biopharmaceutical companies that may be approached, after securing the invention with a patent.

During the second phase of technology assessment (see later in this chapter), the TTO attempts to evaluate whether the disclosed invention is patentable, i.e., whether it is novel, useful, and nonobvious. Furthermore, because of the special ethical issues surrounding biotechnology applications (previously mentioned in Chapter 2), biotechnology patentability needs also to be assessed. In some cases, the discovery is not as significant or nonobvious, yet it may eventually become a trade secret, transferable to an interested biopharmaceutical manufacturer on a license. In such case, a confidentiality agreement is signed, and a licensing agreement may materialize, without the existence of a patent.

When the above prerequisites are satisfied, the TTO proceeds into the third phase, namely, patenting of the invention (see Chapter 2). The patenting process may be initiated by the appropriate in-house patenting lawyers, or be assigned to a collaborating law firm, specializing in IP management. Furthermore, the same law firm may be assigned to monitor patent adherence by the licensee or patent infringement by a competitor, and also prosecute any infringements, given the mandate by the academic institution.

A special issue arises in the cases where the academic institution's department involved in the invention had been under research assistance from either a state (e.g., Cancer Prevention and Research Institute of Texas; http://www.cprit.state.tx.us/index.html), or a government (e.g., NIH; http://www.nih.gov), or a patient society (e.g., American Lung Association; http://www.lungusa.org), or even a biopharma company. In such cases, the academic institution would have signed detailed research agreements with all funding partners, guaranteeing confidentiality, describing the personnel involved and facilities used, and also describing the fate of IP potentially discovered during the funded research process. Usually, external research funding does not award automatic patenting rights to the sponsors, but, instead, gives them priority access to scientific announcements or publications arising from such research, and also the rights to first refuse a resulting patent, i.e., decide first whether to license the resulting patent for a mutually agreed fee.

Technology Transfer Offices

Most academic institutions and government research funding agencies now have a dedicated TTO involved in the process of commercializing inventions discovered by the institution's or agency scientists. As previously described, these offices oversee the six-step process and are also involved in determining whether an invention is novel, useful, nonobvious,

TABLE 3.5   Productivity of Harvard's Office of Technology Development

	2006	2007	2008	2009
Invention disclosures	180	217	295	277
New patent applications filed	169	147	170	172
U.S. patents issued	35	43	55	45
Licenses	11	24	26	36
Total licensing revenue (MM)	$20.9	$12.5	$21.1	$12.4
Start-up companies	6	6	12	8
Industry sponsored research agreements	12	22	42	37
Collaboration agreements	7	3	4	9

Source: Courtesy of Harvard's Office of Technology Development, Cambridge, MA, http://www.techtransfer.harvard.edu/mediacenter/annuals/stats/

and patentable by the major patent offices mentioned in Chapter 2. As far as their organizational structure is concerned, they are either an in-house academic department, or a not-for-profit academic spin-out involved in commercializing the institutional inventions, maximizing their returns, and returning these proceeds to the institution for funding its future research activities.

According to the Association of University Technology Managers (AUTM: http://www.autm.net/FY_2007_Licensing_Activity_Survey.htm) during the Fiscal Year 2007, there were

- 19,827 disclosures received by organizations

- 5,109 licenses and options signed

- 3,622 patents issued

For a snapshot of an actual academic TTO performance, please review the productivity of Harvard's TTO summarized in Table 3.5.

THE BAYH–DOLE ACT

In 1980, the U.S. federal government enacted the Bayh–Dole Act, which has since played a vital role in commercializing the inventions produced at U.S. academic institutions with public funding. In summary, the Act awarded the rights to academic inventions to the universities themselves. In turn, the academic institutions started negotiating the out-licensing of their inventions to private companies, which then invested large amounts of money in bringing these inventions, among which there were monumental biopharmaceutical discoveries, to the marketplace. This process allowed the invention-producing institutions to flourish, set up TTOs, capitalize on their inventions, and secure long-term royalties from private companies, which in turn produced more R&D at the institutions. The U.S. government also benefited by strengthening its academic base, its national innovative capacity, and its patent productivity, attracting private funds from around the world in a positive innovation spiral. Finally, as the biopharmaceutical industry is concerned, it quickly recognized the commercial potential of those inventions, gained exclusive licenses to commercialize them, and became one of the most research-intensive, forward-looking, and innovative business sectors, not only among the U.S. economy, but a significant global industry, bringing numerous biotherapeutics to the market place and improving the quality of life of millions of patients along the way.

The Bayh–Dole Act is part of the U.S. Code regarding patent law, Title 35, Part II, Chapter 18, Paragraph 200 (http://www.law.cornell.edu/uscode/35/200.html), and has also been implemented in the Code of Federal Regulations (C.F.R.) containing general and permanent rules and regulations published in the Federal Register, Title 37, Chapter IV, Part 401: "Rights to inventions made by non-profit organizations and small business firms under government grants, (http://www.access.gpo.gov/nara/cfr/waisidx_02/37cfr401_02.html) contracts, and cooperative agreements." The 109th U.S. Congress has in fact recognized the great contributions of the Bayh–Dole Act on December 14, 2005 with a "Sense of the Congress Resolution." The impact of the bioindustry–university partnering can be assessed in the Biotechnology Industry Organization (BIO) 2009 press release that follows.

Impact of Bioindustry–University Partnering Example: BIO Releases New Study Showing Industry/University Partnerships Critical to U.S. Economy
    WASHINGTON, D.C. (Wednesday, October 28, 2009)—"A study released today by the Biotechnology Industry Organization (BIO) provides first-of-its-kind data on the importance of university/industry research and development partnerships to the U.S. economy. The study of university technology licensing from 1996 to 2007 shows a $187 billion dollar positive impact on the U.S. Gross National Product (GNP) and a $457 billion addition to gross industrial output, using very conservative models. "It has long been believed that the Bayh–Dole Act, which permits and encourages industry to partner with research universities to turn

federally-funded basic research into new and valuable products, is a critical factor in driving America's innovation economy. Indeed, because of this inspired piece of legislation, the U.S. leads the world in commercializing university-based research to create new companies and good, high-paying jobs throughout the country," stated BIO President & CEO Jim Greenwood. "This new study provides the evidence to back up that belief."

Before the passage of the Bayh–Dole Act in 1980, inventions arising from the billions of taxpayer dollars invested annually in university research remained largely on laboratory shelves and were rarely commercialized because of restrictive patenting and licensing practices. This situation changed with passage of the Bayh–Dole Act, which allows university inventors to patent their discoveries and license them to commercial partners with maximum flexibility and limited federal bureaucracy. As a result, the biotech revolution was born, turning inventions into products that are improving public health, cleaning our environment, and feeding the world.

Other key findings of the study include: University-licensed products commercialized by industry created at least 279,000 new jobs across the U.S. during the 12-year period; The annual change in U.S. GDP due to university-licensed products grew each year, illustrating that the impact of university patent licensing grows even more important each year.

Source: Courtesy of BIO Press Release, Washington, DC, October 28, 2009, http://www.bio.org

TECHNOLOGY ASSESSMENT

We have previously described that the technology transfer process for an invention follows the six steps: (1) invention disclosure, (2) technology assessment, (3) patenting, (4) licensing, (5) testing, regulatory approval, and finally, (6) commercial launching and marketing.

Technology assessment is the in-depth analysis and evaluation of a new technology, comprising an indispensable part of the subsequent technology's commercialization. In the case of a new biotechnology application, it comprises of several thorough steps, namely, patentability (based on novelty, usefulness, nonobviousness, and ethical), legal, research, clinical, manufacturing, regulatory, financial, and commercial. Each process step requires the inputs of specialized databases and in-house and external

experts, the existence of standardized and objective processes, procedures, and measuring tools, and finally a robust decision-making process
that will allow the beneficial, efficient, and expeditious evaluation of each
technology and its subsequent commercialization steps. Furthermore,
technology assessment needs to be open, reproducible, thorough, objective,
and unbiased, giving the evaluating potential licensee a 360° view of the
invention under the microscope.

Due Diligence

Technology assessment is often called "due diligence," a process of evaluation of potential investments mandated by the U.S. Securities Act of 1933,
following the occasionally worthless investment advice given to unsus-
pecting investors by financial analysts before the financial crash of 1929.
Ever since, the process of a thorough evaluation of every given aspect of
operation for a company looking for external investments has been copied and standardized for every single product or company assessments,
especially in the case of biotechnology inventions, requiring a thorough
analysis and evaluation before commercialization. In the next few pages,
we further elaborate on some of the biopharmaceutical due diligence components. An overview of the technology assessment process is presented
by Figure 3.2.

Furthermore, Figure 3.3 gives an overview of the parallel processes of
opportunity versus accessibility evaluations for a given biopharmaceutical
licensing target currently undergoing clinical trials.

In summary, due diligence is a process of information gathering and
evaluation, including both confidential and public information. It is a
two-way process, although the buyer's (licensee's) is frequently more thorough than the seller's (licensor's). To be valuable, it must be completed
before conclusion of any deal. Typically, the formal process begins when
parties showing serious interest, confidentiality agreement in place, and
outline commercial terms have been discussed, or even agreed ("subject
to due diligence").

Biopharma Due Diligence Components
Assessing the Idea
Study the invention disclosure. What is the intracellular/extracellular
target? What are the target physiological systems? What is the mechanism of action? What would its potential effects on human disease be?
Is it patentable—novel, nonobvious, and useful? Is it ethical? What is the

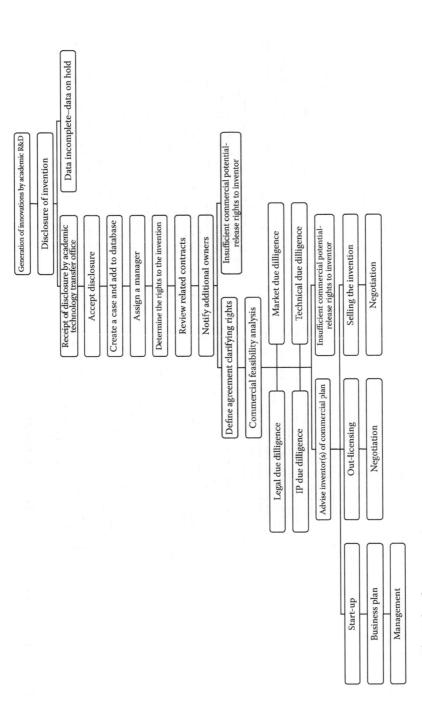

FIGURE 3.2 The technology assessment process.

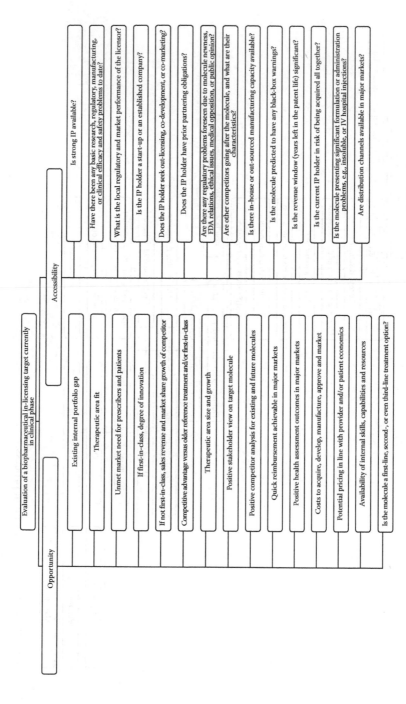

FIGURE 3.3 Opportunity versus accessibility of a licensing target.

current stage of development? Are the required tools, techniques, in vitro and animal models, or bioassays developed? If not, how long would it take to develop them? What would prominent disease researchers or clinical experts have to say about the invention? Has it been disclosed already to friends, colleagues, media, or the public? Are there prior references (art) in written or electronic form? Does the invention possess the freedom to operate? If not, who holds the missing rights? Would it make practical, therapeutic, ethical, and financial sense to patent it?

Due Diligence—Pre-Visit

In the process of a biopharma company assessing an academic pharmacological invention, the company personnel should record all potential issues for discussion during their first on-site visit, for example, CMC (chemistry, manufacturing, and controls), preclinical, clinical, regulatory, financial, commercial, and legal.

First Interview with Inventor

How did the idea come about? What did critical experiments show? What do experimental data (e.g., HPLC or bioassay) show exactly? Why does the inventor believe this is patentable? What is the current patent status? Has the invention been announced or published before? What would be its future diagnostic/therapeutic applications, which indications, monotherapy or combination, what patient groups? What is the expected magnitude of diagnostic/therapeutic effect? Which experimental processes are needed for the invention evaluation? Which scientists would the inventor recommend as potential evaluators? Are there any scientific secrets hidden from the patent applications? Is the inventor committed in validating the invention's functionality? Would the inventor be "mobile," should the biopharma need her/his expert services? What are the next steps in the patenting process?

Due Diligence—Patentability

Basic requirements are novelty, nonobviousness, usefulness, ethical base, protection of human species, as well as the environment. Extensive literature search (free and paid) is essential. Extensive patent search (free and paid) is also mandated. Higher requirements are freedom to operate and broad scope (e.g., not only applicable on Drosophila mitochondria). Who are the legal professionals managing the patent application process? Which are the patent offices where the application was submitted?

Was there a significant geographic region missed? Were the patent claims broad enough? What is the patenting time frame? Are there any additional patent applications underway?

Due Diligence—Legal

The basic issue here is whether there is any patent or other legal issue preventing further development of the patent by the in-licensing biopharma. For example:

What about the inventor? Is she/he respectable, published, and in good standing with students, colleagues, the department, and the university? Is there any indication the inventor did not act alone, did not include someone in the license application, copied the work of someone else, or has already published this work before? Did the inventor have legal access to the facilities, reagents, devices, and methods used during the invention process? Does the inventor have all required licenses to reproduce the material (e.g., she/he is a properly trained and board-certified physician, or does she/he have a license for radioactivity handling, etc.)? Was the inventor's research funded by government or another entity? Do they hold patent rights (unlikely), or rights of first refusal (possibly against us), or rights of first publications (barring us from doing so in the future)? Are there any pending litigations against the inventor, for example, from a former graduate student, or an employer?

What about the Patent Applications or Issued Patents?

What is the patent strength? If not strong, are there any additional trade secrets available? Even if patent is challengeable, can an additional period of regulatory exclusivity (see Chapter 2) prolong its life? What is the patent freedom to operate? Who is presently holding the licenses we lack? Would they be interested in giving us a license-to-operate, or would they block us? What is the patent's freedom to exclude others from copying? Did it come from a patent pool, co-owned by others? Are there any competing patent applications under review? Can they beat us to the finish line? Is there any patent litigation pending against us? What are its proponents? Which are its claims and how do we manage the challenge? Do we have the financial resources to raise a battle?

Due Diligence—Clinical: Is the Product Safe and Effective in Humans?

What is the global clinical trial program? What were the results of trials completed, and what are the primary/secondary endpoints of ongoing or future trials? What was the quality of clinical trial centers and primary investigators chosen? How many patients have been included in the trials, and what is the statistical power of these trials? Were the primary and secondary endpoints chosen properly? Were the endpoints clearly met? How do the pharmacodynamic and pharmacokinetic results look like? Are there any skeletons in the closet? What is the emerging dose range in humans? Can it be safely and practically administered? Will it lead to good patient compliance?

Furthermore, what was the efficacy of the product? Is it statistically different from placebo or other comparators? How does it compare to the "reference" treatment modality? Will it be used as monotherapy or combination? Will it be first-line treatment or, unfortunately, only second- or even third line? What was the product safety? Was the animal safety profile reproduced in humans, or were there any unexpected findings? Did it lead to a high number of patient withdrawals? Were there any unexpected patient deaths, potentially associated with the product? Will the product require any damaging "black box" warnings, or cumbersome postapproval patient monitoring? What was the side effect profile? Were there any annoying or unbearable side effects? How was the patient quality-of-life (QoL) affected? How will this finding play in reimbursement and formulary discussions? What was the opinion of healthcare personnel, patients, and their carers toward the treatment?

Due Diligence—CMC: Can a Product Be Made
Is the process acceptable by the relevant regulatory authorities? Is it technically feasible? Is the process easy, transferable, validated, and scalable? What are the manufacturing capital requirements? Is the existing manufacturing facility FDA-validated? Are the raw materials validated by their manufacturer (regulatory, quality, and customs-wise)? Are the quantities guaranteed? Is their manufacturer respectable, experienced, financially stable, and in a politically stable environment? What are the manufacturing risks involved? Can they be monitored and managed? Are the estimated costs-of-goods (COGS) acceptable? Do these COGS lead to a sellable and reimbursable proposition? How many major pharmaceutical markets would accept such a sales proposition? If we in-license the product, who will undertake the development costs? Can they be shared, as well as the risks? Does the inventor hold any necessary scientific/process secrets? Will these be shared? Is the inventor still interested in the project, would she/he be available as a consultant, or even become our employee?

Due Diligence—Regulatory

What is the probability of regulatory approval in the major markets (United States, Europe, and Japan)? Was the observed efficacy and safety statistical significance the ones required? Have all required clinical trials been programmed, completed, summarized, and submitted? What are the planned indications, dosages, and formulations? What is the expected summary of product characteristics (SmPC) and the associated patient information leaflet (PIL)? Are any damaging "black box warnings" expected? What is the time frame for approval? Can we expect any beneficial additional exclusivity (such as those described in Chapter 12)? What are the complete contents of ALL regulatory submissions to ALL regulatory agencies to date? What is the progress of regulatory negotiations to date, and what are the still pending issues to be resolved? Have our patents and manufacturing facilities declared to and/or validated by the regulatory agencies?

Due Diligence—Financial

Does the product strategically fit with our existing portfolio? What are the estimated capital expenditures and COGS? What are the estimated populations of total patients, total patients diagnosed, total patients under treatment, and total patients compliant with treatment? What is the treatment duration, what is the expected price, and degree of reimbursement? Who are the existing and future competitors? What is the forecasted market share based on the comparison of features between all treatment comparators? What is the effective patent life or exclusivity periods expected? What is the total sales potential over the product's life cycle? Will the product reach blockbuster potential (see Chapter 13)? Is there a planned development program for additional indications, combinations, dosages, and formulations that will expand its sales potential? What are the planned product's sales, marketing, general and administrative costs? What is the bottom-line product profitability? Is the profitability worth the in-licensing, R&D, and marketing efforts?

Due Diligence—Commercial

Who are the target prescribers, and do we have an established relationship with them? What are the product's unique selling points (USPs)? What is our brand name and components (see Chapter 8)? Is the product's project plan progressing nicely? Is the business plan thorough and realistic? How do we prepare the product, the company, and the market for this product? Who will become the scientific spokespersons for our product? What kind of sales and marketing activities do we plan? How are these distributed among all target audiences, e.g., prescribers, regulators, healthcare personnel, patients, patient associations, families, media, and the general public? What is the expected product pricing? What is our reimbursement strategy? What is our global distribution strategy? How much will it cost us?

Technology Assessment Report

The results of all due diligence evaluations summarized above will eventually be included in a detailed technology assessment report that will be presented to relevant management for a final licensing decision. This report will comprise of the following components: (1) executive summary, (2) technology overview, (3) patentability overview, (4) patent status, (5) overall legal status, (6) clinical overview, (7) chemistry, manufacturing, and controls overview, (8) regulatory overview, (9) financial overview, (10) commercial overview, (11) business plan, (12) project plan (with important endpoints to be met along the way), (13) testimonials and references, (14) recommendations, and (15) accompanying documentation (photocopies and complete digital archive of everything listed above—several blue-ray disk-size).

Technology Transfer Example: Oxford University's Isis Innovation

Isis Innovation, the University's wholly-owned technology transfer company, was founded in 1988, and has pioneered the successful commercial exploitation of academic research and invention. It is now the most successful university technology transfer company in the UK, filing, on average, one new patent per week. More than 60 Oxford spin-out companies have been formed, beginning with Oxford Instruments in 1959, which today is a global leader in advanced instrumentation, employing over 1,500 people in 16 countries. Its products are used world-wide for scientific research, analysis and healthcare, and the company has been listed on the London Stock Exchange since 1983. The combined value of Oxford's spin-out companies has reached £2 billion, using quoted market capitalisations and investor valuations for unquoted companies. The creation of these new spin-out companies benefits local economic development and has created many new jobs in the region. The companies have spun out from a variety of departments and are developing a broad range of innovative products and technologies, including: drugs technology based on the body's natural biological response to oxygen deficiency (Reox, 2003); artificial high performance fibres based on the principles used by spiders and insects (Spinox, 2002); realistic character animation for games and films based on biology and computer science (NaturalMotion, 2001); or test strips which give instant diagnoses from a single drop of blood (Oxford Biosensors, 2000).

Source: Courtesy of Oxford University, Oxford, U.K., http://www. ox.ac.uk/enterprise/innovation/knowledge_transfer.html

LICENSING PROCESS

Having reviewed the technology transfer and technology assessment processes, let us now study the overall licensing process, from start to finish. This process comprises of five critical parts, namely, (1) search and identify, (2) evaluate, (3) value, (4) negotiate, and (5) sign. In particular, valuation will be seen through the often varying sights of the licensor, licensee, and even the inventor, the three main players involved.

In-Licensing: The Players

The licensor is typically an academic research institution. As soon as their TTO identifies a new patentable invention, they undertake all the necessary steps to secure the patenting rights for the institution, and also find potential licensees for the commercialization step. Their priorities are (1) securing the patenting rights, (2) identifying a well-respected and financially strong licensee, (3) maximizing the potential value of the royalties, (4) re-administering those royalties to future research, (5) strengthening the research capabilities of the inventing lab and recognizing the inventor (tenure, salary, chairmanship), and also (6) publishing, when appropriate, and increasing the university's scientific publication citation mark.

The licensee is typically a biotechnology start-up. Having secured the patent rights for their own biotechnology process/tool/product, they have now identified that they need additional freedom to operate for a certain rate-limiting R&D step. Their contacts with the proper TTOs has alerted them to an emerging technology at the institution above, and they have previously spoken to the inventor through the obvious scientific conference routes. Their priorities are (1) conducting a thorough technology assessment for the invention; (2) securing the patent rights in advance of their competitors, most preferably exclusively; (3) minimizing the size of the royalties; (4) securing the cooperation of the inventor and the dissemination of critical lab scientific secrets; (5) establishing a long-term relationship with the institution and setting up an advisory board; (6) attracting potential investors for their technology acquisition; and (7) maximizing the speed of the technology commercialization.

The inventor is typically the director of an academic lab, e.g., the monoclonal antibody unit within the department of molecular immunology at the School of Life Sciences. Their priorities are (1) scientific recognition from peers within the school, as well as the immunology field around the world, (2) securing the patent rights for the school, (3) maximizing the grant support for their lab, (4) attracting additional scientific talent to the lab, (5) training the biotech's research lab on various aspects of the invention, and (6) securing the first publication rights for their invention.

In-Licensing Criteria

We have previously described the intense nature of technology assessment for a potential in-licensing candidate. The criteria used can be company-specific, so that all in-licensing opportunities fit well with company's long-term objectives. For example, a biotechnology company may be looking for (1) autoimmune field, (2) rheumatoid arthritis in particular, (3) anti-TNF mechanism, (4) biological, (5) preclinical compounds at least 6 months from first-in-man trials, proof-of-concept completed in two major RA animal models, high therapeutic index, long half-life, beneficial side-effect profile, and (6) clinical compounds entering phase II, practical dose range defined, well tolerable and safe, solid pharmacodynamic and pharmacokinetic data, to be used as first line, monotherapy treatment. Manufacturing process in place with yield further improvable, COGS acceptable, and potential pricing at 15× COGS, shelf life more than 2 years.

Licensing Negotiations Essentials

Licensing negotiations come into play when patent rights seem secure and an interested potential licensee has been identified. These negotiations are equally thorough and intensive with the technology assessment phase, and must eventually lead to a "win–win" situation, where both licensing parties seem content, secure, financially rewarded, non-competing, collaborating, and willing to bring this invention to commercialization.

While the negotiation details would fill a dedicated book, we only focus on certain essentials, namely, the license breadth, the mutual risk involved, as well as the type of payment agreed.

The breadth of license describes where the invention can be used by the licensee. For example, one candidate molecule coming from a discovery platform, or all of them; one indication applicable, or all; one formulation possible, or all; one dosage strength, or the whole spectrum; monotherapy only, or in combination too; first-line or second-line too; together with other treatment modalities (e.g., radiotherapy), or solely pharmacological; all types of treatment settings, or only in nephrology units; all prescribing physicians, or only specialists; exclusive rights or not.

Important aspects to be considered are as follows: (1) What are the mutual needs? (2) Does the licensor have commercialization plans of its own? (3) Is the licensee experienced and strong enough to undertake full portfolio responsibility? (4) Are other parties interested in sharing the rights? (5) And if exclusive, what happens if the licensee loses interest or changes priorities along the commercialization plan (see Chapter 14)? As far as the geographic rights are concerned, the licensor needs to think of the following: Where is the product launched? Does the licensee have a true global presence? Would it be appropriate to divide regional rights across regional licensees with stronger presence? Should the licensor keep the home market for itself? Does the licensee plan to create local subsidiaries or sublicense to local representatives? Can global marketing campaigns be implemented efficiently? Are the regional prices similar? How do we control parallel imports, i.e., a local wholesaler buying cheap and re-exporting the product to a foreign market eroding the local licensee's profits? Do we want a global multinational everywhere, or do we keep local markets belonging to the so-called rest-of-world (ROW, meaning outside the United States, Europe, and Japan) for local companies?

Another issue mentioned above is the degree of mutual risk accepted. For example, is it an exclusive, global, and outright out-licensing over all future commercialization phases, or does the licensor wish or the licensee demand a more cooperative and less risky deal? For example, what happens if the invention never materializes to a new biopharmaceutical and the product is not approvable? Or what if the licensee is so imposing that the miniscule royalties promised fall far short of the actual sales of the product? In either situation, maybe the licensee or the licensor ought to have decided to proceed alongside up to certain milestones, or throughout the product's life cycle, with varying rewards, based on the respective risks and costs undertaken. For example, if the licensor is willing to contribute up to 20% of all R&D costs, they may be entitled to higher sales royalties upon commercialization. On the other hand, if the product does not get approved, the licensee may have saved significant R&D costs from total value destruction.

The type of payment involved is another sensitive negotiation issue. For example, is a down payment demanded, are other advanced payments guaranteed along certain milestones, what is the win–win royalty rate, who undertakes the costs of development, sales and marketing, and how are monies to be paid. That is, is actual cash exchanged, are licensee stocks offered in place of cash, does the licensee agree to invest in licensor equity too (in a deal involving two companies), etc.

To close the negotiation essentials subject, do not forget the ever-important clawbacks, that is, what happens if something goes wrong? How are milestones monitored objectively, how are product sales captured, who is responsible, who reimburses whom, what are the mutual communication channels, how are differences resolved, what courts are applicable, which side has termination rights, and what happens to those patent rights at the base of all this.

Closing the Deal

Having negotiated the deal components over a long period, closing the deal is still not an easy task. We have previously mentioned win–win, the mutual needs and priorities, as well as several negotiation essentials. All negotiations need to conclude in an efficient manner, since (1) mutual priorities may shift along the way, (2) the deal's momentum may gradually diminish, (3) key personnel may leave, (4) a competitor may capitalize on the delay, (5) a new invention may be the indication's "killer," (6) pricing and reimbursement changes may turn the invention unprofitable, or even (7) the licensee's share price may drop abruptly reducing the deal funding potential. Thus, closing the deal should focus on understanding each side's needs, having optimal communication, resolving differences in a productive manner, making mutual concessions, and rushing to the finish line.

There are five elements of the essence in all biotechnology licensing deals: needs—regulations—conflicts—payments—timing. First, where does each side need to be in 10 years down the line, i.e., with the product launched and profitable, secure, and sharing or not? Second, would the antitrust, financial, regulatory, and ethical authorities agree to all deal aspects? Third, what if the two sides have a conflict, and how best

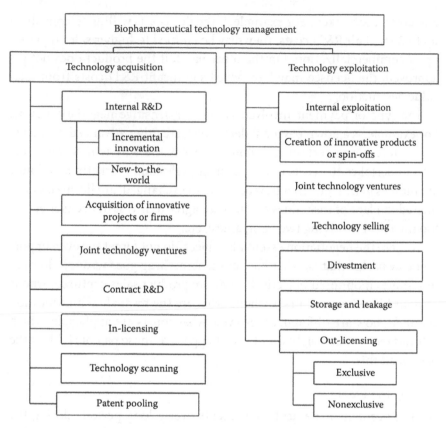

FIGURE 3.4 Technology acquisition and exploitation strategies. (Adapted from Granstrand, O. and Sjölander, S., *Res. Policy*, 19, 35, 1990.)

to overcome it? Fourth, how much is to be paid, in what form, and who bears the risks and rewards? Fifth, how long does it take start to finish, biotechnology can NOT wait. When all the above seem disturbingly difficult, we'd better look at prior healthcare biotechnology success stories, for example, RITUXAN and Stanford University, or NEUPOGEN and Sloan Kettering Hospital.

Figures 3.4 and 3.5 describe the critical technology acquisition and exploitation strategies, as well as the in-licensing process, respectively.

Types of License

There are various major types of biotechnology licensing deals. For example, an exclusive license allows only one entity to commercialize the invention in any indication or geographic region. A nonexclusive license gives the right to a licensee but also retains the right to give another license to

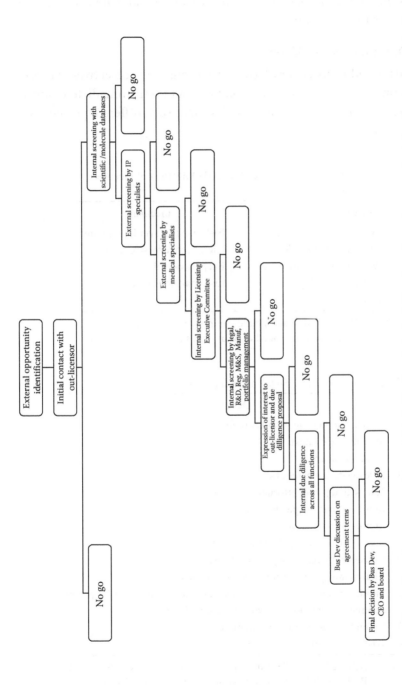

FIGURE 3.5 The in-licensing process. (From Malek, E., Bench to bedside: Oncology drug product development and target commercialization. University of Colorado Technology Transfer, Boulder, CO, PowerPoint Presentation, April 2005, https://www.cu.edu/techtransfer/. With permission.)

an additional party. Additionally, a sole patent gives the right to a licensee and prevents the issuance of another license on the same invention to any other parties in the future.

Financial Objectives of Licensing

The licensor and licensee may have similar long-term objectives concerning the commercialization of an invention, but their immediate financial objectives may be far apart. Table 3.6 describes such different perspectives for either side.

TABLE 3.6   Which Are the Financial Objectives of Licensee and Licensor?

Licensee	Licensor
Slow cash/late investments	Fast cash (recover investments)
Risk avoidance/late deal	High licence fees/royalties
Low licensee fees/royalties	Keep ownership
Product ownership	Risk sharing/early deal
Exclusivity	

Note: Progress: find acceptable compromises that motivate both parties to work together. Win–win situations are possible.

TABLE 3.7   Important Steps in Pricing a Patent

	Description
1	Check whether the patent is in force
2	Identify the context
3	Read the patent
4	Investigate the patent's scope
5	Talk with a patent attorney
6	Inquire about the patent's validity
7	Inquire into blocking patents
8	Investigate foreign patent protection
9	Consider the remaining life of the patent
10	Analyze any prior royalties paid for the patent
11	Inquire into any actual or threatened litigation involving the patent
12	Estimate a demand curve for the patented item
13	Do an income-approach valuation
14	Write the patent valuation report

Source: Adapted from Cromley, J.T., *J. Account.*, November 2004, Posted at: http://www.journalofaccountancy.com/Issues/2004/Nov/20StepsForPricingAPatent.htm

Pricing a Patent

Patents are IP that may need to be appraised for accounting, tax, litigation, and transactional purposes in situations that include sales of businesses and company mergers (which might require valuing portfolios of inventions). Table 3.7 lists some important steps in pricing a patent.

For a licensing process example see the STANFORD University OTL, STANFORD University, Stanford, CA, http://otl.stanford.edu/about

QUESTIONS

1. What is described by Rogers' diffusion of innovations' model? How does this apply to biopharmaceuticals?
2. What are some of the innovation models used by biotechnology companies today?
3. Describe common examples of product, process, management, and marketing innovation in the biopharmaceutical industry.
4. Which are the four basic commercialization questions for biopharmaceutical products, as adapted from Kotler's commercialization model?
5. What is the process of biopharmaceutical product commercialization? Describe each phase in brief.
6. What are the major advantages and disadvantages of biopharmaceutical licensing? Defend either side of the argument in a debate.
7. Which are the major methods and steps of the biotechnology transfer process?
8. What is the biopharmaceutical due diligence process? Describe its component in brief.
9. Which are the biopharmaceutical licensing essentials?
10. What are the important steps in pricing a biopharmaceutical patent?

EXERCISES

1. Pharmaceutical and biopharmaceutical companies are implementing fundamentally different models of R&D innovation. Describe 10 examples of different models announced by various companies.
2. Ever since 1982, there have been numerous life-saving biopharmaceutical innovations launched in the marketplace. Provide 20 different examples of innovative therapeutic classes introduced along the way.

3. Academic technology transfer offices have played an important role in healthcare biotechnology commercialization. Identify five examples of academic TTOs that have helped commercialize a biopharmaceutical product. Compare their practices.

4. Provide 10 examples each for public (free), as well as proprietary (subscription) biotechnology licensing resources that can play a significant role in biopharmaceutical licensing.

5. What role has the Bayh–Dole Act played in healthcare biotechnology commercialization? How do major biotechnology industry associations and universities value its long-term impact?

6. A big pharma organization is embarking on in-licensing a promising biopharmaceutical currently in phase II clinical trials. What regulatory and financial parameters need to be assessed before proceeding into final licensing negotiations with the biopharma start-up?

7. Identify the different in-licensing criteria used by five biopharmaceutical companies in their licensing efforts.

8. When partnering with a larger organization, biopharmaceutical start-ups are looking for various criteria. Describe what some organizations are offering under the title "why partner with us in biopharmaceutical development."

9. There is a plethora of financial arrangements used in biopharmaceutical licensing. By using publicly available web resources, describe some of the most commonly used models.

10. Provide a detailed example of a biopharmaceutical in development as valued by industry analysts. What methods did they use in their valuation? Be specific.

REFERENCES

Association of University Technology Managers (AUTM), 2008. *Licensing Activity Survey FY2007*. Deerfield, IL, http://www.autm.net/FY_2007_Licensing_ Activity_Survey.htm

AUTM, Deerfield, IL, http://www.autm.net/FY_2007_Licensing_Activity_Survey. htm

Betz, U.A.K., 2005. How many genomics targets can a portfolio afford? *DDT* 10(15): 1057–1063, August 2005.

Bills, K., 2004. A guide to licensing biotechnology. *Les Nouvelles* 39: 86–94, June 2004.

BIO Press Release, October 28, 2009, Washington, DC, http://www.bio.org

Cromley, J.T., 2004. 20 steps for pricing a patent. *Journal of Accountancy*, November 2004. Posted at: http://www.journalofaccountancy.com/Issues/2004/Nov/ 20StepsForPricingAPatent.htm

Ernst & Young, 2009. Beyond borders: The global biotechnology report 2009. Boston, MA: E&Y.

Genentech, South San Francisco, CA, http://www.gene.com/gene/about/corporate/history/

Granstrand, O. and Sjölander, S., 1990. Managing innovation in multi-technology corporations *Research Policy* 19: 35–60.

Kotler, P. 1994. *Marketing Management: Analysis, Planning, Implementation, and Control.* New York: Prentice Hall.

Malek, E. 2005. Bench to bedside: Oncology drug product development and target commercialization. University of Colorado Technology Transfer, PowerPoint Presentation, April 2005, https://www.cu.edu/techtransfer/downloads/news/presentations2005/BenchtoBedside.ppt

Oxford University, Oxford, U.K., http://www.ox.ac.uk/enterprise/innovation/knowledge_transfer.html

Rogers, E. M. 1995. *Diffusion of Innovations.* Fourth Edition, p. 35, Simon and Schuster, New York, NY.

Stanford University OTL, Stanford University, Stanford, CA, http://otl.stanford.edu/about

Yale University Office of Cooperative Research, 2010. New Haven, CT. Posted at: http://innovators.yale.edu/commercializing.asp (Accessed on July 10, 2010).

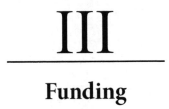

Funding

III

Funding

## CHAPTER 4

Biofinance

Most biotechnology companies are young companies developing their first products and depend on investor capital for survival. According to BioWorld, biotechnology attracted more than $24.8 billion in financing in 2007 and raised more than $100 billion in the five-year span of 2003–2007.

Source: Courtesy of BIO, Biotechnology industry facts, Washington, DC, November 16, 2008, http://www.bio.org

A RMED WITH A PATENTED biotechnology invention, a biotechnology start-up is faced with a long, uphill, arduous road to a biopharmaceutical product approval by regulatory agencies, its commercial launch, and eventual company profitability. The exact steps of this company's road to profitability will be presented in detail in the following chapters. The present chapter will focus on the huge financing needs of this start-up, throughout its life cycle, which are presently and conservatively estimated to be over $800 million.

These funds are required due to the fact that a very lengthy and resource-hungry research and development phase needs to be completed efficiently, while a sole product candidate will result after the preclinical screening of thousands of candidates, and the subsequent clinical testing of at least 10 of them, on average. Overall, the R&D phase may require in excess of 10 years in duration, and hundreds of specialized personnel, as well as expensive tools, processes, and facilities need to be financed throughout this period on external financing. The skills and processes required to attract this scale of external financing will be discussed further below.

BIOFINANCE IN NUMBERS

The sources and scale of biotechnology financing in the advanced bio-pharmaceutical markets (United States, Europe, and Japan) are monitored in detail by specialized financing or consulting companies, such as the likes of Ernst & Young, Burrill & Company, and BioWorld. Additional sources of financing information are the various stock markets, the relevant biotechnology industry associations, the financial news agencies, as well as biotechnology companies themselves. According to Burrill & Company (2009b) "financings and partnering deals collectively brought

TABLE 4.1 Biotechnology Financing during 2008 in the United States, Europe, and Canada (in $ Million)

	2008			% Change over 2007		
	United States	Europe	Canada	United States	Europe	Canada
IPO	6	111	0	−99.5	−89	−100
Follow-on and other offerings	8,547	1115	271	−42	−77	−61
Venture financing	4,445	1369	207	−19	−15	−41
Total	12,998	2595	478	−39	−66	−55

Source: Courtesy of Ernst & Young, *Beyond Borders—Global Biotechnology Report*, E&Y, Boston, MA, 2009.

TABLE 4.2 U.S. Biotech Financings for 3Q 2009 (in $ Thousands)

	Q1 08	Q2 08	Q3 08	Total	Q1 09	Q2 09	Q3 09	Total
Public								
IPO	6	0	0	6	0	0	94	94
Follow-ons	701	312	693	1,706	579	1,464	1,507	3,550
PIPE's	370	203	308	881	302	431	638	1,371
Debt	1622	360	408	2,390	2651	1,505	1,065	5,221
Private								
VC	837	1007	1085	2,929	1486	849	759	3,094
Other	20	226	20	262	31	23	60	114
Total	3556	2108	2514	8,178	5049	4,272	4,123	13,444
Partnering	3091	4141	2962	10,194	4761	8,018	9,390	22,169
Grand total	6647	6249	5476	18,372	9810	12,990	13,513	35,613

Source: Courtesy of Burrill & Company (2009b), Press Release, San Francisco, CA, October 1, 2009, http://www.burrillandco.com/news–2009.html

TABLE 4.3   Biotechnology Stock Indices between August 14, 2008 and March 9, 2009

	High	**Low**
Amex Biotechnology Index (BTK) Closing	886.57 (August 14, 2008)	541.77 (March 9, 2009)
NASDAQ Biotechnology Index (NBI)	930.98 (August 14, 2008)	608.34 (March 9, 2009)
Dow Jones Industrial (DJIA)	11,782.35 (August 14, 2008)	6,547.05 (March 9, 2009)

in $30 billion for U.S. companies in 2008 with over $10 billion through financings and $20 billion in partnering capital. The IPO window closed early in the year and only Bioheart managed to IPO, although it only raised about $6 million."

Tables 4.1 through 4.3 describe the healthcare biotechnology financing status as late as the third quarter of 2009, and the recently declining fate of the industry financings due to the global recession of financial markets around the world, following the 2007–2008 housing bubble in major markets.

THE FINANCING LIFE CYCLE

In a typical biotechnology start-up scenario, a young pharmacology PhD working at an academic institution comes up with a new method of gene manipulation. Obliged, he reports that to the university's TTO, and if all goes well, the TTO proceeds with a patent application. While the patent is pending, the scientist contacts a team of friends at other schools, and they all decide to take this invention all the way to commercialization. Over the coming Christmas, they come up with a product concept, and record that on the omnipresent "night club napkin," as the history goes. Immediately after the holidays, they apply to the university's TTO and soon after they succeed in securing their first state seed funds to take the invention further.

Having withdrawn the seed money from the bank, they hire their first lab space at a nearby technology incubator, and write up their first business plan, using help from an old friend with an MBA. When the business plan looks promising, they borrow additional money from family and friends (affectionately called the FFFs—friends, family, and fools) and decide to incorporate their start-up dream with the name Advanced Therapies (AT). Over the next few years, the initial team of 5 grows to 23, they are all working for 16 h a day/7 days a week/52 weeks; some of them become entrenched into personal debt, but have managed to undergo 3–4 private rounds of financing, attracting $250,000 and taken the molecule all the way past the target discovery and validation stage. They now stand before their biggest challenge to date, namely, going public and attempting to raise a large amount of money from international investors in exchange for the sale of AT's equity, but still 8 years from any potential commercial sales. In the last two paragraphs, we have fast-forwarded through years of labor on the way to this start-up's commercialization. Let us now study the important and multiple stages of financing, one step at a time.

Stages of Financing

The financing life cycle of a biotechnology start-up includes several steps that can be distinguished to belong in one of four major stages, namely, seed, early stage, expansion stage, and late stage (see Figure 4.1 and Table 4.4).

Seed/Start-Up Stage Financing

During this stage, AT can only hope for small amounts of money coming from sources that have a vested interest in advancing science, attracting economic development, as well as talent, publications, or fame to the area. These sources usually include the academic institution itself, a not-for-profit interested in advanced therapeutic discoveries, for example, a patient association or a charity, the state government, or even the federal/national

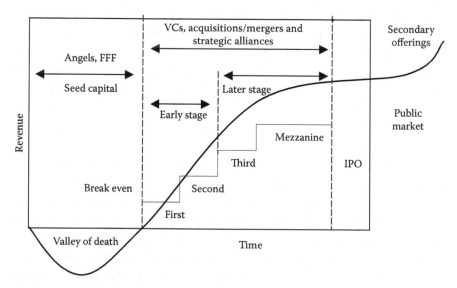

FIGURE 4.1   Start-up financing cycle.

TABLE 4.4 Biopharma Funding Alternatives

Drug Development Stage	Basic Research	Target Discovery and Validation	Drug Design	Preclinical	Clinical Phase I	Clinical Phase II	Clinical Phase III	Approval	Market
Company stage	Pre-seed	Seed	Early stage	Start-up	Mid stage	Late stage			
Company age (years)	0.5	1.0	2.0	3.0	4.0	5.5	7.0	9.0	10.0
Stage duration (years)	0.5	1.0	1.0	1.0	1.5	1.5	2.0	1.0	
Financing round	−1	0	First	Second	Third	Fourth	Bridge	Initial public offering (IPO)	
Risk	Extreme	Extreme	Very high	Very high	High	Moderate	Low	Minimal	
Company valuation ($)	1 million	2 million	3 million	8 million	12 million	20 million	40 million	100 million	
Indicative total funding ($)	200,000	500,000	2 million	4 million	8 million	25 million	10 million	200 million	
Business stage	Unmet need IP developed Lab proof of principle	Business Plan Proof of concept IP validation Doctor interest	Cell assays Small molecules Drug leads Pharmacokinetics Rodent tests	Animal models Scale up Formulation Batch manufacture	First in humans Tolerability Pharmacokinetics Pharmacodynamics	Safety Dose ranging Clinical proof of principle Pharmacodynamics	Safety Efficacy Pharmacodynamics	100,000 page new drug application submitted	Market share capture Long-term safety

(continued)

TABLE 4.4 (continued)   Biopharma Funding Alternatives

Drug Development Stage	Basic Research	Target Discovery and Validation	Drug Design	Preclinical	Clinical Phase I	Clinical Phase II	Clinical Phase III	Approval	Market
Use of funds	Basic and applied research	IP validation	Drug leads tested in rodents	More complex animal models	First-in-human research, clin trial batch manufacture	Safety and dose ranging in patient volunteers	Patient testing, manufacturing, and infrastructure	Application and consultation fees	Market share capture and international expansion
Source of funds									
Entrepreneur			First bold enough to invest, small investment, low expectations for return						
Friends, family, and fools (3 Fs)			Limited funds, based on trust, no expectations for return, may rock relationship						
Angel investors		Limited funds, also offer mentoring and networking, may become interim management							
Government funds	Not paid back, cover salaries and overheads, stifling bureaucracy, and limited availability								

Venture capital (VC)	Offer significant funds, difficult to attract, demanding returns, impose controls, take hold of significant stakes, aim for speedy exit
Asset-based lender	May lend land, office or lab space, may require down payments or guarantees
Equipment lesser	Lease expensive scientific apparatus, require nominal fees over the lease duration
Trade credit	
Factoring	Financial lending based on a percentage of future income, or factoring
Mezzanine lender	
Public debt	Biopharmas collect much-needed capital, without issuing shares or losing control and/or a company stake, but mostly banks require guarantees
IPO	Significant funds to be collected from the public markets, but require large preparation, are costly, and shed large stakes to institutional and/or private investors
Acquisition, LBO	Late-stage option, available to companies wishing expeditious market entry. Require exchanging large stakes in the start-up for tiny stakes in a multinational conglomerate

Note: Shaded areas indicate NOT applicable drug development stages, meaning that funds listed in rows come into effect at certain drug development stages only.

government. The typical amounts involved are in the range of $5,000–$30,000, and usually do not include any guarantees or company equity in exchange, other than the usual scientific publication proving a scientific milestone. Funding sources like this abound for biotech, and their identification and attraction is a must do for the start-up, either through the former TTO office's contacts, or through the Internet.

Early-Stage Financing

At this stage, AT is just entering the target discovery and validation phase. Here, a small number of chemical modifications of a molecular candidate are being tested in a cell assay proving initial efficacy over a reference drug, showing a "proof of concept," that is increased efficacy of molecule AD_THER_51 in cultured neuronal cells. Here, the critical issue is to prove that the intellectual property covered in the patent pending is valid, and that a therapeutic target is defined and validated. AT is now 1 year of age, still far from preclinical or clinical testing, essential personnel are being slowly attracted, and the vast majority of funds are being consumed by R&D. The usual source of funding during this period is venture capitalists (VCs). The funding stage may also be called first-stage financing. An indicative funding figure is $500,000, in exchange for a number of company stocks, usually at discount rates over their nominal value in the order of 40%–50%, taking into account the large risks involved. The stocks may be referred to as Series A Preferred, and at this stage the five entrepreneurs may receive their first small salaries, but lose the overall control of AT, due to their stock dilution below the 50% limit. Here the funding becomes available in installments attached to reaching mutually agreed research milestones.

Expansion-Stage Financing

At this stage, AT has reached its drug design phase, namely, the biochemical modification of the initially promising protein molecule by substituting or adding additional amino acids, their chemical bonds between them, as well as the stereoscopically molecular structure (tertiary structure) in search of a protein molecule that will be able to bind to the previously identified physiological target (e.g., a receptor) maximizing specificity and efficacy, while minimizing unwanted effects. The process involves a lot of expensive computing power, experienced personnel, and knowledgeable pharmaceutical chemists and biochemists in modifying their target molecule accordingly.

When this process is completed, the lead molecules move into the phase of preclinical testing, which includes progressively larger animal models in vivo, and the advanced monitoring of a plethora of preclinical end points regarding pharmacodynamics, pharmacokinetics, dose range, efficacy, tolerability, and safety (short- and long-term). The funding resources required during this stage are significantly bigger than before, and in the range of several millions of U.S. dollars. Funding may be provided by VCs or other "institutional" investors (representing large bank, insurance fund, or hedge fund institutions).

During this expansion stage, we may even identify different subphases. For example, second-stage financing is attracted in order to acquire lab equipment, animals, and facilities and has an investors' exit horizon (see below) of 7 years. Here, investors play a larger role in directing the strategic moves of AT and they are given company stock at discount rates of 30%–40%.

In bridge financing, AT has reached a target pool of three molecular candidates that are planned to enter the arduous phase of clinical research within a year. However, because an initial public listing (IPO; see below) is still several months away, the company may seek bridge funds from the same investors during second-stage or additional ones, in the range of $1 or $2 million. Finally, in a different-case scenario, a competing bio start-up has failed in its animal testing phase, and requires additional funds for the repetition of the drug design phase or the implementation of different animal models, thus seeking the so-called restart financing. Obviously, the bargaining power of the troubled bio start-up is limited, stocks are priced significantly less than the previous financing round, while the investors demand a management change, and strict milestones before undertaking any additional risk. The resulting dilution for the previously existing investors is also significant.

Later Stage

During this stage, AT has probably entered the clinical phase stage, without going to the public financing markets. Phase I clinical trials have defined the acceptable dose range, while interim results from Phase II trials indicate that everything is according to schedule. However, the need for expanding these trials in order to include a larger patient number, together with the hesitation of the young entrepreneurs to go public, has exhausted all previously collected funds, and is calling for a later-stage financing round. The sought-after funds now exceed $10 million;

they may last for another full year of clinical trials and are rarely provided by eager investors. Instead, the financing role is probably taken up by strategic investors, who are willing to contribute significant cash, in exchange for company equity, but also require the right to play a role in the company's strategic decisions, such as the indications and products chosen, the hiring of additional headcount, or the company's relocation into bigger facilities.

Unavoidably, the freedom of the young entrepreneurs to decide on their own destiny is automatically limited, but they are forced to join forces with the strategic partner, who is usually a larger, profitable, and well-established biopharma, a big pharma looking to diversify, or even a private investor with significant personal funds. If the clinical trials proceed according to plan, then an initial public offering (IPO) is soon to be planned, and this brings the imminent exit of most strategic investors. Most of the funds are being spent on the continuation of the clinical trial program. Overall, the major financing stages for biopharmaceutical companies are being summarized in Table 4.5.

TABLE 4.5　Which Are the Financing Stages for Biopharmas?

Risk Type	Characteristics	Financing	Timing Investment	Additional Partners	% Ownership
Early R&D	Proof of principle	Seed financing	$250–600k, 3–6 months burn	Angels, VC, and entrepreneur	20–50
Second-stage R&D	Early in vivo results, prototypes, resolving technical challenges	First round financing	$1–5 million, 1 year burn	VC, Institutional investors	20–50
Execution	Early product development, clinical trials	Early mezzanine	$5–15 million, 1–1.5 years burn	Strategic partners	20–30
Market	Later-stage clinical trials, regulatory and product development	Later-stage mezzanine and IPO	$20–50 million, 2–3 years burn	Public markets	25–35

TABLE 4.6   What Are the Two Most Common Alternatives for Raising Money?

Alternative	Explanation
Debt financing	Debt financing is getting a loan. The most common sources of debt financing are commercial banks and the Small Business Administration (through its guaranteed loan program)
Equity funding	Equity funding means exchanging partial ownership in a firm, usually in the form of stock, for funding. Angel investors, private placement, venture capital, and initial public offerings are the most common sources of equity funding. Equity funding is not a loan—the money that is received is not paid back. Instead, equity investors become partial owners of a firm

Equity versus Debt Financing

We have previously described various stages of biopharma financing, at which several investors have invested their own funds in exchange for AT's stock, which gave them the right to partial ownership of the young biotechnology start-up. In all these instances, the degree of control by the original entrepreneurs has been steadily decreasing, while their company's available funds were repeatedly replenished, and the company's valuation has been rising.

In other cases, the entrepreneurs involved may not wish to give away so soon their brain child's control, through the above-mentioned equity financing. An alternative means for financing is borrowing funds, oftentimes in a much smaller scale than equity financing, without however having to cede control of their company. This alternative financing pathway is called debt- or non-dilutive, since the degree of company ownership (indicated by the personally owned percentage of company's equity) is not diluted by successive rounds of issuing company stocks, which are sold in exchange for equity financing. Both these alternative financing pathways are summarized in Table 4.6, while non-dilutive financing is further presented below.

For a biotechnology funding example see: Amgen Announces the Formation of Amgen Ventures, AMGEN Press Release, Thousand Oaks, CA, November 11, 2004, http://www.amgen.com

NON-DILUTIVE FINANCING

We have previously mentioned that avoiding further equity dilution for AT may be the desire of the company's original entrepreneurs. Furthermore, some of the original investors (VCs and others) may at some point also wish to avoid further dilution, if they believe that the company's directors can either go through some cost-cutting, or if the external offers for additional share dilution do not value the company the same way these investors believe.

For example, a large institutional investor may value AT lower that its existing investors, or they are more risk-averse, or they predict lower market sales of the planned biotherapeutic still in development, or even have doubts about future manufacturing feasibility or the level of COGS. In all these instances, the original entrepreneurs and their initial investors may decide to avoid further dilution, and instead opt for one of the available non-dilutive financing alternatives, as described below.

Licensing

In Chapter 3, we have described the advantages of the licensing option in detail. Why should AT consider the licensing option, instead of taking the molecules under consideration all the way to commercialization? Let us hypothesize that the company is currently in preclinical research of three lead molecule candidates that show promising effects in animal models of autoimmune disease. Theoretically, if clinical trials complete successfully, all three molecules will be approved in treating one or more autoimmune diseases with similar mechanisms of actions, for example, they will be efficacious in rheumatoid arthritis, psoriasis, Crohn's disease, or multiple sclerosis. However, taking all three candidates through intensive clinical testing over thousands of patients belonging to distinct patient populations would require in excess of $500 million. Such an amount of funding would be very difficult to attract, even if the company decides to go public before completing the trials.

As an alternative, however, AT could have decided to sell the commercialization rights to one or even two out of the three molecular candidates, solely for the use in psoriasis and Crohn's disease, while opting to maintain full product rights for the remaining candidate in rheumatoid arthritis and multiple sclerosis, indications with huge market potentials of their own. In this way, the young biopharma would have received significant down payment funds from one or more potential partners, and also have secured future royalties on sales of these candidates that would boost its own R&D well beyond the originally anticipated lead candidate for autoimmune diseases. This way, the company would have avoided the significant equity dilution, would have lowered the risks involved tremendously, would have secured long-term income, and also increased the valuation of the remaining product due to available R&D funds in the bank.

Shared Risk License Models

AT's options may not have been exhausted in out-licensing its two product candidates. For example, not content with losing all future rights on its two lead candidates, the company may have opted for shared R&D efforts, costs, and future profits with another biopharmaceutical partner, or out-licensing rights to a single indication or a single regional market. For example, out-licensing one lead candidate in the field of Crohn's disease, or another candidate in rheumatoid arthritis only outside AT's home U.S.-market would have also provided shared benefits and responsibilities for either biopharma.

The possibilities are endless, and can only be compared thorough company valuations for every existing scenario. Another possibility would be a combined out-licensing to and equity investment by a larger partner into AT, as is often announced in biopharma licensing press releases. Finally, because out-licensing its product rights may incur significant taxes in some national markets, our biopharma start-up may accept an equity investment in lieu of tax payment by its partner.

Royalty Financing

Royalty financing is an alternative financing method to either equity financing or out-licensing. Let us think of our familiar AT having undergone several rounds of financing that have managed to finance all company's operations up to the end of Phase II clinical trials. At this moment, the company is faced with a large Phase III clinical trial program, which has focused on only one molecular candidate in the most promising indication, e.g., rheumatoid arthritis. All prospects of this candidate look extremely promising, while its efficacy and safety observed in Phase II seem far superior to those of commercially available alternative biotherapies. The product's peak sales can now be predicted with more detail, while the company's valuation has recently been upgraded by several financial analysts.

At this point, the start-up's new CFO proposes the option of royalty financing to its board of directors. According to his plan, a well-respected life sciences–focused bank wishes to offer significant financing in exchange for a guaranteed proportion of future sales, say in the order of 20% of future global sales and up to $500 million over the first 5 years of future sales. Taking into account the cost of future money, the bank is offering $400 million upfront, as well as additional contributions, if AT manages to pay the promised royalties to the bank sooner. The outcome has led to increased liquidity, no share dilution, and an accelerated clinical program due to the recently acquired funds. As expected, royalty financing depends on later-stage product valuations, significant projected commercial revenue streams, and several important milestones reached before an investor steps in. Furthermore, it only makes sense, if alternative scenarios are deemed suboptimal by the biopharma's board, for example, an IPO with high dilution, or an out-licensing with very restrictive terms, or even a smaller valuation than the biopharma was hoping for through the public markets.

Royalty Financing Example: ISIS PHARMACEUTICALS

Isis Pharmaceuticals to Receive $24 Million for a Portion of Its Macugen(R) Royalty Rights. CARLSBAD, California, December 21/PRNewswire-FirstCall/—Isis Pharmaceuticals, Inc. (Nasdaq: ISIS) announced today that it has sold a portion of its royalty rights in Macugen & reg; (pegaptanib sodium injection) to Drug Royalty USA, Inc. (DRC) in exchange for aggregate payments of $24 million over the next three years. Under the terms of the agreement, Isis and DRC will share the royalty rights on Macugen through 2009. After 2009, Isis retains all royalties to Macugen. In 2001, Eyetech Pharmaceuticals, Inc., the company developing Macugen, licensed from Isis specific patents necessary to develop, manufacture and commercialize Macugen. Under the license agreement, Isis receives royalties on sales of Macugen and milestones upon the approval of Macugen for new therapeutic indications. Macugen is approved for the treatment of wet age-related macular degeneration and is being investigated in clinical trials for diabetic macular edema. Under the agreement, through 2009 DRC will receive royalties on the first $500 million of annual sales of Macugen Isis and DRC will each receive 50 percent of royalties on annual sales between $500 million and $1 billion. Isis retains 90 percent of all royalties on annual sales in excess of $1 billion and 100 percent of all royalties after 2009. Isis has retained all milestones payable to Isis by Eyetech under the license agreement. Isis has earned $6 million in milestones to date from Eyetech in relation to the development of Macugen. Earlier this week, Isis earned a $3 million milestone payment associated with the marketing clearance of Macugen by the U.S. Food and Drug Administration (FDA) for wet AMD. Also in 2004, Isis earned a $1 million milestone payment from Eyetech associated with Eyetech's filing of a New Drug Application (NDA) for Macugen for wet AMD.

According to the Association of University Technology Managers (AUTM: http://www.autm.net/FY_2007_Licensing_Activity_Survey.htm) during the Fiscal Year 2007, there were:

- 19,827 disclosures received by organizations
- 5,109 licenses and options signed
- 3,622 patents issued

Source: Courtesy of ISIS Pharmaceuticals Press Release, Carlsbad, CA, http://www.isispharm.com

Debt Financing

Borrowing money from a willing financial institution is another financing option for biopharmas. Unfortunately, it comes with its own caveats. First, it carries a significant amount of risk, since the riskiness of modern biotechnology may bring a start-up into the risk of administration, that is, a court-ordered expert administering all its financial obligations, whereas company creditors are given priority over the company's shareholders or employees. Second, the debt option comes into play usually after a biopharma has already commercialized its first product, has a steady revenue stream, and wishes to expand further with the help of debt financing, and thus is not an option for early-stage companies. Third, increasing the company's debt leverage may limit its possibilities for potential in-licensing or merger and acquisition opportunities.

On the other hand, as mentioned above, debt financing is not dilutive and is not subject to taxation. As with every AT competitor out there, the rule of thumb is that their board of directors and an able finance department should constantly evaluate several financing scenarios, and compare them with each other using a variety of benchmarks and models, on their way to a better company valuation, less dilution, and fewer risks involved along the way.

Venture Debt

As previously mentioned, wealthy VCs may offer equity financing to early-stage biopharmaceutical start-ups. Nevertheless, their offer is dilutive; they require significant participation into the company's strategic decisions, and mandate an early exit in the form of a planned IPO. Instead, a biopharma may request an alternative funding option from the VCs, namely, that of venture debt. In such a deal, VCs offer the company a credit line in the order of $20 million, and require significant interest, far in excess of regular business financing rates, that may reach 15% or above, payable every month, over a set period. Once again, the non-dilution is a positive alternative; however the cost of venture debt has to be compared with other forms of financing, either dilutive or non-dilutive.

Convertible Debt

An alternative method of debt financing is called convertible debt. In this scenario, AT may decide to issue a convertible bond, that is, borrow money from interested investors who are given the right, if the company's share price surpasses a certain predefined level, to convert this debt into company's equity at a certain time point in the future. The conversion rate is mutually agreed to be lower that the reached share price, giving an added incentive to potential investors to capitalize on the firm's rising stock valuation. Because of the upside potential, the debt interest is less than the previously mentioned debt financing option.

Be careful! If the company's share price fails to rise over the planned level, and even falls on the back of negative clinical trial news, the suddenly diminished stock valuation may inhibit the biopharma from repaying its debt on time, with severe consequences. Obviously, a company is warned to conduct its own valuations very realistically and also do everything in its power to maintain its share price over a certain limit, before it reaps any benefits from choosing such a funding alternative. This fact indicates to potential convertible debt investors that the company stands behind its projections, and sends a positive signal to the healthcare biotechnology marketplace.

SEED FUNDING

Seed Funding Sources

We have previously described the struggles of AT's founders in securing a small amount of personal funds necessary for the company's incorporation and initial operations. Based on personal savings, credit card debt, consumer loans, or even second and third house mortgages, the personal funds initially gathered soon run out as the biotechnology's startup's research and development efforts get into gear. At this moment, the company is still very young and untested and venture capital or other types of funding are significantly difficult to attract. The usual method of additional funding needed for initial laboratory setup and in vitro testing is attracting seed money from either academic, state, or private sources in order for the start-up to secure basic facilities, resources, and personnel. In most cases, academic institutions license out their IP to the investors themselves, who are also assisted in their initial efforts with limited seed money from the university. In other cases, state, federal, or national funds are available to secure the venture, in exchange for technology commercialization, know-how and job creation, and also private funds later attracted into the state.

The amount of seed funds is usually in the range of few tens of thousands of U.S. dollars, while the sources abound and are usually identified through academic TTOs, or the Internet. For example, the University of California (http://universityofcalifornia.edu/), the University of Oxford, United Kingdom (http://www.isis-innovation.com/), the U.S. National Institutes of Health (http://grants.nih.gov/grants/guide/index.html), the European Investment Bank (http://www.eib.org), and the European Investment Fund (http://www.eif.org) are some of the institutions offering seed funding to biotechnology entrepreneurs. Seed funding is characterized by large discount rates (in excess of 60%) due to the high risks involved, is usually constructed as a convertible debt, is taken up almost entirely by R&D expenses, and is also attached to diluting the start-up's board of directors with investors' representatives who may even overtake the board at this early point. On the other hand, the seed investors are experienced bioentrepreneurs and may offer valuable input to the young and inexperienced start-up team. Seed financing may occasionally need to be extended if the start-up organization needs additional R&D time to prove a biotechnology product's proof of concept. In this case, the funds attracted are called start-up financing, carry a smaller risk, offer a smaller discount (down to 50%), and are usually attached to invaluable input from the investors.

BUSINESS ANGELS

Business angels, as their title describes, are investors who appear between the seed- and venture capital funding phases of a start-up, and offer their much-needed "angel" funds in support of the critical first R&D steps of the start-up, during a make-or-break period of testing and proof-of-concept attempts. These individuals are interested in investing their disposable income in young promising companies, with a higher risk-profile, which on the other hand may eventually reward them with significantly higher returns than what a large capitalization public company could offer. The angel investment is typically attached to company stock or convertible debt. The amounts of money involved in biotechnology investing are larger than seed, but lower than venture capital, usually in the range of $1 million. The angel investors' willingness to invest in early-stage companies has historically covered a large percentage of biotechnology companies before they reached public markets, with total amounts that are even comparable to the much larger, but less available venture capital in either the U.S. or European markets.

Angel Investor Characteristics

Angel investors tend to invest their personal wealth in technology areas they know well, often their previous area of expertise. Their incentives are not solely personal gain, but oftentimes they are after the excitement that surrounds a new biomedical innovation, the critical nature of initial strategic decisions, the camaraderie that develops among entrepreneurs and investors, as well as the opportunity to guide younger entrepreneurs in their initial business life. Angel investors occasionally pool their resources together and set up angel networks, so that (1) they spread their investments across various technologies, (2) they publicize their capabilities across a wider audience, (3) they share early-stage company information, (4) they maintain a closer contact with academic institutions, and (5) they attract a larger number of proposals for bioentrepreneurs-to-be.

The vehicles used for their activities are wide publicity, frequent interaction with innovative institutions, business plan competitions, innovation awards, and entrepreneurship conferences where they tend to meet and interact with promising entrepreneurs. Today, angel investing is not only about offering financial assistance in exchange for convertible start-up debt. It is also about competing with other angel networks, VCs, giant pharma and biopharma, or banks and other institutions for the best innovations offering the highest possible returns. Table 4.7 summarizes the common characteristics of angel investors active in biotechnology commercialization efforts, while Table 4.8 presents the main reasons for angel involvement in risky biopharmaceutical enterprises.

Criteria and Return on Angel Investments Sought

We have previously described how early-stage companies are in need of significant financial resources before they reach a demonstrable "proof of

TABLE 4.7   What Are the Common Characteristics of Business Angels Investing in Biopharmaceutical Development?

1   Private individual investing own wealth in early-stage businesses AND own expertise and network of contacts
2   Investment €25,000–250,000
3   Willing to share their managerial skills, specialist knowledge, and networks
4   No sector preference
5   Often prefer to invest in their region of residence
6   Seeking profit, but also fun
7   Usually total investments below 25% of wealth
8   Minority share in the business—entrepreneur should stay in control
9   Can become involved in the business ("active Angel") or not ("passive Angel")

TABLE 4.8   Which Are the Main Reasons for Investor Involvement in Biopharmaceutical Enterprises?

1   Eventually take control of the business
2   Support regional development
3   My involvement is essential for the business
4   Ensure that the management work in line with my interests
5   Receive a higher return on investment
6   Help the management
7   Help small businesses develop

concept" that can then be presented to VCs or large financial institutions for larger funds. Before such early demonstration of efficacy and safety can be produced, there are very limited sources of funding, in addition to the three Fs seen above. Therefore, the scarcity of funding opportunities, together with the riskiness of such endeavors at this early stage of development can only be matched with a much higher rate of promised returns to those offered by more established and less risky businesses.

Typically, angel investors risking their personal funds in early-stage biotechnology enterprises demand rates of return in the area of 10 to 20 times the investment after a mutually agreed early exit, in the form of the company going public through an IPO, or being acquired by a larger organization before it even reaches commercialization. Such a seemingly exorbitant rate of return can only be validated by taking into account the small percentage of biotechnology innovations ever reaching commercialization, or the high degree of start-up failures even before reaching the coveted clinical trial phase. In summary, when risk is the "name of the game," higher returns are justifiable in the world of biotech commercialization.

TABLE 4.9   What Criteria Are Business Angels
Using in Selecting Biopharmaceutical Investments?

1 Current and comprehensive business plan
2 Strong and committed management team
3 High growth/scalable/strong business forecast
4 Developed product/service with sales
5 Angel involvement welcome
6 Realistic pre-money value
7 But entrepreneurs' qualities are most important

As far as the criteria for evaluating a potential biotechnology investment by angel investors are concerned, classical efficacy and safety endpoints for any given biopharmaceutical candidates may not be available yet at that stage of development. Instead, a scientifically sound but business-savvy plan, coupled with the scientific caliber and publications of the entrepreneurial founders' team will probably tip the scale in favor of such risky investments at an early stage. Additional criteria for selecting an investment are listed in Table 4.9.

In Figure 4.1, a top-level, long-term view of a biotechnology start-up's arduous path to commercialization has been presented. It becomes evident that several rounds of financing, over the 10 year-long R&D effort need to materialize, before the company secures a successful public offering (IPO) and finally commercial sales income. Very often, the basic research and preclinical phases become protracted while difficult bioassay, animal model, or biomanufacturing issues need to be resolved. In addition, when entering the clinical testing phase becomes a more distant dream, significant venture capital in the range of several millions of U.S. dollars are not easily secured and then the dream of commercialization becomes even more distant.

Faced with this emerging trend in bioscience product development, several angel investor networks have recently considered investing into more advanced stages of development. This fact is also due to the decreasing rate of biopharma R&D productivity, the emergence of large VC funds focusing on later-stage investments, as well as the increasing competition among angel networks. For these reasons, angel investing may now be found in early clinical phases, making the need for larger angel funds to be pooled, and more complex and prolonged R&D projects to be screened and selected. Table 4.10 provides selected angel industry statistics during 2007.

TABLE 4.10   Angel Industry Statistics, 2007

Investment Values in Euros	European Union	United States
Networks	297	245
Estimate number of angels	75,000	250,000
Investment per round	165,000	210,500
Total estimate invested annually	3–5 billion	20 billion
Total invested by VC annually in seed (EVCA data)	4 billion	20 billion

Source: Courtesy of EBAN, ACA, Center for Venture Research. EBAN: Ixelles, Belgium, EBAN Presentation, http://www.eban.org/

Biotech Angel Investing in Numbers

Kansas City, Missouri, May 18, 2009—Angel group leaders report in a recent survey by the Angel Capital Association (ACA) that average investment activity per group declined by nine percent in 2008 from 2007, although several angel groups actually increased investments because they see new opportunities during the recession. The survey also found that as the recession lengthened, predictions for 2009 changed: between November 2008 and April 2009, a higher percentage of those surveyed forecast overall decreases in activity this year, but the percentage of respondents predicting more investment also increased. Survey data for the ACA Angel Group Confidence Report was collected from leaders of ACA member angel organizations in March and April 2009 and is an update to a November 2008 survey on the impact of the recession on angel groups and predictions for 2009.

According to survey responses, the average group investment per deal in 2008 ($276,918) was about four percent larger than the 2007 average, but the average number of investments per group (6.3) was about 14 percent less than in 2007. Total funding per group in 2008 averaged $1.77 million and was nine percent lower than the $1.94 million 2007 per group average. As of September, 2008 ACA has 165 member angel groups and another 22 organization as affiliates throughout North America. These angel groups: Fund approximately 700 new companies each year, and have an on-going portfolio of more than 5000 entrepreneurial companies throughout the United States and Canada. Have as their members about 7000 high-net-worth individuals, all of whom are "accredited investors" under

SEC guidelines, with a net worth of at least $1 million, an annual income of at least $200,000, or both. Many, if not most, have a net worth many times that minimum requirement.

Source: Courtesy of ACA Press Release, Kansas City, MO, May 18, 2009, http://www.aca.com

For a biotechnology-focused business angel example see: BUSINESS ANGELS NETWORK, BIOTECHNOLOGY IRELAND, Press Release, Dublin, Ireland, September 21, 2009, http://www.biotechnologyireland.com

VENTURE CAPITAL

Moving along the AT's financing life cycle, its young entrepreneurs may now be faced with the start of a large preclinical testing phase. During this phase, their lead candidates need to be proven with the use of more advanced animal models, for example, moving from the tiny rodents into rabbits, dogs, pigs, or monkeys, in which prior research, either in-house or external, has developed disease models that are essential for testing the candidates in their planned indication. For such a huge effort to be undertaken, a new animal facility needs to be leased, experienced personnel to be recruited, new laboratory equipment to be installed, and hundreds of tests to be conducted, monitored, and analyzed. The whole testing phase has been estimated at $4 million.

Looking into the available resources, the company's founders realize that the last angel investment has left them with another 6 months' cash burn, and that an additional financing round is soon to be conducted. The company's eye sights are now fixed on large regional investors, who have pooled their resources into an organized investment vehicle, commonly known as venture capital or VC. In particular, several wealthy individuals, a few banks and a pension fund have pooled significant funds together, and have set up a company (structured as a partnership or limited liability company), which now employs dedicated and experienced personnel, capable of evaluating and selecting through several competing biotechnology innovations.

The VC firm, having received AT's business plan proposal, will evaluate their intellectual property, the scientific and managerial skills of its entrepreneurs, will ask independent experts to validate the biotechnology innovation involved, and will finally compare the anticipated rate of return with that of hundreds of other innovations. Having selected them, the VC firm will then offer to invest into their start-up in exchange for a significant equity stake into the company, and several other critical demands. For example, to be represented into the company's board, to be given a significant proportion of voting rights, to influence the strategic direction of the company, and also to negotiate an expeditious public stock offering that will give them the right to sell their company stake at a large premium. On the other hand, the VC partners will offer the young start-up much needed supervision, strategic advice, additional skills, industry networking, financial acumen, and experienced decision-making guiding the start-up through the rough seas of commercialization. VC is an investment alternative that has played a critical role in biotechnology commercialization since its inception during the 1970s. Today, it is still providing an essential financing role, although it is unavoidably related with the global state of the economy, and the availability of funds for risky early-stage investments.

Venture Capital Funds

As previously discussed, a VC fund is set up by wealthy individuals or institutional investors who initially commit to contribute a set amount of money. After its legal incorporation (mostly as a limited partnership), the fund attracts financial and management experts to run its daily operations. The fund's employees then initiate their most important functions. These are (1) networking in the financial community, (2) networking in the academic/entrepreneurial community, (3) attracting capital for investment, (4) attracting innovative investment proposals, (5) evaluating and choosing the most promising proposals, (6) funding those proposals and becoming actual participants and consultants into the respective projects, and finally, (7) programming an IPO where they sell their acquired start-up shares at a significant premium.

VC funds are initially set up by declaring their target capital to be raised, for example, $1 billion, and later spend few months to several years in attracting its investors. When all the planned capital is secured, the fund is said to be closed and a set period of fund life then begins, usually 10 years. During the fund's life cycle, the subsequent few years are spent in attracting and valuing innovative proposals, the middle years are spent participating in those promising biotechnology investments, while the final remaining years before the fund's expiration are spent in calling IPOs and selling their stakes for a profit. Those profits may then be invested in setting up subsequent funds, with new technology targets, bigger capital, or different investors. The idea behind the fund's limited life cycle is based on changing market conditions, a call for urgency by investors and start-ups alike, the need for an early exit from the investment while a biopharma's share price can suddenly rise by leaps and bounds (e.g., when their first product is approved by regulatory authorities), and also a need to avoid reaching the maturity phase of any biopharmaceutical enterprise (see Chapter 12). Figure 4.2 details the usual modus operandi of any venture capital fund.

Venture Capital Investment Criteria

As far as the investment criteria being used by VC firms in deciding whether to invest in promising biotechnology start-ups are concerned, emphasis is given on the following set of criteria:

- Intellectual property: strength, patents sought and received, freedom to operate, threat of litigation

- Concept: mechanism of action, physiological target, applicable indications, orphan exclusion, unmet medical need, new biological entity (NBE), size of the market, existing competitors, other treatments in development, estimated peak sales

- Entrepreneurs: innovators still on board, sound scientific profile, scientific publications and their citation indices, management attracted, prior start-up/commercialization/approval/IPO experience, personal funds invested

- Major R&D milestones reached, current financial status, rate of cash burn, manufacturing method with good yields and COGS, anticipated pricing

- Years to approval and commercialization, planned exit, scientific and management experts available to help

This set of criteria may occasionally expand to assess new mechanisms, new molecules, new indications, new manufacturing methods (e.g., transgenics), or new exit strategies, as needed.

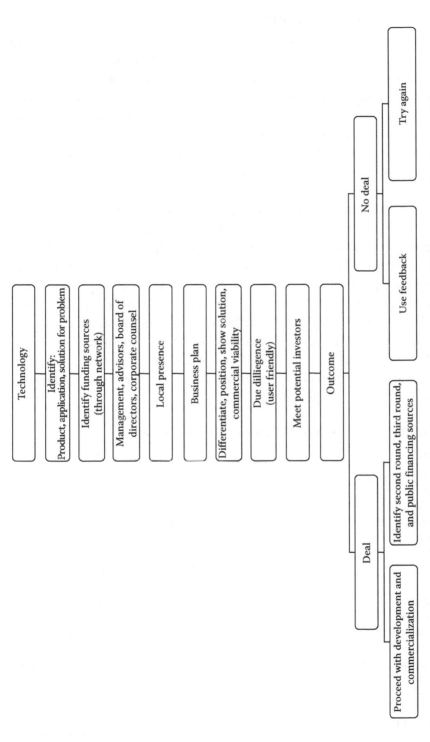

FIGURE 4.2 How does venture work? (Courtesy of Burril & Company, San Francisco, CA, www.burrillandco.com.)

How Are VCs Compensated?

In the previous paragraphs, we have described how a VC fund is set up, where investors commit to a finite amount of investments each, while the limited partners take care of daily operations, the identification of innovative ideas, their valuation, etc. These limited partners are further incentivized to produce a significant return for the capital they manage through a mixture of management fees and interest on the capital. Let us see how this works.

The management fee, usually in the region of 2%, takes care of the payment for daily operations, office and equipment lease, personnel salaries and travel, publicity, road shows, valuations, expert fees, etc. On the other hand, an interest on the profits of the venture capital managed is an incentive to attract as much capital as initially anticipated, and then identify the most promising opportunities and race to invest in them, so that the capital is multiplied in value. Such interest, usually in the range of 20% of the fund's profits, is a significant incentive to maximize the fund's value. The remaining 80% of the fund's profits is returned to the investors, at the end of the fund's life cycle. In the biotechnology business, an anticipated annual rate of return of a life-sciences VC fund is usually in the range of 25%–35%. Of this, management fees and taxation will bring it down to an annual net return of approximately 22%. Let us see how this looks in numbers, as illustrated in Table 4.11.

TABLE 4.11   A Life-Sciences Venture Capital Fund's Returns

Year	1	2	3	4	5	6	7	8	9	10	Total
Funds invested (billion)	1.00										
Annual gross RR (%)	30	30	30	30	30	30	30	30	30	30	30
Fund valuation	1.30	1.69	2.20	2.86	3.71	4.83	6.27	8.16	10.60	13.79	17.92
Valuation multiple	1.3	1.7	2.2	2.9	3.7	4.8	6.3	8.2	10.6	13.8	17.9
Annual net RR (%)	22	22	22	22	22	22	22	22	22	22	22
Total fund value (billion)	1.2	1.5	1.8	2.2	2.7	3.3	4.0	4.9	6.0	7.3	8.9
Net return (billion)											7.9

Now, let us hypothesize that a San Francisco-based life-sciences VC fund has managed to secure a University of Stanford's biotechnology innovation, and invested funds at an early stage. The fund's relationship with the innovators has gradually grown closer, while the respective valuations have gradually been rising. Well into the fund's 10-year vested period, another innovation appears from MIT. This time around, another Boston-based VC fund races to secure the new innovation. Luckily, the SF-based fund reaches maturity and the Californian biopharmaceutical firm announces an IPO, which goes extremely successfully with the public markets returning a hefty rate of return to the fund. Rich with the newly acquired funds, the SF-based fund reaches the end of its life cycle, and the satisfied investors look for another investment. Unfortunately, the MIT innovation is now taken by a competitor fund, leaving them in the lookout for several years to come.

To prevent such an occurrence and missing out on large biotechnology innovations that only come around every few years, the West Coast investors now announce the creation of a series of funds, each guaranteed with significant funds that will run successively to its other, and look across different stages of product development (early stage versus late stage), as well as across different technology platforms (e.g., monoclonal antibodies and growth factors), as well both in the United States and Europe. By doing so, the investors now secure their presence in several future therapies, and in companies young or mature, across the Atlantic. The multiple funds created may even belong to a fund of funds, which is proactively planned to play a significant role in future biotechnology commercializations.

In the paragraphs above, wealthy investors are described to pool their funds together, set up a new VC fund, and attract innovative life-sciences business proposals. More recently, the well-tested and proven VC model has been imitated by more risk-averse individual or institutional investors, even some that have a multiple role, in the biotechnology commercialization process (e.g., as both innovators and investors). The following list summarizes some of the entities active in biotechnology VC funding:

- Private: professionally managed, return on investment focused, and may bring network, business advice, credibility, for example, Kleiner Perkins Caufield & Byers (http://www.kpcb.com/)

- Corporate: manage risk, distribution networks, product R&D, operational skills, and spinouts, for example, Novartis Venture Fund (http://www.venturefund.novartis.com/)

- Academic: intellectual property, spinouts, for example, Harvard Capital Group (http://www.harvardcapital.com/)

- Government: create new jobs and grow economy, offer cash, tax incentives, in-kind, stem brain-drain, for example, the Maryland Venture Fund (http://www.choosemaryland.org/businessresources/pages/MarylandVentureFund.aspx)

When it comes to venture capital from pharmaceutical companies, the list of big pharma companies setting up biotechnology-focused VC funds has been steadily growing over the years. These funds offer biotechnology start-ups not only an opportunity to raise critical funds for their survival and eventual commercialization, but also the added incentives of therapeutic area expertise, freedom to operate in-house, regulatory assistance, strategic focus, opinion-leader contacts, and many others. The list below includes several high-profile industry-backed, life-science venture funds.

According to McKee (2009), Amgen, Genentech, and Pfizer all have corporate investment funds located in, and active in investing in California. EMD Serono invests an early-stage fund alongside a strategic fund allied with the MS Society, "Fast Forward"—blends corporate and philanthropic strategies. The Pfizer Incubator http://www.thepfizerincubator.com combines funding with access to laboratory facilities in San Diego, with another facility mentioned for the Bay Area and one for Philadelphia. The funding commitment is $50 million. Lilly Ventures operates out of Indianapolis and Roche Venture Fund (Basel) has invested in 25 companies in 10 countries.

Biotech Venture Capital Investment in Numbers

Venture capital investment in biotechnology is being monitored by VC industry associations, as well biotechnology-related consulting or investment firms. In the first category, valuable sources of VC information include the U.S. National Venture Capital Association (http://www.nvca.org/), the British Venture Capital Association (http://www.bvca.co.uk/home), the European Private Equity and Venture Capital Association (http://www.evca.eu/), and the Australian Private Equity and Venture Capital Association (http://www.avcal.com.au/). In the second category, we distinguish Ernst & Young (http://www.ey.com), Burrill & Company (http://www.burrillandco.com/), Deloitte Recap (http://www.recap.com/), and PricewaterhouseCoopers MoneyTree Report (https://www.pwcmoneytree.com). A brief snapshot of

TABLE 4.12   What Were the Venture Capital Investments in Biotechnology
Companies during 1999–2008? (in $ Million)

1999	2000	2001	2002	2003	2004	2005	2006	2007	2008
2008	4171	3439	3236	3669	4268	3916	4576	5217	4528

Source: Courtesy of NCVA, *NVCA 2009 Yearbook*, Fairfax, VA.

the life-sciences venture capital investment during the recent years is provided
by the sources mentioned above, in the following paragraphs and in Tables
4.12 and 4.13.

As reported by NVCA, venture capital under management in the United
States by the end of 2009 decreased 11.9% from the 2008 level and more
than 35% from its reported peak in 2006. This decrease is not unexpected
and is the result of anticipated fallout from the technology bubble burst
around the millennium. The industry managed $179.4 billion at year-end
2009 compared with $203.7 billion a year earlier. As with contractions in

TABLE 4.13   Total Venture Capital Investments in the Life Sciences, 2007,
(in $ Million)

Country	VC Investment	% among 25 Countries Total	Country	VC Investment	% among 25 Countries Total
United States	5507.0	68.3	Japan	68.2	0.85
Canada	462.3	5.73	Finland	30.4	0.38
France	388.1	4.81	Austria	20.6	0.26
United Kingdom	341.1	4.23	Italy	19.1	0.24
			Norway	12.8	0.16
Germany	293.6	3.64	Ireland	7.5	0.09
Sweden	220.1	2.73	Portugal	3.3	0.04
Switzerland	120.1	1.49	Hungary	3.0	0.04
Australia	117.9	1.46	Poland	1.2	0.01
Belgium	100.1	1.24	Greece	0.4	0.01
Spain	97.7	1.21	Czech Republic	0.1	0.00
Korea	96.1	1.19			
Denmark	77.9	0.97	Luxembourg	0.0	0.00
Netherlands	75.4	0.94			

Sources: Courtesy of OECD, based on data from Thomson Financial, PwC, EVCA, and
National Venture Capital Associations, Paris, France; van Beuzekom, B. and
Arundel, A., 2009. *OECD Biotechnology Statistics 2009*, OECD: Paris, May 25,
2009, (http://www.oecd.org/dataoecd/4/23/42833898.pdf). With permission.

Note: Venture capital is limited to investment in seed, start-up, early development and
expansion stages. Later-stage replacement and buyout investments are excluded.

other industry metrics, the capital under management decline is specifically the result of the large amount of capital raised during 2001 and earlier being replaced by smaller new funds in recent years. All indications are that some additional contractions are ahead. With 2009 fundraising 1/7 the amount raised in 2000, the industry has returned to a more traditional size band. At the end of 2009, 794 firms managed 1188 funds, down from peaks of 1023 firms in 2005 and 1883 managed funds in 2001. Headcount similarly declined from 8892 at the end of 2007 to 6828 at the end of 2009.

Source: Courtesy of NVCA, *NVCA 2010 Yearbook*, Fairfax, VA.

On the other side of the Atlantic, EVCA (2010) has reported that investments by European private equity and venture capital firms amounted to €73.8bn in 2007, and approximately 5,200 European companies received private equity investments (Table 4.13).

In May 2004, the European Venture Capital Association (EVCA) (http://www.evca.com) published an assessment of how favorable the tax and legal environments of 25 European countries are for private equity and venture capital, and for promoting entrepreneurship. This found that the United Kingdom, Ireland, and Luxembourg have the most favorable regimes, with Greece, Netherlands, Portugal, and Belgium in the next group. Finland, Germany, Austria, and Denmark had the least favorable environments.

The MoneyTree Report is a quarterly study of venture capital investment activity in the United States (see Table 4.14). As a collaboration between PricewaterhouseCoopers and the National Venture Capital Association based upon data from Thomson Reuters, it is the only industry-endorsed research of its kind. Its report for the period of Q1 2005 to Q4 2009 is shown in Table 4.14.

For a VC funding example in biotechnology see: PACIFIC BIO-SCIENCES, Menlo Park, CA, Pacific Biosciences Press Release, July 14, 2008. http://www.pacificbiosciences.com/

EXIT STRATEGY

Exit Options

We have previously discussed how an aspiring biopharmaceutical start-up vies for several rounds of private financing, including the substantial VC round, which hopefully brings the start-up at the dawn of extensive clinical trials, or specifically Phase III, with its demanding patient numbers

TABLE 4.14 The MoneyTree Report

Quarter	Total VC Investment	Return Rate (%)	Number of Investments	Quarter	Total VC Investment	Return Rate (%)	Number of Investments
Q1 2005	$763M	1.66	82	Q3 2007	$1145M	2.49	112
Q2 2005	$1205M	2.62	104	Q4 2007	$1305M	2.84	138
Q3 2005	$1058M	2.30	105	Q1 2008	$1051M	2.29	135
Q4 2005	$978M	2.13	105	Q2 2008	$983M	2.14	123
Q1 2006	$928M	2.02	99	Q3 2008	$1210M	2.64	121
Q2 2006	$1335M	2.91	129	Q4 2008	$1090M	2.37	118
Q3 2006	$1158M	2.52	109	Q1 2009	$646M	1.41	90
Q4 2006	$1169M	2.55	127	Q2 2009	$947M	2.06	90
Q1 2007	$1521M	3.31	110	Q3 2009	$905M	1.97	104
Q2 2007	$1327M	2.89	134	Q1 2009	$763M	1.66	82

Source: Courtesy of The MoneyTree Report, https://www.pwcmoneytree.com/MTPublic/ns/index.jsp

and large finances. At this point, three supplemental forces are driving the start-up into the public financing markets. First, the private investors holding significant equity stakes into the company wish to capitalize on the Phase III momentum, which has skyrocketed the company's valuation, an ideal point for a fast and rewarding exit during the company's fast-advancing prelaunch phase. Second, the company is in need of significant funds to enroll and monitor thousands of patients in dozens of clinical trial centers across the world. Finally, the public stock market exchanges have been informed about the promising Phase I or Phase II results, and based on the biopharmaceutical R&D productivity model, are willing to invest significant funds before the company launches its promising new therapy.

At this ideal financial intersection, the company is faced with two major "exit" scenarios, i.e., the means by which private investors sell their stock portfolio to new investors, and they invest in new early-stage opportunities. These scenarios involve either the IPO of company stock through a stock exchange listing, or the sale of company to a larger equity, usually in the form of a big pharma or established biopharma player. We will examine these two options in detail below. Very often, the biopharma start-up will meet unanticipated challenges in its commercialization pathway, for example, persisting bioassay problems, manufacturing difficulties or disappointing yields, significant side effects, and others. When faced with these challenges, the planned R&D time immediately gets prolonged, new funds are required to overcome these obstacles, and the whole company sustainability gets in question. When additional financing rounds are the only option, the doubts about the commercial feasibility of the whole projects are raised, while new investors are more difficult to convince. Therefore, it is in the biopharma's best interest to minimize risks, accelerate exit, and minimize the share dilution from potential new investors. Table 4.15 summarizes the strategies to either shorten the time to market, or minimize VC equity, as proposed by YALE University's TTO.

IPO Option

The IPO option has been biotechnology's Holy Grail ever since its inception in 1978, with the then incorporation of Genentech. This mad race to commercialization has been previously immortalized in business titles describing the race "from bench to bedside" or "alchemy to IPO." During

TABLE 4.15   Strategies to Accelerate Exit and Minimize Dilution

Shorten Time to Market	Minimize VC Equity
License in later-stage compound	NIH and NCI
Acquire later-stage product	Venture philanthropies
Reengineer generic compound	DARPA
Reformulate marketed compound	Partner with large pharma or medtech
Pursue product with shorter test period	State funds: CT Innovations, Pennsylvania
Pursue disease with smaller patient	Country funds: Scotland's Co-Investment
size for smaller clinical trial size	Fund; France's Premier Jour @ Genopole
Partner with large pharma or medtech	University funds

Source: Courtesy of Constance Mckee, i2 Grants Associates, Woodside, CA.

this period, however, neither the number of bioscience companies going public, nor the amount of funds secured through their IPO has been steadily rising. The reasons for such discrepancy are either the gradually reduced R&D productivity or the occasional global financial recessions, including the severe financial storm which started in late 2007 and is still raging while this book is being written.

According to Burrill & Company, the market for biotech IPOs has slowed greatly since its peak 4 years ago. Fortunately, the slack has been picked up by large pharmaceutical companies that are struggling to fill their drug pipelines as their established blockbuster products are coming off patent and facing the threat of competition from generics. Since 2005, over $60 billion has been invested in biotech company acquisitions by the pharmaceutical industry. This trend rose to new heights in the summer of 2008 when Roche offered to purchase for $44 billion the remaining 44% of the shares of Genentech it did not already own. In 2007, 8 of the 17 new chemical entities approved by the FDA had been licensed or acquired from biotech ventures by large traditional pharmaceutical companies earlier in their development.

Acquisition Option

An alternative exit for a biotechnology start-up is being acquired by a larger pharmaceutical or biopharma company. Once again, the start-up secures the financial resources to commercialization, a strategic partnership between the big pharma R&D/regulatory/marketing muscle and the biopharma's entrepreneurial model is created, and the founders are rewarded with impressive monetary returns, either in cash that can be used for a new start-up, or shares in the merged company. On the other hand, the big pharma acquires critical biotechnology know-how, retains a team with important expertise, supplements its own product portfolio, and may even use this acquisition as a stepping stone toward a complete business model change into the exciting new world of biopharmaceutical innovation.

Exit Financial Scenarios

In a planned IPO exit scenario, the biopharma's top management is being replaced by seasoned biopharma executives who have previously taken other companies public, and are very articulate in discussing with institutional investors or the financial media about the merits of the innovative technology under commercialization. While the IPO process itself will be discussed below, here we will only describe the equity ratio of the initial entrepreneurs being finally diluted under the 10% mark, but simultaneously making them "paper millionaires," i.e., owners of a significant fortune tied to the company stock which has been upwardly re-valued during the IPO process. Other stock holders include the company's core personnel holding stock portfolios (mostly allocated to them as free share options which have vested over the years of their tenure with the company; usually under 10%), and finally private investors and VCs who own over 80% of the company just before taking it public.

Exit Option under Distress

A special financial scenario exists in case the biopharma has failed to meet its R&D milestones, for example, because the biopharmaceutical under development has been found not statistically significantly better than the comparable reference treatment, or because an unexpected side effect (e.g., carcinogenicity in mice) has threatened its commercialization effort. In similar cases, the company's valuation drops precipitously, leaving the founders with the unavoidable liquidation scenario. Under this scenario, the company decides to sell its IP rights, its laboratory facilities, equipment, animals, or reagents, and out of these proceeds try to satisfy numerous stakeholder demands, either lenders, investors, providers, founders, or employees. Under a liquidation scenario, accounts payable are paid off first, then the court-appointed liquidation supervisors, later the institutional lenders, and later the preferred share holders. As far as the common share stock holders are concerned (usually the inventors, friends, family, and…fools), they are left last in the claims priority list, often leaving them without any reimbursement at all. Needless to say, this very scenario has kept the entire AT's board awake several nights to date.

For a biopharma liquidation example see: NEOSE TECHNOLOGIES, Neose Technologies Press Release, Horsham, PA, September 18, 2008. http://www.neose.com

INITIAL PUBLIC OFFERING

Reasons for an IPO

An IPO refers to the issuance of a previously chosen number of equity shares by a biopharmaceutical company, priced at a certain level, and listed at a public stock exchange for any interested investor, individual or institutional, to purchase in anticipation of future profit. The basic consequences of such a listing are (1) share dilution for the previous investors (company founders, employees, and external investors), (2) raising of significant funds from new investors, (3) share price increase if there is strong interest from potential new investors, and (4) an increased transparency and reporting from the company being listed.

Let us study an IPO closer. A biopharmaceutical start-up company seeks to be listed in a public stock exchange when in need to attract significant amounts of money (hundreds of millions of U.S. dollars) in order to proceed with expensive clinical trials, or to build large manufacturing facilities, or even to plan a global product launch and the subsequent creation of several foreign company subsidiaries. Such a listing will only become successful if (1) it holds a strong IP portfolio, (2) the company has previously reached a proof of concept, (3) it has previously attracted several respectable investors, (4) its product portfolio has a large valuation, and (5) regulatory approval, a profitable pricing, and the required reimbursement can predictably be achieved. The basic reasons for a biopharmaceutical public stock exchange listing are summarized in Table 4.16.

IPO Underwriters

Returning to our beloved AT, the company has decided to set up an IPO, in order to attract funds for its Phase II/III program of a new biopharmaceutical. In order to do so, the top management needs to retain the services of external experts, namely, one or more investment banks who

TABLE 4.16   What Are the Main Reasons That Motivate Biopharmaceutical Firms to Go Public?

Reason 1	Reason 2	Reason 3	Reason 4
It is a way to raise equity capital to fund current and future operations	An IPO raises a firm's public profile, making it easier to attract high-quality customers, alliance partners, and employees	An IPO is a liquidity event that provides a means for a company shareholders to cash out their investments	By going public, a firm creates another form of currency that can be used to grow the company

will serve as the IPO's underwriters, i.e., its overseeing intermediaries, as well as other experts, such as law firms active in the field of securities law in the country(ies) where the stock exchange(s) chosen is based. In order to do so, AT decides to issue 1,000,000 common shares, which in addition to the already issued 200,000 will dilute the founders' equity to fewer than 10% and those of preexisting investors to a similar percentage. Later, the IPO underwriter, together with the company, will proceed through a very thorough valuation (see later in this chapter), which may value the company at $600 million (based on forecasted product sales of the existing product portfolio). Based on these facts, shares could be priced at $500 each (600,000,000 valuation/1,200,000 shares issued). Armed with this information, the two sides decide to list AT's shares at $450, thus giving the potential investors an obvious incentive to purchase.

The next step is to offer these shares to potential investors around the world. Here, the IPO underwriter approaches a number of large institutional investors (e.g., investment funds, mutual funds, pension funds, or wealthy private investors). In an effort to sell the shares, both the underwriters and the company's top management (CEO, CFO, R&D head, marketing head, scientific affairs, and public affairs) embark on an around-the-world "road show" where the largest potential investors get to meet the management and hear about the exciting prospects of AT, within a limited pre-IPO period of time. In addition, biotechnology media, consulting firms, industry blogs, and scientific media are privileged to preliminary R&D results indicating the proof of concept, dose ranges, as well as the company's business plan.

After the potential investors express their initial interest, the underwriter gets to negotiate with them the number of shares they are interested in. Previously, the underwriter has made a deal with AT, which may exist

TABLE 4.17 How Do Financial Analysts and Portfolio Managers Conduct In-Depth Research of a Biopharmaceutical Company?

Meeting with management	Sell-side conferences
Medical/industry conferences	Sell-side research
Talking to doctors	Company Web sites
Company analyst days	Looking at the "smart money"
Talking to other investors	

in a variety of forms, for example: (1) to purchase all shares from AT and then resell them to investors, (2) to do all it can to sell their shares, or (3) attempt to sell all shares, and if not return them to AT. In addition, AT may decide to place their shares themselves directly to investors, or even conduct a "reverse auction," often called a "Dutch auction," where shares are offered at an initially high price, which is then gradually lowered until all of them find an interested buyer.

The IPO underwriters may even purchase some of AT's shares for themselves, while they are usually reimbursed by keeping a share of the share sale profits, usually around 6%–7% (included in the share price and offered by AT). If they fail to secure institutional investors, they may even tap their retail investors, while they are often given a permission by the biopharma to increase the number of offered shares by as much as 15% (in AT's case up to 1,100,000 new shares issued) in order to cover any increased demand. As anticipated, both the IPO underwriter and the approached institutional investors rely on the advice and recommendations of their in-house financial analysts and portfolio managers, as well as external experts in order to evaluate the prospects of AT's listing. Several biopharmaceutical companies, in an effort to persuade additional investors in the future, list the external financial analysts who monitor their stock closely. Table 4.17 summarizes the most commonly used criteria for such an evaluation.

Biotech IPO Activity in Numbers

The recent status of biotechnology IPOs can be seen in Tables 4.18 through 4.20, using data from Burrill & Company or the U.S. National Venture Capital Association.

For an IPO example see: HUMAN GENOME SCIENCES announces proposed public offering of common stock, Human Genome Sciences Inc., Rockville, Maryland, HGSI Press Release, July 27, 2009, http://www.hgsi.com/quarterly-results/2.html

TABLE 4.18   Biotech IPOs Completed during
2000–2008

Year	Number of IPOs	IPO Financings ($ Million)
2000	66	6490
2001	7	440
2002	4	445
2003	7	456
2004	29	1701
2005	17	819
2006	19	920
2007	28	2041
2008	1	6

Source: Burrill & Company, *Biotech 2009—Life Sciences: Navigating the Sea of Change,* Burrill and Co., San Francisco, CA, 2009a. With permission.

TABLE 4.19   What Was the Total Offering Size of Venture-Backed IPOs in Biotechnology during 1999–2008? (in $ Million)

1999	2000	2001	2002	2003	2004	2005	2006	2007	2008
328	4085	335	331	440	1436	782	855	1315	0

Source: Courtesy of NVCA, *NVCA 2009 Yearbook,* Fairfax, VA.

TABLE 4.20   What Were the Valuations of NVCA-Member VC-Backed Biotechnology Companies during 1995–2008? (in $ Million)

Average Valuation	Max	Upper Quartile	Median	Lower Quartile	Min
64.4	864.0	91.8	42.1	16.0	0.1

Source: Courtesy of NVCA, *NVCA 2009 Yearbook,* Fairfax, VA.

POST-IPO (FOLLOW-ON) FUNDING

Following its IPO, AT manages to secure a large amount of money, which is sufficient to take the company all the way through clinical trials and its regulatory applications to the United States, Europe, and Japan. Now faced with the prospects of international expansion, setting up subsidiaries, establishing the required product stocks, and hiring large numbers of foreign sales and marketing professionals, AT is considering another round of public financing, often called "follow-on" or "secondary" offering. Such an offering may be dilutive or non-dilutive, as described below.

Dilutive Funding

In a dilutive follow-on placement, additional new company shares are to be issued, and sold in the public markets, bringing in fresh cash that can be useful in a variety of ways. For example, AT may expand internationally, or build a more sophisticated and bigger manufacturing plant, or build additional plants around the world, or hire a bigger sales force, or acquire a promising start-up, or decide to diversify vertically (i.e., purchase a distributor, or specialty pharma company—see Chapter 11), or even repay a bank debt with high interest. Obviously, the dilutive nature of such a placement may bring opposition from existing investors; however, the long-term plans can easily outweigh the dilution with further sales, profits, and valuation.

Non-Dilutive Funding

In the previous chapters, we have described how an IPO Underwriter reaches out to institutional investors before a planned IPO stock sale. During this process, a mutual or pension fund may decide to purchase 100,000 AT shares, for a sum of $50 million each. Two years later, a stock market decline, or a new pension regulation may force either companies to sell their AT stock holdings in the stock exchange, by going through a non-dilutive placement. In this scenario, the funds attracted from the sale do not come into AT's bank accounts, and the number of existing shares remains unchanged (no dilution). The secondary offering may, however, offer a big pharma a significant percentage of AT shares, or another major investor a say into the company, forcing a new board of directors' formation, or even the ousting of AT's underperforming management (hopefully not).

Types of Follow-On Funding

According to the specific nature of the use of the secondary offering's proceeds by the biopharma, we may distinguish the following types:

- Acquisition financing: AT acquires a minority stake in another biopharma.

- Acquisition for expansion: AT acquires a Chinese pharmaceutical company, in order to get firm flooring into China's emerging market.

- Management/leveraged buyout: When AT agrees to be acquired by a big pharma company, a dedicated employee team decides to invest their personal funds and those coming from a secondary offering in order to take AT into a new direction.

- Recap/turnaround: As a last-ditch effort, AT decides to hold a secondary offering, in an effort to save it from looming bankruptcy and find funds for clinical trials in a new indication.

For a follow-on public offering example see: INSPIRE Pharmaceuticals, INSPIRE Pharmaceuticals Press Release, Durham, NC, August 10, 2009, http://www.inspirepharm.com/

BIOTECH VALUATION
Why Is Valuation Needed?

As with AT above, its IPO pricing and subsequent gathering of much-needed funds for its first product commercialization were based on a thorough company valuation, giving its potential investors a realistic measure of its R&D feasibility and commercial success in the future. Valuing a biotechnology company may be required for attracting investors and employees, preparing for an IPO, undergoing merger or acquisition negotiations, intracompany reporting, financial analysis by its external analysts offering investment recommendations, reporting to financial authorities, competing with other companies for an IP asset, being involved in litigation, etc.

Biotechnology portfolio valuations are essential through the company life cycle, indispensable even if the company is private, perpetually repeated, and occasionally disputable between two negotiating parties, hence their precise and realistic nature are constantly under review. The simplest method for a product/project/company valuation is the discounted cash flow (DCF) method, where all future cash flows are estimated and then discounted backward (annually reduced by the existing interest rates) in order to give a present valuation. The obvious disadvantage of such a method is that it ignores the strategic consequences of managerial decisions, taking, for example, overly conservative or risky decisions that may lead the company to varying future cash flows. This disadvantage has lately been minimized by the use of financial modeling that allows scenario playing or the evaluation of different options, subjects which are being discussed below.

Qualitative Valuation

In the absence of essential historical data, or comparable competitive portfolios, or as just a preliminary valuation screening, financial analysts may use qualitative criteria in order to compare biotechnology products, projects, or companies themselves. In using such a method, every single portfolio parameter is qualitatively evaluated and compared with the characteristics of other, better known products (reference treatments) or companies (fully developed biopharmas). For example, what are the biopharma's vision—mission—values (see Chapters 8 and 9), who are the management team, how big is the market and what are the unmet medical needs that the company's products can satisfy, what are the product characteristics and potential advantages. In addition, which is the product strategy (segmentation—targeting—profiling—branding—sales—marketing), what about the product's distribution, pricing and reimbursement, how will it be protected after patent expiration, and so on. Here the evaluation essentials are thorough examination of every aspect of the business, definition of major product/company attributes and their objective ranking, benchmarking against the competition, and thorough understanding of the business model. For a more detailed portfolio valuation, though, a quantitative valuation is mandated.

Quantitative Valuation

There are three accepted valuation methodologies that utilize the cost, market, and income as the bases: close analysis of other methods or "new" methods detailed in the ever-growing literature on IP valuation reveals that they are usually variations or improvements over these basic methods. The existing approaches to biotechnology portfolio quantitative valuations are being summarized in Figure 4.3.

Cost Approach

Let us return to our dream biopharma called AT, which has been the brainchild of four pharmacologists, its founding members. The innovators have labored for 4 years while working as postdoctoral associates at a major academic institution. Having conceived an innovative idea, they contacted the academic TTO, applied for patent, and secured the rights to their invention creating a spin-off, which is none other than AT. Following some early-stage financing rounds, the company is now in search of significant venture capital, in order to enter the preclinical phase for their

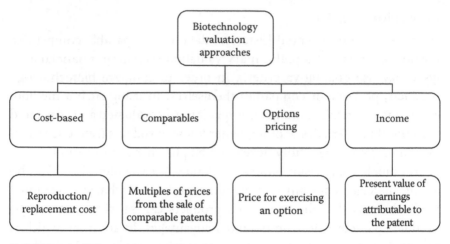

FIGURE 4.3 Valuation approaches.

most promising biopharmaceutical candidate molecule. The VCs, however, are hard to convince. The biopharmaceutical is still a long way from even entering clinical trials, the molecule would comprise a new therapeutic entity, and there are no similar products in the marketplace. The main component of their business proposal that is still missing is a valuation for their technology. The four entrepreneurs then run to the institution's business school library and come up with a valuation approach that might help them, namely, the cost approach.

The cost approach attempts to value the existing intellectual property that is based on a USPTO patent already showing beneficial effects in vitro and small animal models, by estimating the total costs to replace the future commercial availability of the IP under review. In other words, the question is if the innovation was to be tested at another academic institution over another 4 years, and the respective scientists went through the same process of patenting and spinning a company out, and then taking the innovation through the same basic and early in vitro research tests, how much would it take to reach that while taking into account the appearance of competitors and their negative effects on valuation. The cost approach is expressed by a plain mathematical formula:

$$FMV = CRN - PD - FO - EO$$

where the "fair market value" (FMV) would be equal to cost of new replacement (CRN) less physical depreciation (PD), functional obsolescence (FO), and economic obsolescence (EO).

Market Approach

The market approach seeks to identify market transactions involving biotechnology intellectual property and deduct the current innovation's value by looking at similar innovations in such transactions. In other words, let us hypothesize that 10 years before AT was incorporated, another biopharma named Pharmacon was incorporated and has since taken its first biopharmaceutical to commercialization, in the same indication with AT, what is the value Pharmacon commanded for its biopharmaceutical when it out-licensed it to Pfizer? Or, if that biopharmaceutical was never out-licensed on its own, how much was the whole of Pharmacon sold for when it merged with Eli Lilly, and what partial value out of Pharmacon can be attributed down to the specific biopharmaceutical under review?

In essence, the market approach is very similar to valuing real estate, where the house being sold is being compared with similar houses sold at the vicinity over recent years. What happens though, if a similar sale of biotechnology IP was never recorded or did not become public? In this case, AT's entrepreneurs can look at the stock exchange for current market valuations of similar biopharmaceutical companies which have already been through a successful IPO. The complete market value of such a comparator is its current capitalization, some of which is due to tangible assets (e.g., land, buildings, offices, labs and their equipment), while the remainder is attributed to various IP, a part of which resembles AT's own.

Fine, but what happens if the company is owned by a Nobel Prize winner in medicine, bringing fame and goodwill to the company, or the comparator company is majority-owned by a billionaire family with strong connections and lobbying? Obviously, the market approach needs to take these factors into account, and hopefully identify another comparator with a large investor base, a major institutional investor (who has hopefully researched that company in depth), it is actively followed by a number of well-respected independent financial analysts (suggesting a certain degree of scrutiny), it is actively traded at a stock exchange (suggesting no insider trading with the stock), as well as other precautions.

Income Approach

The third quantitative valuation approach that can be applied, namely, the income approach, is based on the theory of discounted cash floor (DCF). In plain words, while AT's innovation is still in preclinical phase, it still requires a significant amount to complete all clinical trials and apply for regulatory approval, while at the same time it needs to overcome all

R&D-associated risks. If it finally enters the marketplace, it will require significant sales and marketing efforts before it reaches its full market potential, after which it will gradually decline, while combating competition-related and other risks along the way. Therefore, if the product's life cycle is accurately forecasted until divestiture, all costs are estimated, all sales income is forecasted, and all risks of failure are taken into account, a thorough valuation picture will emerge, where valuation will constantly rise until the product's peak sales, and will then gradually subside until it gets divested. Furthermore, if you take into account the associated cost of money over the product's life cycle, then you end up with a valuation that can easily be articulated to VCs or validated and improved by experts.

Let us think about this for a while. In order for the income approach to come up with a realistic valuation, we need to take care of three parameters: (1) costs, (2) income, and (3) risks along the life cycle. Costs for R&D are discussed in Chapter 6, those for manufacturing in Chapter 7, and those for sales and marketing in Chapters 8 and 9. As far as the forecasted sales income is concerned, several sales forecasting methods are presented in Chapters 8 and 12. When it comes to risks, Chapters 6 and 14 may be able to guide you in your valuation attempts.

However, if all risks are identified and ranked, how much does a product's valuation gets reduced because of them along the life cycle? There are various methods for dealing with this uncertainty. For example, several parallel DCF estimates may be calculated, according to various risk quantifications and assigned discounts. Another method is the so-called Monte-Carlo simulation, resembling the famous casino playing odds. Here even further optimistic and pessimistic scenarios may be assigned different cash flow values for a multitude of DCFs estimated per product, through the use of sophisticated software.

A relatively new method, the competitive advantage valuation (CAV) claims to address the shortcomings of the above valuation methods. The competitive advantage contribution of an intellectual property asset is defined as the asset's advantages or disadvantages in comparison to an average substitute intellectual property asset.

Valuation of Options

Real-options valuation methods can help assess the value investors are assigning biotech companies. The value of the company is derived from the expected profits of the company's products and the potential for growth of the company into one with many profitable drugs. Real-options valuation methods can be applied to estimate the value of individual projects, which are then used to estimate the value of the whole company.

Decision Trees   Decision tree is a method of modeling decision situations that are characterized by a sequence of subsequent decisions and uncertainties (Eppen et al., 1989). This is typical for long-term R&D projects that consist of multiple stages with certain probabilities of success and which require decisions to be made throughout the life of the project.

For a biotechnology valuation example see: AVEXA and PROGEN merger, AVEXA Press Release, Melbourne, Australia, February 11, 2009, http://www.avexa.com.au

QUESTIONS

1. Which are the main stages of financing of biopharmaceutical start-ups?
2. What are the differences between equity and debt financing for biopharmas?
3. Which are the major methods of non-dilutive financing for biopharmaceutical companies?
4. Which are the main reasons for investor involvement in biopharmaceutical enterprises?
5. What are the investment criteria and return rates sought by angel investors in biotechnology?
6. What are the investment criteria and return rates sought by VCs in biotechnology?
7. What are the major types of entities active in biotechnology VC funding?
8. Which are the main strategies to accelerate exit and minimize dilution in biopharmaceutical start-ups?
9. What are the main reasons and the process for an IPO by a biopharmaceutical start-up?
10. Which are the main types of follow-on funding?

EXERCISES

1. Identify 10 different sources of seed financing for either U.S.- or Europe-based biopharmaceutical start-ups. Describe the size and application process for these financing sources.
2. Two biotechnology entrepreneurs plan to apply for seed funding. How should they prepare a core application file, and what resources may they utilize to assist them?

3. Several pharmaceutical and biopharmaceutical organizations operate biotechnology-focused VC funds. Identify 10 of them and describe their investment criteria and usual investment size.

4. By using publicly available web resources identify one biopharmaceutical product in development for which its manufacturer attracted financing during basic research, target discovery and validation, drug design, preclinical, clinical phase I, clinical phase II, clinical phase III, approval, or post-marketing. Describe the size of that financing round, as well as the collective financing attracted until then during its R&D phase.

5. What are the advantages and disadvantages of dilutive versus non-dilutive financing options available to the AT's founders? Defend either option in a debate.

6. Identify five examples of biopharmaceutical start-ups that have resorted to royalty financing to date. Describe the financial aspects of each deal and explain the method's advantages and disadvantages versus alternative methods of financing.

7. A well-known Internet entrepreneur has been impressed by the promise of healthcare biotechnology and wants to become an angel investor. What are the relevant industry associations, their respective investment focus and size, and how should the new angel proceed?

8. Identify a major biotechnology-focused VC fund. Describe how it is operated, what are its investment criteria, its past successes, and its plans for the future.

9. How does healthcare biotechnology VC investment compare between the United States and Europe? Describe their similarities and differences. How does the smaller side close the gap?

10. Biotechnology valuation is a complex procedure requiring multifaceted expertise and specialized modeling. Identify the major methods and provide a brief example as described by publicly available web resources.

REFERENCES

ACA Press Release, Kansas City, MO, May 18, 2009, http://www.aca.com

Amgen Press Release, Thousand Oaks, CA, November 11, 2004, http://www.amgen.com

AVEXA Press Release, Melbourne, Australia, February 11, 2009, http://www.avexa.com.au

Biotechnology Industry Organization, 2008. Biotechnology industry facts. Posted at: http://www.bio.org/speeches/pubs/er/statistics.asp

BIOTECHNOLOGY Ireland, Press Release, Dublin, Ireland, September, 21, 2009, http://www.biotechnologyireland.com

Burrill & Company, 2009a. *Biotech 2009—Life Sciences: Navigating the Sea of Change*, San Francisco, CA: Burrill and Co.

Burrill & Company, 2009b. Biotech holds up well in the face of financial crisis and market turmoil, Press Release, January 2, 2009.

Burrill & Company, 2009c. Press Release, San Francisco, CA, October 1, 2009, http://www.burrillandco.com/news-2009.html

EBAN, ACA, Center for Venture Research. EBAN: Ixelles, Belgium, EBAN Presentation, http://www.eban.org/

Eppen, G.D., Martin, R.K., and Schrage, L., 1989. A scenario approach to capacity planning. *Operations Research* 37(4) 517–527.

Ernst & Young, 2009. *Beyond Borders: The Global Biotechnology Report 2009*. Boston, MA: E&Y.

European Private Equity & Venture Capital Association (EVCA), 2010. Key facts and figures. Posted at http://www.evca.eu.publicandregulatoryaffairs/default.aspx?id=86 (Accessed on October 2, 2010.)

HGSI Press Release, Rockville, MD, July 27, 2009, http://www.hgsi.com/quarterly-results/2.html

INSPIRE Pharmaceuticals Press Release, Durham, NC, August 10, 2009, http://www.inspirepharm.com/

ISIS Pharmaceuticals Press Release, Carlsbad, CA, http://www.isispharm.com

McKee, C., 2009. Business of biotech 7. Yale Biotechnology & Pharmaceutical Society, 30 March–2 April 2009, PowerPoint presentation. Posted at: http://www.yale.edu/ybps/businessofbiotechnologyprogram2009/BOB7_FINAL_19Mar2009.ppt

Neose Technologies Press Release, Horsham, PA, September 18, 2008, http://www.neose.com

NVCA, *NVCA 2009 Yearbook*, Fairfax, VA.

NVCA, *NVCA 2010 Yearbook*, Fairfax, VA.

Pacific Biosciences Press Release, Menlo Park, California, July 14, 2008.

The MoneyTree Report, https://www.pwcmoneytree.com

van Beuzekom, B. and Arundel, A. 2009. OECD Biotechnology Statistics 2009 (http://www.oecd.org/dataoecd/4/23/42833898.pdf). OECD: Paris, May 25, 2009.

## CHAPTER 5

Biopartnering

Corporate partnering has been critical to biotech success. According to BioWorld, in 2007 biotechnology companies struck 417 new partnerships with pharmaceutical companies and 473 deals with fellow biotech companies. The industry also saw 126 mergers and acquisitions.

Source: BIO, Biotechnology Industry Facts, Washington, DC, Nov. 16, 2008a, http://www.bio.org

IN CHAPTER 4, WE IDENTIFIED several financing methods, some of them dilutive and others not. Among the non-dilutive ones, one of the most important factors for biotechnology start-ups on their path to commercialization is partnering. Partnering among biotechnology companies, from now on biopartnering, is a long-term commitment between two or more business entities who agree to combine their resources in pursuit of a common goal. Biopartnering is based mainly on two premises: (1) it is very challenging, long, resource consuming, and risky for a biotechnology start-up to reach commercialization, and (2) biopartnering aims to produce synergy between the two biopartners, that is the combined capabilities and resources from the partnership to exceed the sum of the capabilities and resources of each party. Other obvious advantages over angel, VC, or IPO financings are the avoidance of dilution, as well as the avoidance of risks associated with financial recessions and the subsequent, euphemistic stock market "corrections."

VARIOUS BIOPARTNERING DEALS

A variety of biopartnering deals are presented below. These vary from plain research and development agreements or patent pooling, to more risk-sharing agreements, such as co-development, co-marketing, or co-promotion agreements, to product out-licensing, or even to mergers and acquisitions of one entity by another. Respectively, the financial terms involved vary from no exchanges, to one-time payments, to future royalties, to minority equity investments, to majority acquisitions, or even the merging of all assets existing on either side. Once again, the four overlying factors for biopartnering are (1) synergy-seeking, e.g., shared know-how, or leaner organizations, (2) non-dilutive financing, (3) risk-sharing, and (4) intellectual property validation.

BIOPARTNERING IN NUMBERS

There are a variety of information sources on biopartnering, including several consulting firms (see Chapter 4). On October 29, 1982, the U.S. Food and Drug Administration (FDA) approved the marketing of Humulin, a human insulin made artificially with gene-splicing techniques. The product was initially developed by scientists at the City of Hope National Medical Center in Duarte, California, and Genentech Inc. in South San Francisco who first succeeded in producing it in the laboratory. Genentech later partnered with Eli Lilly and Company which applied to the FDA and subsequently launched the first biopharmaceutical commercially. According to BioWorld, in 2007 biotechnology companies struck 417 new partnerships with pharmaceutical companies and 473 deals with fellow biotech companies. The industry also saw 126 mergers and acquisitions. Biotechnology attracted more than $24.8 billion in financing in 2007 and raised more than $100 billion in the 5-year span of 2003–2007 (BIO, 2008a,b).

Strategic Alliances

While the number of strategic alliance transactions involving U.S. biotechnology companies in 2008 remained fairly consistent with prior years, the potential value of strategic alliances increased to a record level of almost $30 billion. This was driven mostly by an increase in the potential value of biotech–biotech deals, which increased more than 50% to $9.7 billion. The disclosed up-front payments in these transactions, in the form of license payments and equity investments, totaled $3.7 billion, providing an important source of capital for current operations.

TABLE 5.1   Biotechnology M&A Examples during 2008 (U.S.$ Billion)

Pharma/Biotech	Roche/Genentech	44
Biotech/Biotech	Invitrogen/Applied Biosystems	6.7
Pharma/Specialty	Shionogi/Sciele	11
Diagnostics	Roche/Ventana	3.4
Meditech	Fresenius/APP Pharma	3.7

Source: Burrill & Company, *Biotech 2009—Life Sciences: Navigating the Sea of Change*, Burrill & Co., San Francisco, CA, 2009. With permission.

M&As

US companies accounted for 42% of acquiring companies and 41% of targets in global biotech M&A deals over the 2003–2008 period. UK companies were the second most active as acquirers and targets. 4% of M&A deals since 2003 have been valued at more than $500m, while 70% were for less than $100m. The average deal value for the five year period was $94m. Figures are based upon the 378 M&A deals during this period for which values were disclosed. Marketed products and technology access continue to be the key drivers of M&A. Of recent M&A deals, 46% have been founded upon targets with commercialized products, while 34% were geared to harness technology platforms. Cash is the main payment mechanism for M&A deals. Of the 50 most recent deals for which values are known, 54% were cash-only, while a further 18% were for cash and future milestone payments. M&A will be an important source of future company growth. 45% of respondents to a proprietary Business Insights survey expect over 20% of their company's future growth to stem from M&A.

Source: Courtesy of Business Insights, *Biotech M&A Strategies: Deal Assessments, Trends and Future Prospects*, London, U.K., 2008.

According to E&Y (2009), on the biotechnology M&A front, 2008 was a strong year for the U.S. biotech industry. There were 53 transactions involving U.S. biotech companies, with a total value of more than U.S. $28.5 billion, a record for any single year.

Table 5.1 provides selected biotechnology M&A examples during 2008.

STRATEGIC PARTNERING

Why Big Pharma Needs Biotech

Big pharma companies have been relying heavily on the blockbuster model, namely, putting large sales and marketing resources behind their products in hopes of maximizing their commercial potential and reaching blockbuster status—over a billion US$ yearly sales (for more on blockbusters see Chapter 13). However, the blockbuster model has lately been losing its appeal for the following reasons: (1) the rate of pharmaceutical R&D productivity has gradually been decreasing, (2) the period of innovator market exclusivity has also been decreasing, (3) healthcare costs have gradually been rising putting a strain on blockbusters' commercial potential, (4) several blockbuster withdrawals have highlighted the risks associated with relying too heavily on blockbusters, (5) blockbusters are faced with severe sales declines due to the introduction of generic copies after their own patent expiration, and (6) several blockbuster companies have seen their fortunes decline and eventually became acquired due to the loss of blockbuster income.

In fact, it is easy to identify several blockbuster pharmaceuticals by reading through the pharmaceutical company annual reports and comparing the blockbuster contribution with total company sales. This trend has also been replicated by biopharmaceutical blockbusters, which are just losing their patent protection and are now faced with generic competition, by the so-called biogenerics or biosimilars (see Chapter 13). Even if no company products ever reach blockbuster status, there are several other risk signs for biopharma company sustainability:

- High percentage of total sales in the company's domestic market

- High percentage of total sales in-licensed from multinational big pharma

- High percentage of sales from co-marketed and/or co-promoted products

- High percentage sales from off-patent products

- High percentage of sales from products with short patent life remaining

- No replacement products for those going off-patent soon

- A company blockbuster in the marketplace under FDA review asking for the addition of special warnings on its packaging

- Plethora of low revenue products

- Revenue not focused in key therapy areas

- Low investment in R&D

- R&D investment not focused in established therapy areas

- Poor pipeline

Examples of some of the most commercially successful partnered bio-pharmaceuticals include Aranesp, Avonex, Epogen, Intron-A, Neupogen, Procrit, and Remicade.

Advantages:
Faced with the above risk factors, biopharmaceutical and pharmaceutical companies alike have embarked on huge business development efforts in search of biopartnering deals that would (1) give them freedom to operate, (2) supplement their product portfolios, (3) attract much needed capital, (4) mitigate their risks, and (5) offer much needed synergies. Major biopharmas and big pharmas have business development departments with over 1000 professionals, constantly looking for the "next big thing." Let us now review biopartnering's major advantages and disadvantages in more detail.

Some of the most frequent advantages are described in Table 5.2. Figure 5.1 summarizes the multiple synergies found in biopartnering deals.

Disadvantages:
Biopartnering is not always recommended, while even when selected is not devoid of disadvantages. Some of the most frequent ones are described in Table 5.3.

Building versus Buying versus Partnering

Biopartnering is one of the ways of value creation, the others being going it alone (building), or purchasing (buying) an IP right, a tool, a bioassay, an animal model, etc. All of these alternatives have their own advantages and disadvantages, a summary of which is presented in Table 5.4.

Building presents the following advantages: the biopharma becomes a technology leader or pioneer (e.g., Genentech), it holds the patent rights, it creates a core business, and it captures a competitive advantage. On the other hand, externally *acquiring* a technology is recommended when a biopharma lacks the necessary freedom to operate, when time is of the essence (due to impending competition, or regulatory changes), when there is no in-house expertise, or when market leadership needs to be captured within a limited period of time. Finally, the *partnering* option is ideal when a biopharma races against time, it needs to reduce risk, it needs to leapfrog the competition, it needs to adapt to special market conditions (e.g., foreign regulations and market conditions), or when customers are only looking for the best therapeutic alternative, which cannot be achieved in-house.

TABLE 5.2   Major Advantages of Biopartnering

Advantage	Description
Autonomy	Avoidance of dilution, prevention of bankruptcy
Capital costs	Huge capital projects before commercial sales difficult
Capital market access	Partnering with big company is an investment criterion
Capitalization increase	Partnering is an immediate capitalization booster
Competitiveness	Increased share-of-voice and prescriber capture
Cost synergies	Reduced development, manufacturing, marketing cost
Credibility, legitimacy, validation	Regulators, prescribers, patients, investors, employees
Distribution synergies	Foreign agent or specialty pharma add value
Economies of scale	Combined manufacturing or marketing is cost-effective
Exit	Out-licensing may prevent IPO dilution
Growth	Launching with a partner increases market share
Innovation	Shares ideas, personnel, and know-how give boost
Intellectual property protection	Big biopharma muscle is sometimes essential
International access	Keeping domestic market and out-licensing foreign ones
Knowledge transfer	Co-development enhances knowledge transfer
Management expertise	Big pharma assisting small biotech with strategy
Manufacturing synergies	Outsourcing offers less capital costs and higher yield
Marketing synergies	Increased hospital, prescriber, and patient knowledge
Medical specialty relationships	Medical specialty expertise offered by partner
R&D synergies	Parallel development, avoidance of ground-zero delays
Regulatory expertise	Japanese company submitting to FDA with U.S. partner
Therapeutic area presence	Lack of commercialization mandates therapeutic area expertise

For a strategic partnering example see: NeoTherapeutics and GPC Biotech, NeoTherapeutics Press Release, Irvine, CA, October 1, 2009, http://www.neot.com

EARLY-STAGE DEAL MAKING

Faced with a mounting cash-burn rate and preclinical milestones that cannot easily be met, Advanced Therapies' entrepreneurs are considering either seeking for a venture capital partner, or out-licensing

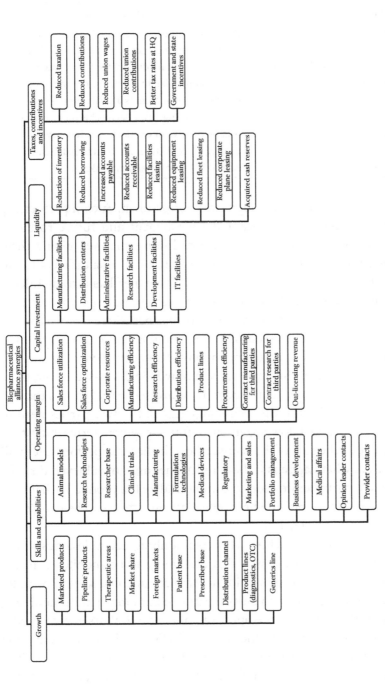

FIGURE 5.1 Sources of synergies in partnering. (Adapted from Bertoncelj, A., Value creation in mergers and acquisitions, University of Cambridge, Institute for Manufacturing, Cambridge, U.K., Symposium Proceedings, http://www.ifm.eng.cam.ac.uk/cim/symposium2008/08proceedings/16%20-%20Andrej%20Bertoncelj.pdf, 2008.)

TABLE 5.3   Major Disadvantages of Biopartnering

Disadvantage	Description
Flexibility loss	Partners may raise opposition in strategic issues
External scrutiny	Before partnering comes extensive due diligence
Future financing round difficulties	Small investors are discouraged by corporate ones
Co-dependency	A partner may fail to deliver or run out of business
Costs	Business development is a costly proposition
Confidentiality	After partnering, trade secrets become obsolete
Intellectual property loss	A large co-developer may turn adversary
Organizational disruptions	A merger/acquisition may lead to redundancies
Reputation damage	Partnering may be seen as weakness

their technology to a larger biopharma across town. Such a partnership will not only secure a significant down payment and future royalties, but will also become available in a non-dilutive manner, giving them the required resources to pursue another technology in a different therapeutic field. The selected biopharmaceutical partner has already offered to in-license the IP rights for a given indication, or even partner with Advanced Therapies in a more cooperative manner where the two companies will share resources, responsibilities, and risks in codeveloping their innovation all the way to regulatory approval and commercialization.

While the nature of this early-stage deal will be discussed below, there are two significant issues that need to be addressed. First, should the bigger biopharma in-license the technology rights, the two parties need to commonly agree about down payment or future payment terms, milestone achievement on the part of the licensee, how the licensee performance will be measured, what happens if these milestones are not achieved (i.e., the licensee fails to further develop or commercialize the product), what happens to the IP at the end, and how potential conflicts are to be handled in such negative case scenarios.

Second, if the licensee achieves the commonly agreed milestones within the agreed time periods, how is this deal going to be monitored in the future, how are royalties to be paid, how are commercial sales to be independently monitored, how do the two parties commonly handle the arising issues along the way (e.g., pre-approval, pricing, reimbursement or side-effect issues), and which are the communication and conflict-resolution pathways between the two parties. Eventually, if the alliance achieves all its goals, the two parties may even further their collaboration, by collaborating again on another molecule, or this time codevelop it, or the original

TABLE 5.4   Build, Buy, or Partner?

Value Generation →

		Disadvantages	Advantages
Risk Generation ↑	**Build**	Product development risks Financial risks Market switching risks Development costs Switching costs Longest time to market Ignored external opportunities Legacy costs You cannot build everything from scratch	Highest degree of control Ownership of IP Avoiding goodwill costs Highest profit opportunity Strongest branding Thorough knowledge Years to prepare and optimize Building internal know-how Opportunities for outsourcing income
	Buy	Cost of acquisition Cost of integration Cost of restructuring Cost of borrowing Need for asset sale (e.g., OTC division) Ignored internal opportunities Risk from biased due diligence (e.g., CEO influence) Internal resistance to change Long-term toxicity risk Anti-competition risks	Intermediate time to market Ownership of IP Fast acquisition of skills and capabilities Can trade noncore for core resources Technology leap forward Can enter foreign market with an impact Immediate increase in revenues and profits Can acquire promising R&D portfolio
	Partner	Minimum control Bureaucracy of big pharma partners Lack of procedures in start-ups Difficult alliance management Time-consuming communications Difficult to break up Problems if partner goes under Cost of integration Lower gross margins	Shortest time to market Capturing the synergies Strongest market presence More economical than buy option Tried and tested Lowest switching costs Higher credibility Improved access Future partnering opportunities

Source: Adapted from Jaiya, G.S., Integrating Business and Intellectual Property Strategy, WIPO, Geneva, Switzerland. PowerPoint presentation, Posted at: http://www.wipo.int/edocs/mdocs/sme/en/wipo_kipo_kipa_ip_ge_08/wipo_kipo_kipa_ip_ge_08_www_109875.ppt, 2008.

licensee becomes a major shareholder in the licensor. Additional forms of biopartnering will be discussed in the following paragraphs.

Licensing versus Co-Development

We have just mentioned AT's dilemma on whether to pursue an out-licensing deal or seek a more cooperative co-development deal. Out-licensing will give it an immediate down payment, will secure future royalties over the biopharmaceutical candidate's life cycle, will avoid equity dilution, while it provides them with sufficient means for developing a second technology in another indication. Original biopharmaceutical companies formed in the late 1970s or throughout the 1980s decided that out-licensing was an appropriate way of securing those much-needed R&D funds, and out-licensed not only their first or second biopharmaceuticals but entire product portfolios, avoiding the competitive commercialization arenas, setting up their own sales and marketing organizations, or competing against big pharma in large indications.

Later, as commercial royalty income started flowing into their financial departments, additional funds were available for late clinical trials, and instead of out-licensing their products at an early stage, they opted to apply to the regulatory authorities themselves, and launched in the U.S. market with a specialized in-house team, while out-licensing the international commercial rights to the product to a big pharma player, for example, Amgen and Genentech choosing Roche or Eli Lilly as their partners. Later on, in stage three of the biopharmaceutical industry evolution, the pioneer biopharmas became financially independent and opted to be fully independent while setting up foreign subsidiaries in major international markets (e.g., Japan, Germany, United Kingdom, Spain, Italy, and France) that would launch their new products into those markets, while out-licensing the rights for Latin American or the so-called rest-of-the-world markets.

In other situations, biopharmas did not out-license their future products to major pharmaceutical players, but instead negotiated co-development agreements whereby both parties would share IP, resources, expertise, and contacts in achieving product approval. This scenario exposed the biopharmas to larger capital requirements and risks, but allowed them to maintain commercial rights even after regulatory approval, when they either split the therapeutic indications approved, or the geographical regions, or they even co-marketed or co-promoted the approved biopharmaceutical (see below). The early technology alliances or the profit- and risk-sharing co-development deals are compared in Table 5.5.

TABLE 5.5   Partnership Strategy: Two Types of Alliances

Alliance Type	Timing	Goal
Early technology access	Early stage (years 1–3)	Secure revenues to:
Provide product to partners to pursue well validated, intractable targets		Fund development of company's technology platform
Do not engage in extensive optimization		Commence investment in internal pipeline
		Screen product against many types of targets
Co-development/profit-share	Later stage (years 4–7)	Share risk/reward of bringing forward initial clinical candidates
Partner half of company pipeline to jointly develop optimized leads		
Retain 50/50 co-development, co-promotion rights		

Early-Stage Deal Example: PTC Therapeutics

SOUTH PLAINFIELD, N.J., September 2, 2009—PTC Therapeutics, Inc. (PTC) today announced an exclusive research collaboration and licensing agreement with Roche for the development of orally bioavailable small molecules utilizing PTC's technology called Gene Expression Modulation by Small-molecules (GEMS™). The collaboration focuses initially on four CNS disease targets to be jointly selected. Under the terms of the agreement, Roche will make upfront cash payment of $12 million and fund PTC's research efforts. Subject to achievement of several successive milestones, there is the potential for PTC to earn up to $239 million in research, development, regulatory, and commercial milestone payments per target. PTC would also receive up to double digit royalties for all products resulting from this collaboration. Roche has the option to add four targets to the collaboration across therapeutic areas, for additional cash payments.

Source: Courtesy of PTC Therapeutics Press Release, South Plainfield, NJ, September 2, 2009, http://ptct.client.shareholder. com/releases.cfm

MERGERS AND ACQUISITIONS

The modern healthcare biotechnology industry would not be the same today if it were not for the ubiquitous merger and acquisition activity throughout its history. Merger is defined as the operational and financial fusion between two previously independent and comparable business entities into a larger, combined organization. On the other hand, acquisition is defined as the absorption of one of these business entities by the other, in a manner that the larger organization prevails and imposes its control over the smaller entity (evolution of the species in the business world). According to Dealogic (2008), global M&A activity reached $4.4 trillion in 2007 and the volume of deals in 2007 was 21% higher than in 2006. Besides growing in their number, the size of individual deals rose to unprecedented levels where some mega deals have already surpassed a hundred billion dollar value (all industries studied).

Motives behind M&A

Motives driving the frenzy of biotechnology M&As in the recent years are multiple, and most of them have already been described as the two partners seek to capitalize on the advantages of biopartnering detailed above. In summary, various synergies, economies of scale, enhanced credibility, access to new products and markets, market share capture, knowledge transfer, vertical integration and diversification, or replacement of products under expiring patents have been some of the major reasons driving the M&A trend.

The partnering advantages named above are only a part of the biotechnology M&A story. Unfortunately, other, more debatable or subjective factors have also played a significant role behind some of the M&A deals. For example, managerial ambitions to create the industry's biggest conglomerates or efforts to invest stagnating cash reserves, or attempts to evade a company's maturity phase (see Chapter 12) have also been responsible for some of the industry's M&A moves. It has also been suggested that the list of motives behind M&A's occasionally borders to the mundane, namely, the efforts of the chairman of the board or the chief executive officer to personally take their companies through the biggest mega deal to date, or even retire "with a bang," and be rewarded with a huge personal monetary reward, which is the prevailing scenario in case a company is being acquired. Despite the debatable nature of some of the associated motives, biotechnology M&As remain a valuable engine of industry regeneration, challenging of the status quo, and growth. The remaining paragraphs focus on that positive aspect while the paragraphs dedicated to alliance management and implementation attempt to steer the M&A decision toward its most rewarding strategy and planning.

Merger

We have just mentioned that a merger is an operational and financial fusion between two previously independent and comparable entities. Let us take this definition into the biotechnology world. Two independent biopharmas have managed to survive years of risky and expensive R&D, eventually succeeding in having their first biopharmaceuticals approved and launched into the marketplace. Having marketed and sold their products across the world they now find themselves, respectively, in similar therapeutic areas (e.g., both are active in neurology, one in multiple sclerosis and the other in Alzheimer's), with similar organizational bases (approximately 3000 employees, each), struggling to commercialize their newest innovations which are turning hard to come by, and fighting larger big pharma competitors with presence in more neurology indications (e.g., Parkinson's, schizophrenia, and depression). The two CEOs meet at the annual U.S. BIO conference, and over a dinner cocktail the idea of merging comes to the table.

When back to their San Francisco and Boston HQs, respectively, they assign a core team of trusted business development professionals to work together on the road to merging. Nine months later, with a swift common press release, the two CEOs announce their companies' merging, and list the following advantages: development and marketing economies of scale, patent pooling, presence in more therapeutic areas and foreign markets, as well as a new focus in commercializing a new Parkinson's medication together. The following day, analysts and investors alike appreciate their combined focus and economies of scale, and lead the two companies' share prices to an all-time high, of almost 35% over their premerger highs.

The above scenario has appeared again and again in the healthcare biotechnology world. Let us look further into the details. The new company will have a combined name, respective investors will turn in their shares in exchange for shares in the new entity, one CEO will remain on the job (usually the most promising, active, younger, and stock-market friendly), while the other CEO will become the conglomerate's chairman of the board (usually the most senior, experienced, strategic, and respected). The new company will refocus its R&D efforts across three centers of excellence (namely, a basic research center close to Stanford University, a target discovery and validation center close to MIT, and a third preclinical excellence center just outside Oxford, United Kingdom).

The commercial organization will now comprise of three independent business units (namely, multiple sclerosis, Alzheimer's, and Parkinson's), foreign subsidiaries will combine in new offices while there will be two main manufacturing facilities across the Atlantic (both scalable and more risk-averse). As a result, the new company now has a wider indication base, increased know-how, larger presence in every market where it operates, reduced risk, increased capital base, reduced cost base, increased R&D budgets, increased share of voice among the world's neurologists, and increased competitiveness against their big pharma opponents. According to either side, a new, more promising era has just begun.

Classification of Mergers   Biopharmaceutical mergers can be classified according to the nature of the merging companies. For example, the merging of a biotechnology company buying another firm is called a *horizontal* merger, since both companies stand side by side (horizontally) within the same industry. The merging of a biopharma buying a contract biomanufacturer in order to increase its in-house manufacturing capacity is called a *vertical* merger, since the two companies stand vertically to each other in the industry value chain pyramid, usually depicted as a "strategy/R&D/manufacturing/sales and marketing" river flowing downstream. The merging of a biopharma with an infant milk formula manufacturer is called a *concentric* merger, since both companies are in the consumer healthcare business. Furthermore, the merging of a biopharma with a candy manufacturer would be a *conglomerate* merger, since the two companies operate in different industries.

There can also be *reverse* mergers, for example, when a biotechnology start-up is eager to become public but cannot wait until all IPO preparations and processes are complete. In such a case, the biopharma may select to purchase a failing pharmaceutical company which is publicly listed, and thus automatically gain access to public investors who will now be interested in purchasing the stock of the failing entity now representing a biotechnology promise. Occasionally, a biopharmaceutical powerhouse that is focused on certain central nervous system (CNS) indications discovers a new molecule that may hold therapeutic potential in a non-CNS indication. Not wishing to out-license its molecule, the management decides to go through a *demerger* or *spinout*, indicating the splitting of the company's shares in two new share entities, where the spinout is given certain buildings, laboratories, employees, and intellectual property, and will from now on be individually listed in the stock exchange as a new biopharmaceutical entity, a spinout of the original biopharma.

Occasionally, an established biopharma may be interested in merging with a competitor, for example, within the field of diabetes. Under such a scenario, the two competing manufacturers of biosynthetic insulin may end up commanding a 90% market share of the insulin market in a given market, a fact that may discourage competition and free market practices. This scenario will be under the watchful eyes of local antitrust authorities, such as the European Commission (see http://ec.europa.eu/competition/), the U.S. Department of Justice (http://www.justice.gov/atr/), and the U.S. Federal Trade Commission Bureau of Competition (http://www.ftc.gov/bc/index.shtml), who may decide to block this merger.

Another way of classifying biopharmaceutical mergers is the fate of the acquirer's earnings per share (EPS) following the merger. EPS is a part of a company's profit which is allocated to an individual outstanding share of common stock. If the acquirer's investors see the merger as a promising development, the company's EPS will rise immediately after the announcement, thus labeling the merger as an *accretive* merger. On the other hand, if the acquirer's investors see the merger as a nonstrategic, unwanted distraction, then the EPS will fall, making the merger a *dilutive* one. This is the reason for which the financial media tend to report the fate of the merging companies' EPS following a merger announcement.

For a biotechnology merger example see: GPC Biotech-Agennix, GPC Biotech, Martinsried/Munich (Germany), GPC Biotech Press Release, February 18, 2009, http://www.agennix.com/index.php?option=com_content&view=article&id=70%3Agpc-biotech-and-agennix-announce-proposed-merger&catid=8%3Apress-releases&Itemid=56&lang=en

Acquisition

An acquisition, or corporate takeover, is the buying of a younger, smaller biopharma by a larger, more established and mature company. Biopharma acquisitions can be rewarding, offering synergies, access to markets, competitiveness, credibility, and other rewards. However, a large proportion of all sectoral acquisitions often turn into disappointments for management, employees, customers, and investors, for reasons ranging from difficult integration due to resistance to change, lack of communication, strategic re-focusing, etc. Therefore, the issue of alliance implementation and management becomes strategically important and will be further discussed later in this chapter.

In an acquisition, the acquirer purchases the shares of the target company, thus gaining control over all its assets, tangible or intellectual, as well as all its liabilities, for example, loans, fines, future risks, etc. The latter may often derail a biopharmaceutical acquisition, for example, due to a previously unforeseen clinical trial side effect that reduces the approvability of a major drug candidate belonging to the acquired company. Because of the high likelihood of such "mishaps" occurring, the acquirer may offer to purchase certain company assets from the acquired company, for example, excluding a problematic product, manufacturing plant, or subsidiary. This issue then becomes the subject of intense negotiations, but also raises regulatory and tax issues for the two sides.

Types of Acquisition   Biopharmaceutical takeovers may be *friendly* or *hostile*. In the first case, the management of the acquirer approaches that of the smaller company and makes a friendly offer to buy it for cash, or shares, or a combination of both. In the opposite case scenario, the larger company is eyeing the purchase of a competitor, which however is struggling to remain independent. In this case, the acquirer makes a hostile, public offer for all competitor's public shares at a set share price, which usually contains a significant premium over the current share price (in excess of a 30% premium). The public investors (some of them institutional) then declare their interest in the hostile takeover, eventually surpassing the required percentage. Their decision tips the scale for the subsequent takeover, and obviously the replacement of the smaller company's board which were refusing the merger in the first place (hostile meant exactly that).

Another type of acquisition is the purchasing of a larger company that has recently either faced severe challenges and was slowly being forced out of the market, or another that sold its major assets to a third company and retained its company and product brand names as its last assets. These brand names may hold value for the latest acquirer, who decides to purchase them and revamp its own operations in a transaction called *reverse* acquisition.

Mergers and acquisitions have been observed between two pharmaceutical companies, a big pharma and a biopharma, or two individual biopharmas. Table 5.6 contains examples of these three types that have been announced during the running decade.

In addition, a plethora of biopharmaceutical M&As were announced during 2008, a small collection of which is summarized by Ernst & Young in Table 5.7, from their 2009 Beyond borders global biotechnology report.

For a biotechnology acquisition example see: Fovea Pharmaceuticals Fovea Pharmaceuticals Press Release, Paris, France, October 1, 2009, http://www.fovea-pharma.com/news1.htm

TABLE 5.6   Mergers/Acquisitions and Partnering

Big Pharma/Pharma	Big Pharma/Biotech	Biotech/Biotech
Bayer AG/Schering AG	AstraZeneca/MedImmune	Gilead/Myogen
$19.9 billion	$15 billion	$2.5 billion
Merck KgaA/Serono	Abbot/Kos	Genentech/Tanox
$12.9 billion	$3.7 billion	$900 million
UCB/Scwartz Pharma	Eli Lilly/Icos	Illumina/Solexa
$5.4 billion	$2.1 billion	$500 million

Source: Burrill & Company, Biotech 2007: A Global Transformation, Purdue Discovery Lecture Series, West Lafayette, IN, 2007. With permission.

TABLE 5.7   Selected 2008 U.S. Biotech M&As

Company	Location	Acquired Company	Location	Value (U.S.$ Million)
Takeda	Japan	Millennium	New England	8800
Life Technologies	San Diego	Applied Biosystems	SF Bay Area	6700
Eli Lilly	Indiana	ImClone	New York State	6500

Source: Courtesy of Ernst & Young, Beyond Borders: 2009 Global Biotechnology Report, E&Y, Boston, MA, 2009.

ALLIANCES

What Is a Strategic Alliance?

We have previously described in detail the nature of biopharmaceutical mergers and acquisitions, where two previously independent entities decide to combine their assets in pursuit of a common goal. In other situations, these two entities continue to share a common goal, but wish to remain independent. They instead decide to form an alliance, where they mutually contribute tangible and/or intangible assets in pursuit of a common goal, while they remain independent and mutually control their own assets.

The list of assets that may be shared in a biopharmaceutical alliance is long. For example, the two companies may share intellectual property (patents, trademarks), research methodology and tools, manufacturing plants, distribution networks, regulatory and opinion leader contacts, lobbying resources, sales and marketing organizations, financial assets, know-how, and a multitude of others. Strategic alliances share three major elements, namely, (1) a common goal, (2) intangible and/or tangible assets, and (3) risks involved in the combined effort. The two parties are drawn together in pursuit of synergies, access to markets, credibility, and other advantages we discussed in the beginning of this chapter. Any given alliance involves a given deal structure, an illustrative example of which is presented by Figure 5.2.

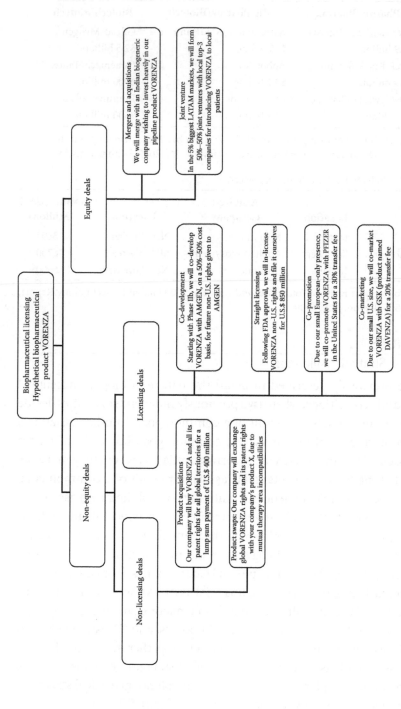

FIGURE 5.2 The deal structure in the biotechnology industry. Includes hypothetical biopharmaceutical product scenario by D. Dogramatzis. (Adapted from Maleck, K. and Pollano, F., Financial aspects of licensing. BioGeneriX. Powerpoint presentation presented at PLCD-Meeting, Berlin, Germany, October 2003. Posted at www.biogenerix.com/publications/PLCDLicensing.pdf (accessed on October 2008).)

Reasons for a Strategic Alliance

The reasons behind biopharmaceutical alliances are multiple. They usually revolve around four major components, namely, revenue buildup, cost minimization, time minimization, and risk minimization (see Table 5.8). It is exactly these individual reasons behind each publicly announced biopharmaceutical alliance that are evaluated by financial analysts and investors, leading to immediate alliance-member share price movements, indicating the expected value from the alliance as evaluated by the markets. As previously mentioned, the final outcome is not always as originally planned, and this is due to problematic alliance implementation and management.

Strategic Alliance Formation Process

The biopharmaceutical alliance formation process is comprised of three major steps, namely, (1) strategy development, (2) partner assessment, and (3) contract negotiation. Let us study these processes in detail.

TABLE 5.8   What Are the Major Reasons for Seeking an Alliance?

Return—Revenue build-up:	Cost:
Incidence, prevalence and treatable patients, price (outcomes, comparables, pharmacoeconomics), reimbursement issues, market potential and market share (competition), penetration and market dynamics (uptake, growth, expansion, competition, etc.), competition, profit and loss pro forma, breakeven and profitability, product life cycle, valuation (NPV, ROI, IRR)	Preclinical proof of principle, preclinical regulatory, requirements, clinical trial (by phase), process development—scale up, COGS, launch, channels—distribution, marketing and sales, third party licenses, milestones and royalties
Competitors, market analysis: size, growth, penetration, share, cycle, price and reimbursement	
Time:	Risk:
Stage of development, size and duration of each clinical trial, patient pool and accrual rates, nature of indication	Extraordinary hurdles (e.g., manufacturing), intellectual property, freedom to operate, capital requirements, opportunity costs, probability of success, competition, SWOT analysis
Demand—patient need—uptake, time to filing and launch (country-by-country), market penetration and share saturation, time to breakeven and profitability	

Source: IBM Global Business Services—IBM Institute for Business Value, Learning the Biopartnering Game—How to Achieve More from Your Biotech Alliance, IBM Global Business Services, Somers, NY, 2004. With permission.

During strategy development, the individual alliance members determine an internal organizational gap that makes the pursuit of a strategic goal on their own practically impossible, resource- and time-consuming, or risky. This gap may be due to lack of intellectual property, or know-how, or research tools, or manufacturing capacity, etc. The gap and its resulting problems identified suggest the pursuit of such a goal in collaboration with an equally interested and capable partner. The alliance scenario is evaluated by top management, which in turn decides it is to the benefit of the organization and gives the go-ahead to the business development department to investigate this possibility.

In the second step, the business development department uses a variety of partner identification tools to identify and evaluate potential partners. For example, they rely on industry contacts, use public and proprietary databases, study the potential partners' web pages, and also attend specialized biopartnering conferences in search of interested parties. Having identified a large number of potentially interesting entities, they then further evaluate their mutual compatibility, strategic fit with their own company, past history, credibility, financial stability, alliance goals, potential exclusivities, existing conflicts, available resources, willingness to collaborate, and a plethora of specialized factors. Having reduced the potential partners to a short list of three to five companies, they then embark on a thorough, strategic, standardized, and objective due diligence process which exposes all advantages and disadvantages of all these potential collaborations. Their ranking is then evaluated by all interested departments, including R&D, manufacturing, regulatory, sales and marketing, financial, legal, and business development that eventually identify the ideal partner to be approached.

In the final stage of alliance formation, contract negotiations between the two parties are initiated, with detailed communication processes, timelines, and deliverables, where potential conflicts are eliminated, mutual concessions are made, and a final contract is produced. The alliance contract is once again screened by legal and top management departments on either side, hopefully resulting in an alliance agreement to be commonly announced through a press conference and press release.

Strategic Alliance Types

Strategic alliances in the biotechnology industry may acquire a number of different forms. A *joint venture* can be a biopharmaceutical alliance where the two parties decide to create a new business entity pursuing their common goal. The new entity is equipped with resources (intangible/tangible) coming from either side and issues shares that belong to either party according to their degree of investment.

In an *equity strategic alliance*, one of the alliance members purchases shares in the other company, allowing it to pursue a commonly set goal, and thus sharing into the costs and risks of the technology to be developed. In other cases, as an added incentive for the smaller biopharma, it may be given a small number of shares belonging to the larger alliance member, as an indication of shared strategy and credibility/validity of the common project.

In a third alliance variant, the *non-equity alliance*, one member of the alliance is investing an amount of money into the second member, without gaining any equity in return, but instead opting for future rights to commercialization, exclusive markets (usually overseas), or development into additional indications of its own. Finally, a *global strategic alliance* involves two biopharmaceutical partners who decide to commonly market and sell a new biopharmaceutical across the world, either co-promoting the product (two companies marketing one brand name), or co-marketing it (the two companies marketing a different brand name of the same product), or one company selling and marketing, while the other is locally distributing it, etc. In similar arrangements, two companies may divide the global pharmaceutical markets among themselves, normally split among four regions, namely, the Americas, Europe, Japan, and the rest of the world, where each retains exclusive rights in some of the four regions. These arrangements mandate the existence of two global biopharmaceutical companies, with respective central and local organizations, prior presence, government contacts, prescriber contacts, and sales and marketing expertise in the chosen areas.

For a biotechnology alliance example see: NeuroSearch and Janssen NeuroSearch Press Release, Ballerup, Denmark, August 17, 2009, http://www.neurosearch.com

BIOTECHNOLOGY ALLIANCES IN NUMBERS

There are various organizations that monitor the announced biotechnology alliances globally, including Ernst & Young, Burrill & Company, and the UNU-MERIT. UNU-MERIT (http://www.merit.unu.edu/) is a joint research and training center of United Nations University (UNU) and Maastricht University, The Netherlands. UNU-MERIT provides insights into the social, political, and economic factors that drive technological change and innovation.

According to UNU-MERIT CATI, their database collects information on strategic alliances by domestic and multinational firms for technology transfer or joint research in biotechnology from announcements or articles in newspapers and professional journals, many of which are in English. Whether or not an alliance is made public and subject to a newspaper report will depend on the interests of the partners and the importance of the alliance to readers. Therefore, the UNU-MERIT CATI database is likely to exclude small alliances and those that the partners do not wish to publicly disclose. In addition, the database favors publications in English and consequently alliances from English-speaking countries such as the United States are likely to be overrepresented. Results are only available by major countries or regions: the United States, Europe, Japan, and non-triad (NT) countries (involving a country outside the previous three countries or regions). The number of alliances has increased from 45 in 1990 to 526 in 2006 (see Table 5.9).

For the last 3 years for which data are available (2004–2006), 1396 biotechnology alliances were included in the UNU-MERIT CATI database. An alliance can include firms from two or more of the four countries or regions, or it can only include domestic firms. The share of alliances that involved one or more partners from the United States reached a peak in the late 1990s. The United States accounted for 86.1% of the 519 biotechnology alliances between 1997 and 1999, compared to 71.3% of the 1396 biotechnology alliances between 2004 and 2006. Between 1997–1999 and 2004–2006, the share of alliances involving European firms increased from 46.2% to 49.7% and the share of alliances involving Japanese firms increased from 8.1% to 10.0%. The largest increase is for alliances involving firms from NT countries. This share

TABLE 5.9   Number of Biotechnology Alliances for Research or Technology Transfer, 2000–2006

	2000	2001	2002	2003	2004	2005	2006
United States	165	274	219	274	277	358	360
Europe	91	171	177	178	197	217	280
Japan	9	17	41	28	32	54	53
Other	22	48	56	52	50	75	96
Total	200	355	332	368	389	481	526

Source: UNU-MERIT CATI database, Maastricht, the Netherlands, April 2009; van Beuzekom, B., and Arundel, A., *OECD Biotechnology Statistics 2009*, OECD, Paris, http://www.oecd.org/dataoecd/4/23/42833898.pdf, May 25, 2009. With permission.

TABLE 5.10   Selected 2008 U.S. Biotech Alliances

Company	Location	Partner	Location	Up-Front License Payments (U.S.$ Million)	Potential Value (U.S.$ Million)
Genzyme	New England	ISIS	San Diego	175	1900
Celgene	New Jersey	Acceleron	New England	45	1871
GlaxoSmithKline	United Kingdom	Archemix	New England	21	1428
Genzyme	New England	Osiris	Mid-Atlantic	130	1380

Source: Courtesy of Ernst & Young, Beyond Borders: 2009 Global Biotechnology Report, E&Y, Boston, MA, 2009.

more than doubled, from 7.3% of all alliances between 1997 and 1999 to 15.8% of alliances between 2004 and 2006 (van Beuzekom and Arundel, OECD, 2009. With permission.)

Selected 2008 U.S. biotechnology alliances, as listed by Ernst & Young in their Beyond borders 2009 global biotechnology report are shown in Table 5.10.

JOINT VENTURES

We have previously described the nature of joint ventures, originating from two alliance partners who set up a new—joint—venture in pursuit of a common goal. The joint venture can be equally owned (50%–50%), or reflect various degrees of ownership between the two parties. In most of the biotechnology industry cases, joint ventures involve the collaboration between a global biotechnology company with a local company active in an international market, whereas the two parties agree to share resources in order to better capitalize on this market's growth opportunity. In such an agreement, the IP owner has the global commercial rights to a biopharmaceutical brand, whereas the local company has superior local market knowledge, prior therapeutic area expertise, regulatory and reimbursement authority contacts, established opinion leader and prescriber relationships, as well as patient, media, and public awareness, making it a more locally suited candidate to capture the planned market share.

There are two major issues making the formation of foreign biopharmaceutical joint ventures (JVs) a sensitive issue. First, the creation of such JVs may be mandatory in order for a multinational company to enter the local market, such as in the case of China and India, and previously Japan). Second, a JV mandates the temporary transfer of brand names, trademarks, and know-how from the originator to the local partner, making the resulting JV often the subject of legal conflict, in case the multinational company decides to discontinue the local JV in exchange for its own subsidiary. In several cases, local partners claim that they are suddenly deprived of future earnings, or that they were not given sufficient time to recuperate their investments in the JV's infrastructure, requesting from local courts (where they hold better contacts) huge compensations or additional local product rights. Unfortunately, biopartnering was never meant to be easy to implement, monitor, and manage, and thus thorough local market knowledge, legal expertise, and prescriber contacts need to be always secured by the multinational before any change in local strategy is envisaged.

For a biotechnology joint venture example see: Advanced Cell Technology and CHA Biotech, Advanced Cell Technology Press Release, Worcester, MA, December 30, 2008, http://www.advancedcell.com

CO-DEVELOPMENT AND CO-PROMOTION DEALS

When the biopharmaceutical industry first originated in the late 1970s, start-up biotechnology companies struggled to collect personal funds from the inventors themselves and later venture capital financing to support their initial clinical trials. Faced, however, with a new-to-the-world technology proposition, an arduous clinical trial program, and huge investments needed to commercialize their biopharmaceutical inventions, they opted to out-license their initial product candidates to financially strong, and well-established pharmaceutical companies. The model of biopharmaceutical–pharmaceutical collaboration in the commercialization of biopharmaceuticals continued for many years, until the resulting royalties from their outsourced products allowed the pioneer biopharmas (Genentech and Amgen) to initially retain U.S. commercial rights for their second generation products, and later retain global rights for their inventions.

In the almost 30 years of healthcare biotechnology commercialization that have followed, several biopharmas have changed their research and development models into more cooperative, resource- and risk-sharing models, whereas the start-up biopharmas would seek co-development agreements from their bigger, established partners. This model, in return, would give them a bigger say in strategic decisions, would allow them to retain commercial rights for both their native and foreign markets, and would later thrust them into the commercial pharmaceutical markets with their increased requirements, regulations, but also rewards. The first decade of the twenty-first century has seen the emergence of such collaborative agreements in research and development, and also in the sales, marketing, and distribution of the newer biopharmaceuticals. Let us now review some of these deals in more detail.

Shared Responsibilities

As expected, additional rights, privileges, and financial rewards in biopharmaceutical alliances come attached to further complexities, strategic dilemmas, costs, and risks, especially for the less-established and financially strapped biotechnology start-ups. For example, co-development agreements come attached to significantly higher R&D costs, associated risks of failure, or risks of facing regulatory approval delays. In addition, co-marketing or co-promotion agreements necessitate the creation of foreign sales and marketing structures for the young biopharmas, as well as local market knowledge and contacts, local government lobbying, significant company brand-building efforts, as well as large global and local marketing campaigns.

Thus, the decision to seek a cooperative alliance is a strategic one that can only be made possible if the biopharma gains access to detailed market information, market intelligence and modeling tools, local contacts, and significant prelaunch financial resources. In addition, significant risk mitigation strategies, such as product portfolio balancing, international market prioritization, joint ventures with local companies, and insurance policies also need to be in place in advance of major expansions.

Co-Promotion

In biopharmaceutical co-promotion agreements, the marketing authorization licensee agrees to have its product co-promoted by a partner, under the same brand, at the same price. The reasons for doing so are multiple: (1) increased share of voice versus the competitors, (2) other in-house, resource-limiting product priorities, (3) emphasis on specialist prescribers (e.g., neurologists) while the partner focuses on general practitioners (family physicians), and (4) co-promotion into additional prescriber groups, where the product licensee does not have a presence. In addition, (5) lack of indication experience, where the product licensee wants to be associated with the co-promotion partner's huge customer awareness, (6) lack of foreign market experience provided by a local co-promotion partner with better expertise, knowledge, and insider contacts, (7) lack of size when a small European licensee attempts to enter the huge U.S. market, (8) risk-mitigation if a foreign promotion may not be widely accepted (e.g., "morning-after pill" in a religious market), and (9) increased credibility, visibility, and employee morale.

In co-promotion agreements, the partner is rewarded with a percentage of sales revenue, plus selective marketing costs, as well as promotional materials paid by the authorization holder, and free training. Nevertheless, a co-promotion agreement is not devoid of potential problems. For example, the co-promotion partner is to be reimbursed by the marketing authorization holder for all sales originating from the partner's promotional efforts, which are very difficult to pinpoint. In such cases, the following means may be used:

- Co-promotion done in rural areas where the authorization holder does not have access

- Co-promotion done in selected indications for each side

- Co-promotion done in selected prescriber targets (e.g., hospital versus private)

Co-Marketing

When biopharmaceutical companies have their new products approved, they often apply for several different brand names and pay the respective regulatory fees for the individual approval of each of them. This practice gives them the right to employ the services of co-marketing partners (either domestic or foreign) who acquire the rights to one of the approved brands by paying a percentage of their own sales revenues back to the original authorization holder. The co-marketing strategy differs from the co-promotion strategy above in the following aspects:

- Product sales are easily attributed to either partner.

- The two partners may choose their own marketing campaigns.

- The two partners bear their own sales and marketing expenses.

- The two products may even command a different price level, usually attached to additional services (homecare, etc.), where allowed.

- The original authorization holder may not wish to have its brand diluted by signing a less-established or even generic partner.

- The authorization holder may hold the additional branded products as a bargaining chip with other manufacturers (exchange of licenses for portfolio building).

- The authorization holder may wish to approach a different segment with a different brand proposition.

- Finally, the two or more co-marketing partners may be competing for the same prescriber customers, unless specifically stated otherwise in their mutual agreement.

Distribution Agreement

When a biopharma finally succeeds in having its biopharmaceutical approved, it needs to set up sales, marketing, and distribution structures to support its launch. While supply chain management will be further discussed in Chapter 11, we will for the time being focus on the biopartnering agreements that are often behind such distribution arrangements.

While attracting, selecting, and hiring the sales and marketing teams, as well as other administrative functions are a large task, they do not require the significant resources required in order to set up a distribution network from scratch. For example, to start with, a biopharma would have to lease well-equipped, refrigerated, monitored, and secure distribution facilities, possibly additional local hubs, distribution robots, a fleet of small warehouse vehicles, a larger fleet of refrigerated trucks, experienced drivers and supervisors, mobile monitoring equipment, special packaging, dedicated IT infrastructure, and others. While these supply chain activities and tools are good to be internal, it often takes a large investment, significant risks, time-delaying permits, and other regulations that necessitate the outsourcing of distribution in several markets.

Distribution agreements describe the responsibilities of two sides in detail: define the market boundaries, distribution timelines, temperature monitoring and other responsibilities of the distribution partner, the method of reimbursement for their services, etc. Major issues to be commonly agreed are the following: authorized representatives, packing, premises and storage, product rejections, recalls, returns, quality assurance and validation, adverse reaction reporting, customer complaint handling, marketing literature distribution, queries, technical tests, jurisdiction in case of conflicts, and notices of agreement termination.

Co-Development and Co-Marketing Example: PharmaMar and Taiho Pharmaceutical

Madrid, March 30th, 2009. PharmaMar SA (Grupo Zeltia, ZEL.MC) and Taiho Pharmaceutical CO., LTD. today announced a license agreement covering the development and commercialization of PharmaMar's lead anti-tumor compound, Yondelis®, for the Japanese market. Yondelis® (trabectedin) is a novel anti-tumor agent of marine origin discovered in the tunicate Ecteinascidia turbinata. In September 2007, it received marketing authorization from the European Commission for the treatment of advanced or metastatic soft tissue sarcoma. In 2008, registration dossiers were submitted to the European Medicines Agency (EMEA) and Food and Drug Administration (FDA) for Yondelis® administered in combination with DOXIL®/Caelyx™ (pegylated liposomal doxorubicin) for the treatment of women with relapsed ovarian cancer. With this agreement, Taiho receives a license to develop and commercialize Yondelis® in Japan, and PharmaMar receives an initial payment of one billion yen (¥1,000,000,000), as well as future payments in addition to double-digit royalties on sales. All development and marketing costs of Yondelis® in Japan will be covered by Taiho.

Source: Courtesy of PharmaMar Press Release, Madrid, Spain, March 30, 2009, http://www.pharmamar.com

LOOKING FOR A PARTNER

During the second stage of the alliance life cycle, the partner of choice locates the resources it needs from other companies. According to Deck et al. (2006), Roche's disease-area strategy teams rely on "finders," well-trained individuals who have a deep knowledge of disease areas, high internal credibility, and who are closely connected with the company's research organization. These "finders" identify opportunities for new treatments—more than 1500 each year. A larger cross-functional team then analyzes each opportunity to see if it is scientifically and commercially viable and aligned with the company's overall strategy.

While partners of choice expend great effort to find the right companies, they also want to be "found" by others. How? By demonstrating

TABLE 5.11   Alliance Target Summary

Target	Reason for interest
Contacts	What can we offer
Decision makers	Competitive benefits
Corporate profile	Evaluation criteria
Alliance track record	Deal structure
Strategic directions	Timeline
Major events	Next steps

Source: Karlovac, N., Strategic Alliances & Positioning, in
9th Annual NIH SBIR/STTR Conference, Las
Vegas, NV, Larta Institute, 2007. With permission.

that they have the right kinds of expertise, treat their partners well, and are effective at getting results. Table 5.11 presents an alliance target summary.

Finding Potential Partners

Potential partners may be found among those who might have an interest, who have the franchise, who are attempting to break in, who have a need (e.g., patent expiry), who bring expertise/infrastructure, who have money, who are doing deals, who comes highly recommended. You need to search everywhere for ideas, for example, industry contacts, trade press and newsletters, company Web sites and SEC reports, and scientific papers and USPTO. You also have to respond vigorously to leads, for example, initial inquiries, direct proposals, referrals, contacts requests for information, etc.

For a partner looking example see: BIOVITRUM, Stockholm, Sweden, http://www.biovitrum.com, accessed on November 1, 2009.

ALLIANCE IMPLEMENTATION AND MANAGEMENT
Alliance Performance

Changing market conditions, intensified global competition, technological innovation, and increasingly shorter product life cycles mean that companies have to reexamine the traditional methods and strategies for expanding their businesses through M&A. M&A can be understood as a corporate strategy at an international as well as national level to better cope with new global conditions. In the push for rapid organizational growth, billions of dollars are spent each year on M&A but only with mixed results.

Bertoncelj (2008) has previously reported that studies of many scholars suggest that more than half of them fail to produce results; at best they are break-even situations. In the first 4–8 months that follow the deal, productivity may be reduced by up to 50% (Huang and Kleiner, 2004). In addition, Sirower (1997) has reported that a major McKinsey & Company study found that 61% of acquisition programs were failures because they did not earn a sufficient return (cost of capital) on the funds invested.

Alliance Implementation

In the past, many licenses involved mid- to late-stage products, as pharma companies were often more confident that these products would be approved within a short period. Due to the competitive nature of the industry, early-stage deals are formed more often. However, the downside of early-stage alliances is that the chances of product failure are increased. As large pharma companies are facing a shortage of new drugs internally, earlier development projects are required to supplement product pipelines. Another dilemma is that large pharma requires new products to fill a gap more quickly and early-stage deals do not solve this problem. The reality is more early-stage investments in biotech, lowering certainty.

Alternative sources for obtaining new molecules can be an option for big pharma companies, and very often biotech companies are only seen as one option to gain products. Apart from the licensing model, pharma companies are also buying over other companies. Pharma and biotech companies are facing challenging times sourcing and selecting the best partner. Multinational pharma companies no longer dominate the partnering scene. Leading biotech and biopharmaceutical companies are emerging and this places more pressure on the pharma companies when they are seeking to form alliances with smaller biotech companies. A key challenge is therefore that small companies with niche products may not integrate their business with the marketing network of a big pharma company and may work with a partner that has its own skill set and culture.

Alliance Management

Research has shown that approximately half of all alliances in most industries, as well as biotech alliances, fall short of expectations. This can be because of intellectual property disputes and royalty disagreements. Other issues include cultural problems. To a certain extent, biotech companies are more flexible because they do not have the same complexity that a large pharma company has within its organization. This can create cultural problems due to poor communication and lack of understanding in terms of what the real objectives are within both companies. Good alliance management can avoid the number of failures that occur (Mudhar, 2006).

For small and emerging biotech companies, the main issue is that they have no funds to support the business and because of the small, intricate nature of the company, they have a closer bond/link to in-house developments. Effective alliance management would then involve a good alliance, where funding is provided and the partner does not stifle innovation by controlling the relationship heavily (Figure 5.3, Tables 5.12 and 5.13).

For an alliance management example, see: AMGEN, Thousand Oaks, CA, http://www.amgen.com/partners/alliance_management.html

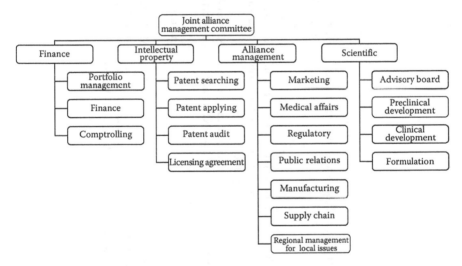

FIGURE 5.3   Typical alliance governance.

TABLE 5.12   How Do You Manage a Biopharmaceutical Alliance?

1	2	3
Organization	**Management**	**Culture**
Business processes	Resources	Trust
Communication	Governance	Attitudes
Infrastructure	Functions	Commitment
Performance management	Legal	Cultural compatibility
		Incentives

TABLE 5.13 There Are Four Aspects of an Alliance That Should Be Measured to Assess Its Productivity

	Input	Process	Output	Outcomes
Stage	Inputs are the resources devoted to the innovation effort	Process transforms the inputs	Outputs are the results of the innovation effort—they are lagging indicators (i.e., after the fact)	Outputs describe quantity, quality, and timeliness—outcomes describes value creation
Measurable elements	Tangible resources: capital, time, software	Creative process: the quality of ideas, conversion rate of ideas into projects	Technology leadership: patents, cites, seminars, licenses	Project profitability
	Intangible resources: talent, motivation, knowledge, brands	Project execution: time and costs of projects under way	New products: number of products, market share, sales	ROI
	External networked customers, suppliers		Business process: BPI metrics	Product value captured
	Innovation systems: recruiting, training, execution, value creation		Market leadership: customer acquisition, customer share	Share price

Source: Davila, T. et al., *Making Innovation Work: How to Manage It, Measure It, and Profit from It,* Prentice Hall, London, U.K., 2005. With permission.

QUESTIONS

1. Which are the main driving forces fueling biopartnering? Which are some of the risk indicators driving big pharma toward more biopartnering deals?
2. Which are the main advantages and disadvantages of biopartnering? Present either side in a debate.
3. A biopharmaceutical company's growth can come from either building, buying, or partnering. What are the main advantages and disadvantages of each approach?
4. What are the main issues driving a biopharmaceutical start-up toward either early partnering or co-development deals? Which were the original biopharma growth models at the dawn of healthcare biotechnology industry?
5. What are the motives behind biopharmaceutical M&A, and what are the similarities and differences between the two approaches?
6. Which are the most commonly used classifications of biopharmaceutical mergers or alliances?
7. What are the major reasons for seeking a biopharmaceutical alliance?
8. Which are the three major steps in the strategic alliance formation process?
9. What are the main characteristics of biopharmaceutical co-development, co-marketing, or co-promotion deals?
10. Which are the four aspects of a biopharmaceutical alliance that should be measured to assess its productivity?

EXERCISES

1. Using publicly available web resources describe five recent examples of pharma/biotech, biotech/biotech, or pharma/specialty biopartnering deals. Provide brief financial data associated with each transaction.
2. Figure 5.1 identifies various sources of synergies in partnering. Using the U.S. BIO member organizations' Web sites, describe examples of synergies as announced by themselves.
3. A biopharma board of directors is split among building, buying, or partnering strategies for future growth. Defend each one of these options in a debate.

4. There were three distinct phases in the historic evolution of biotechnology companies. Which were the reasons for choosing each of those options, and could mistakes have been avoided along the way?
5. By using publicly available web resources, identify three major biopharmas that due to a variety of negative conditions had considered the possibility of getting acquired. Describe how they each proceeded in their search, and whether the final outcome was easily achieved.
6. Biopharmaceutical alliances have had their proponents and critics over the years. Select one example of a successful or a failed alliance, and describe the trials and tribulations that led to either outcome.
7. What are the reasons for seeking a foreign market joint venture, and what issues need to be taken care of by the innovator company before embarking on such a deal? Provide actual examples.
8. There exist numerous financial agreements in biopartnering deals. Identify 10 different financial arrangements and describe a respective example.
9. Describe the strategies, methods, and tools utilized by major biopharmaceutical organizations in finding a biopartner. Provide actual descriptions and costs, where available.
10. Identify a recent major big pharma–biopharma biopartnering deal. Study the case in detail, and describe how the two organizations achieved the optimal alliance management, or less than ideal results.

REFERENCES

Advanced Cell Technology Press Release, Worcester, MA, December 30, 2008, http://www.advancedcell.com

AMGEN, Thousand Oaks, CA, http://www.amgen.com/partners/alliance_management.html

Bertoncelj, A., Value creation in mergers and acquisitions. University of Cambridge, Institute for Manufacturing, Cambridge, U.K., Symposium Proceedings, 2008, http://www.ifm.eng.cam.ac.uk/cim/symposium2008/08proceedings/16%20-%20Andrej%20Bertoncelj.pdf

Biotechnology Industry Organization. 2008a. Biotechnology industry facts. http://www.bio.org/speeches/pubs/er/BiotechGuide2008.pdf

Biotechnology Industry Organization. 2008b. 2007–2008 milestones. Washington, DC: BIO. Posted at: http://bio.org/speeches/pubs/milestone08/2007–2008_BIO_Milestones_WEB.pdf

BIOVITRUM, Stockholm, Sweden, http://www.biovitrum.com (accessed on November 1, 2009).

Burrill & Company, 2007. Biotech 2007: A global transformation. Purdue Discovery Lecture Series. West Lafayette, IN, November 8, 2007. PowerPoint presentation posted at: http://www.purdue.edu/dp/dls/biocrossroads/ppt/burrill.ppt

Burrill & Company, 2009. *Biotech 2009—Life Sciences: Navigating the Sea of Change*. San Francisco, CA: Burrill and Co.

Business Insights, 2008. *Biotech M&A Strategies: Deal Assessments, Trends and Future Prospects*. London, U.K.: Business Insights Ltd.

Davila, T., Shelton, R., and Epstein, M.J., 2005. *Making Innovation Work: How to Manage It, Measure It, and Profit from It*. London, U.K.: Prentice Hall.

Dealogic, 2008. Mergers & acquisitions, M&A Analytics, http://www.dealogic.com

Deck, M., Slowinski, G., and Sagal, M., 2006. Aligning the stars: Using alliance capability to build a constellation of partnerships that deliver, PRTM Article, 01 November 2006. Posted at: http://www.prtm.com/strategicviewpointarticle.aspx?id=1176&langtype=1033

Ernst & Young, 2009. Beyond borders: The global biotechnology report 2009. Boston, MA: E&Y.

Fovea Pharmaceuticals Press Release, Paris, France, October 1, 2009, http://www.fovea-pharma.com/news1.htm

GPC Biotech Press Release, Martinsried, Germany, February 18, 2009, http://www.agennix.com/index/php?option=com_content&view=article&id=70%3Agpc-biotech-and-agennix-announce-proposed-merger&catid=8%3Apress-releases&Itemid=56&lang=en

Huang, C.T. and Kleiner, B., 2004. New developments concerning managing mergers and acquisitions. *Management Research News*, 274(5): 54–62.

IBM Global Business Services—IBM Institute for Business Value, 2004. Learning the biopartnering game—How to achieve more from your biotech alliance. IBM Global Business Services, Somers, NY, 2004. Posted at: http://www.935.ibm.com/services/us/imc/pdf/ge510-3973-02.pdf

Jaiya, G.S., 2008. Integrating business and intellectual property strategy. PowerPoint presentation posted at: http://www.wipo.int/edocs/mdocs/sme/en/ wipo_kipo_kipa_ip_ge_08/wipo_kipo_kipa_ip_ge_08_www_109875.ppt, Geneva, Switzerland: WIPO.

Karlovac, N., 2007. Strategic alliances & positioning, in *9th Annual NIH SBIR/STTR Conference*, February 26–27, 2007 Las Vegas, NV, Larta Institute. Posted at: http://grants2.nih.gov/grants/funding/SBIRConf2007/SBIRConf2007_Karlovac.ppt

Maleck, K. and Pollano, F., 2003. Financial aspects of licensing BioGeneriX. Powerpoint presentation presented as PLCD-Meeting, Berlin, Germany, October 2003. Posted at www.biogenerix.com/publications/PLCDLicensing.pdf (accessed on October 2008).

Mudhar, P., 2006. Key challenges in pharma-biotech alliances and effective management. Frost & Sullivan, 8 May 2006. Posted on: http://www.frost.com

NEOTHERAPEUTICS Press Release, Irvine, CA, October 1, 2009, http://www.neot.com

NeuroSearch Press Release, Ballerup, Denmark, August 17, 2009, http://www.neurosearch.com

PharmaMar Press Release, Madrid, Spain, March 30, 2009, http://www.pharmamar.com

PTC Therapeutics Press Release, South Plainfield, NJ, September 2, 2009, http://ptct.client.shareholder.com/releases.cfm

Sirower, M.L., 1997. *The Synergy Trap: How Companies Lose the Acquisition Game.* New York: The Free Press.

van Beuzekom, B. and Arundel, A., 2009. *OECD Biotechnology Statistics 2009*, OECD, Paris, France, May 25, 2009, http://www.oecd.org/dataoecd/4/23/42833898.pdf

IV

New Product

## CHAPTER 6

Biodrug Research

R&D investment in new medicines by the biopharmaceutical industry was $65.2 billion in 2008, an increase of 3 percent from 2007.

Sources: Courtesy of Burrill & Company, San Francisco, CA and Pharmaceutical Research and Manufacturers of America (PhRMA), *Pharmaceutical Industry Profile 2009*. Washington, DC, March 10, 2009.

BEFORE A BIOPHARMACEUTICAL PRODUCT can be approved by the relevant regulatory authorities for commercial use, it needs to undergo various stages of preclinical (isolated cells, isolated tissues, or animal) and clinical (human volunteers or patients) studies (trials). These studies are conducted by biopharmaceutical companies upon the approval of the clinical trial center ethics committees and later by the health regulatory authorities. The aim of all these studies is to prove that the new biopharmaceutical is safe and effective in a variety of research models (cells, animals, humans) that is superior to comparator products (either fake drug—placebo—or older-generation medicine), or that it improves the quality of life (QoL) of terminally ill patients even if disease cure is not achieved. The preclinical and clinical trials are multiple; they are conducted on thousands of animals/humans, are performed in dozens of research/treatment facilities across the world, employ hundreds of healthcare professionals, and usually require 10 years to complete and hundreds of millions of U.S. dollars. This chapter focuses on the conduct of biopharmaceutical R&D.

GLOBAL BIOPHARMACEUTICAL R&D IN NUMBERS

The main regulatory agencies for the approval of biopharmaceuticals globally are the U.S. Food and Drug Administration (FDA), the European Medicines Evaluation Agency (EMEA), and the Japanese Ministry of Health, Labour and Welfare (MHLW), which will be presented further below. Their biopharmaceutical approval statistics belong to the public domain, and can supply the biopharma industry scholar with valuable insights into the industry's R&D performance. The FDA's tough regulatory standards for new drugs with emphasis on safety and progression-free survival (PFS) benefits had a negative effect on the biotech industry. For incurable cancer, a new drug must show a minimum response rate of 10% and a real prolongation of PFS. There was a decline in new cancer drugs approvals by FDA in 2008.

The FDA approved 21 new drugs in 2008, up from 18 in 2007. In 2008, the FDA approved six new biologics (NME) and new indications for two marketed brands: Arcalyst (rilanocept, Regeneron) bivalent fusion protein for the rare Periodic Syndrome, Cimzia (certolizumab, UCB) mAbs for Crohn's disease Cinryze (Viropharma) complement C1 inhibitor for hereditary angioderma, Nplate (romiplostim, Amgen) peptide for thrombocytopenia, Rocothrom (Bayer, Zymogenetics) rThrombin to control bleeding during surgery, Rotarix (GSK) vaccine for rotavirus gastroenteritis. Furthermore, contract research organizations (CROs; see below) provide insights into the recent trend of pharmaceutical biopharmaceutical companies outsourcing their R&D efforts in order to save time and money, as indicated in Table 6.1.

As far as the R&D investments of the U.S. Pharmaceutical Research and Manufacturers of America (PhRMA) members are concerned, Table 6.2 summarizes their biologics and biotechnology R&D investments during 2007.

TABLE 6.1   Global 2008 Public R&D Market ($)

Total R&D spend = 110 billion	Research = 36 billion/development = 74 billion
	Internal = 73 billion/outsourced = 21 billion

Source: Adapted from COVANCE, Corporate presentation at the *UBS Global Life Sciences Conference*, September 21, 2009, Princeton, NJ, PowerPoint presentation, Posted at: http://ir.covance.com/phoenix.zhtml?c=105891&p=irol-presentations.

TABLE 6.2   Biologics and Biotechnology R&D by PhRMA Member
Companies in 2007

Type	$ Million	% Share
Biotechnology-derived therapeutic proteins	10,075.7	21.0
Vaccines	1,159.9	2.4
Cell or gene therapy	95.3	0.2
All other biologics	796.5	1.7
Total biologics/biotechnology R&D	12,127.4	25.3
Non-biologics/biotechnology R&D	32,178.3	67.2
Uncategorized R&D	3,597.4	7.5
Total R&D	47,903.1	100

Source: European Commission—Commission of the European
Communities, Pharmaceutical sector inquiry final report,
EC, Brussels, SEC (2009) 952, July 8, 2009, Posted at: http://
ec.europa.eu/competition/sectors/pharmaceuticals/inquiry/
communication_en.pdf. With permission.

THE BIOPHARMACEUTICAL R&D PROCESS

Key Steps in the R&D Process of Biological Drugs

A biopharmaceutical's R&D stage is comprised of preclinical and clinical
phases. The first includes target identification, target validation, assay
development, primary screening, secondary screening, lead optimization,
and preclinical studies. The latter comprises of phases I, II, and III. Let's
start from the beginning.

Target Identification

Animal and human diseases have been associated with thousands of patho-
physiological targets, either extracellular or intracellular. For example,
extracellular receptors may be altered, cellular membrane ion-transfer
channels may be blocked, or intracellular genes may be mutated (altered
amino acid composition). Relevant findings are reported by the thousands
in the peer-review scientific literature yearly. Researchers may choose
one or several targets associated with any given disease indication (e.g.,
Parkinson's disease) and further investigate methods of interference with
the pathophysiology of the disease for preventing, alleviating, or curing it.

Target Validation

Having identified and selected a disease target, researchers need to
validate it, that is investigate how and to what degree it is responsible

for disease pathogenesis. For example, if receptors are expressed in mice liver, can a substance interfering with them cause liver disease? Or, if a gene is associated, do disease sufferers all carry it, or are healthy individuals free of it? There are various methods for validating a disease target, for example finding out what the target interacts with, where in the cell it is located, what is the gene coding for the target, what is the protein encoded by the given gene, and what happens if that gene is altered. In pre-genomic (gene unknown) validation methods, we distinguish phage display, yeast-two-hybrid system, expression cloning, and protein pathway studies. In post-genomic (gene known) methods we distinguish single microarray polymorphisms, DNA microarrays, and RNA knockdown.

Assay Development

When a specific disease target is identified and validated, researchers need to develop bioassays in order to test potential drug candidates. These bioassays need to be based on physiological material, which has either been previously extracted from an organism (in vitro or isolated) or is still within a living organism (in vivo). Examples of the first include the rabbit ear artery kept in a tank full of a physiological solution (the author's dissertation thesis model), and of the latter an anesthetized pig receiving drug infusions. A relatively modern assay method is the use of computer models that have been programmed to imitate the body's functions, thus the term in silico (for the computer chips made of silica). The use of these models can potentially save the lives of test animals; however, they cannot imitate the multifunctional tissue interactions of in vivo testing. Ideally, a drug development screen should be cost-effective, fast, accurate, easy to perform, quantitative, and amenable to automation.

Primary Screening

Let's hypothesize for a moment that a given drug bioassay is monitoring vasoconstriction in an isolated animal artery, in vitro. Having predefined that a comparator medicine's human therapeutic dose is causing a drop of pressure by X millimeters of a mercury column, any potential new blood pressure lowering medications can be measured against this level of activity. By testing a large number (thousands and even hundreds of thousands) of chemical/biochemical modifications of a drug candidate in this assay, researchers end up with a number of compounds surpassing that level, which are called "hits" and will be included in further testing.

Secondary Screening

As the complexity of bioassay models used for a drug's screening progresses, drug analogs are sought that will be able to lower blood pressure, while preserving heart, brain, or other organs' functions. Thus, a large collection of analogs may be used in search of those that best cover the required safety and efficacy characteristics of a new medicine, leading to a reduced number of candidates.

Lead Optimization

As the number of promising hits is constantly being reevaluated and reduced, a limited number of those with the most promising attributes is chosen to enter the next phase of studies, namely, preclinical testing in progressively larger animal models. The final candidates (leads) selected possess such molecular structures that give them the highest efficacy, specificity, and tolerability, with the lowest toxicity. These molecular candidates are said to exhibit the optimal structure–activity relationships (SARs) among a large group of molecules originally tested.

Preclinical Studies

When a set of leads has been identified, biopharmaceutical manufacturers need to follow a series of successively more complex animal models, as recommended by the regulatory agencies themselves. For example, a molecular lead will successively be tested in hamsters, rats, dogs, pigs, and monkeys, moving up the evolutionary ladder and as close to human physiology and pathology as possible. In addition, a series of tests will be performed assessing acute toxicity, other tests will assess sub-acute toxicity, and others will assess chronic toxicity, and so on. This process reduces the risk of chronic toxicity manifesting itself years after the initial application into a patient (e.g., gene mutations leading to teratogenicity or cancer). Having completed the series of preclinical tests successfully, the biopharma will finally choose one or two leading drug candidates for studies into humans. For clinical trials to begin, however, all preclinical results need to be collected, analyzed, summarized, and submitted to the regulatory authorities together with an investigational new drug application (IND; see below) that, if approved, will allow them to enter clinical phase I.

Phase I   In advanced animal models (primates) used in preclinical testing, researchers are able to define therapeutic dose, as well as toxic dose levels (the distance between the toxic and effective doses is called therapeutic index and is very important in clinical trial testing). Armed with such information and the IND approval, researchers now invite a small group of healthy human volunteers (approximately 20–80) who are willing to receive gradually increasing doses of the test medication, while various vital parameters are being monitored. The goal of phase I trials is to study drug safety, tolerability, pharmacokinetics, and pharmacodynamics.

Let's review some important definitions here. *Drug safety* is defined as freedom from unwanted drug side effects, i.e., a blood pressure lowering medication causing fainting. *Tolerability* is defined as the distance between the effective dose and the dose at which a human volunteer/ patient decides to discontinue the treatment due to intolerable side effects, e.g., at twice the therapeutic dose nose bleeding causing a trial subject to discontinue treatment. *Pharmacokinetics* is defined as the process by which a drug is absorbed, distributed, metabolized, and eliminated from the body, including the time parameters defining each sub-process. Finally, *pharmacodynamics* is defined as the biochemical and physiological effects of the drug and the mechanism of its action, including the correlation between its actions and its chemical structure. The usual incentives of human volunteers participating into phase I clinical trials are (1) an interest in medical research, (2) a desire to help fellow humans (altruism), (3) free medical assessment, and (4) small monetary rewards (ranging from few hundreds to few thousand U.S. dollars per person). Occasionally, disease patients may be admitted into phase I trials, for compassionate reasons, in case of incurable cancer, AIDS, or other chronic and severe diseases.

Phase II   Armed with phase I clinical trial results, clinical researchers now enroll a larger number of disease patients (40–300) with a dual goal. First, to continue the dose ranging studies in patients until the optimal dosage, route of administration and frequency of administration are determined. Second, to monitor the drug efficacy in the given indication. The efficacy of all test compounds is measured versus previously defined and approved by clinical experts' efficacy objectives, sometimes distinguished in primary, secondary, and tertiary. For example, rheumatoid arthritis medications would be evaluated versus disability indices (primary endpoint), CAT-scan improvements observed (secondary endpoint), or quality of patient life (tertiary endpoint). The efficacy of the drug candidate being tested versus the comparators is expressed in orders of magnitude and relevant statistical significance. Phase II studies are sometimes divided into Phase IIA and Phase IIB. Phase IIA is specifically designed to assess dosing requirements (how much drug should be given), whereas Phase IIB is specifically designed to study efficacy (how well the drug works at the prescribed dose(s)).

Phase III   Phase III clinical trials are the most complex, resource-, and time-consuming of all other preclinical or clinical studies for any given drug candidate. They include several hundred to several thousand patients, at various clinical trial locations, in multiple countries, over a period of years. Having previously defined the optimal dosage and preliminary efficacy, phase III studies focus on studying the drug candidate's efficacy in multiple patient subgroups (women, men, younger age adults, middle-aged, of various races, with concomitant diseases or not, with prior therapy or not—treatment naive—with good adherence or not).

Furthermore, one other aspect of efficacy monitoring is implemented here. The drug candidate is matched versus a fake drug (placebo—containing an inactive substance, usually sugar), or the most widely used disease treatment (reference treatment), and these results are compared for their order of magnitude in response differences, and the order of statistical significance for these differences. The statistical significance is increased as the number of patients with similar results increases. In order to further protect the objectivity of the study, all patients included into the phase III trial are randomized (randomly assigned into one of the three above treatment groups), while their treatment is controlled (versus placebo—or comparator-treatment) in a manner that remains confidential to patients (single-blinded) or patients and physicians alike (double-blinded).

Having completed all stages of the phase III trial, the biopharmaceutical manufacturer who sponsored the trial collects all patient data (in the form of case report forms—CRFs), has them analyzed by specialized statisticians, the results are then reviewed and signed off by a team of clinical experts, and, provided the trial has satisfactorily met all efficacy endpoints, the biopharmaceutical drug candidate is submitted for regulatory approval by the relevant authorities (see FDA, EMEA, and MHLW below). Having obtained the required data for regulatory submission, the study sponsor (biopharma) may continue the trial monitoring for additional data, throughout the regulatory approval evaluation period. During this late phase (sometimes called Phase IIIB), patients who have exhibited disease improvement may agree to remain on the experimental drug until it becomes commercially available, while the sponsor may also shift emphasis into studying further patient subgroups or patients with other indications, collecting data that may be used for the drug's approval into additional indications in the future.

Phase IV   After a biopharmaceutical is approved and commercially sold, large numbers of patients gain access to the new medication. During this phase, medical specialists (investigator-sponsored research) or the marketing authorization holder (biopharma-sponsored research) may opt to further monitor a large number of patients, without any express regulatory approval for doing so. This stage of post-approval clinical trials is called phase IV, or post-marketing. During phase IV, special emphasis is placed on studying the long-term efficacy and safety of the approved medication (e.g., after 10 continuous years on treatment). In addition, special patient populations, which have previously been excluded from phase I–III trials, may now be included, for example pregnant women, the elderly, pediatric, renal patients, and other groups. The benefits of these studies is first the extension of the approved indication to these patient subpopulations (patient benefit), as well as the award of an additional exclusivity period (manufacturer benefit) awarded by the regulatory agencies over and above the traditional 20 year period from patent application to companies who invest in trials for these special patient populations.

During phase IV, it is not uncommon for rare, long-term side effects of the approved medications to manifest themselves, which according to their severity necessitate either the imposition of use restrictions (by way of special warnings on their packaging and attached literature), or even the complete withdrawal of them from the market place, such as in the cases of cerivastatin (Baycol/Lipobay), troglitazone (Rezulin), and natalizumab (Tysabri). Phase IV studies' objectives are: compare to competitor drugs; disease subpopulations; identify new indications; identify new dosing

TABLE 6.3   How Do You Come Up with a Biopharmaceutical Clinical Trial Plan?

Study #	Title/ Objective	Phase	# of Centers	# of Patients	Timelines	Person Responsible
Corporate clinical trials						
Phase IV marketing studies						
Patient registries						
Switch programs						
Patient capture programs						
Patient retention programs						

schema; explore "real-world" effectiveness (e.g., in the office); define effects in special populations (elderly, children, renal); examine impact of concurrent diseases or concurrent drugs; post-marketing surveillance; and drug interactions.

Clinical Trial Planning and Monitoring

As previously described, biopharmaceutical clinical trials are resource- and time-consuming, since they often include thousands of patients, tens of clinical trial centers, hundreds of investigators, at several countries. Their planning and monitoring is the focus of specialized medical experts, clinical research specialists, monitors, statisticians, medical writers, and others. Tables 6.3 and 6.4 provide relevant templates for planning and monitoring such biopharmaceutical global clinical trials. Furthermore, Table 6.5 describes the main focus areas of the biopharmaceutical development process, while Table 6.6 summarizes the biopharmaceutical clinical development process.

Phase IV Study Example: Humira

The January 18, 2008, approval letter for this indication for the treatment of adult patients with moderate to severe chronic

TABLE 6.4   How Do You Monitor Ongoing Corporate Global Clinical Trials?

	Study #1	Study #2	Study #3	Study #4	Study #5
Study code					
Principal investigator					
City					
Hospital					
Country					
Trial center correspondence					
Trial center invoicing code					
Study title					
Study design					
Comparator drug					
Primary endpoints					
Secondary endpoints					
To be included in NDA					
Local drug organization					
Local drug organization Liaison					
Phase					
Max # of patients					
Therapy area					
Company medical Liaison					
Company CRA					
Clinical research organization					
CRO medical Liaison					
External CRA					
Statistician					
Medical writer					
Study progression					
Ethics committee					
First patient enrolled					
Number of patients enrolled					
CRFs collected					
CRFs analyzed					
Interim report					
Patient number completed					
CRF number completed					
All CRFs completed and collected					
Database locked					
Database analyzed					

TABLE 6.4 (continued)   How Do You Monitor Ongoing Corporate Global Clinical Trials?

	Study #1	Study #2	Study #3	Study #4	Study #5
Final report issued					
Major side effects present					
Investigator and support fees reimbursed					
Primary endpoints reached					
Secondary endpoints reached					
Go/no-go decision					
Peer-review articles allowed					
Peer-review articles submitted					
Additional comments					

plaque psoriasis who are candidates for systemic therapy or phototherapy, and when other systemic therapies are medically less appropriate, states: (FDA) determined that Humira poses a serious and significant public health concern relating to increased risk for serious infections. This concern required development of a Medication Guide under 21 C.F.R. 208 in order to prevent serious adverse effects, inform patients of information concerning risks that could affect their decisions to use or continue to use the drug, and/or assure effective use of the drug. To further assess the risks of HUMIRA in the psoriasis population, Abbott committed to conduct a post-marketing prospective, multi-center registry including 5000 adult psoriasis patients treated with HUMIRA in the United States. This commitment was reiterated in the January 18, 2008, approval letter for this new indication. The registry will characterize and assess the incidence of serious adverse events (including serious infections, tuberculosis, opportunistic infections, malignancies, hypersensitivity reactions, autoimmune reactions, and deaths) as well as other adverse events of interest in the study cohort.

Source: Courtesy of Food and Drug Administration Faxed Letter to ABBOTT LABORATORIES, December 16, 2008 RE: BLA# 125057 HUMIRA (adalimumab) Injection, Solution for Subcutaneous use, Silver Spring, MD, http://www.fda.gov

TABLE 6.5 What Are the Main Focus Areas of the Biopharmaceutical Development Process?

1 Discovery and Technology	2 Candidate Molecules	3 Manufacturing Process	4 Indications and Dosages	5 Validate Target Product Profile	6 Regulatory Dossier	7 Regulatory Submissions
Therapeutic area	Academic collaborations	Compare host systems	Valuation of indications	Set regulatory strategy	Understand regulatory requirements	Consult on target product profile
Disease	Intellectual property	Select most efficient host	Select priority indications	Define product positioning	Assemble regulatory file	Share available data
Targets	Lead identification efficiency	Prepare crude preparation	Create target product profile	Design clinical trials	Prepare pricing rationale	Respond to inquiries
In vitro models	Leads identified	Prepare presentation	Identify potential endpoints	Identify trial centers and investigators	Prepare reimbursement rationale	Prepare for manufacturing inspection
In vivo models	Candidates identified	Identify administration route	Run feasibility studies	Run clinical trials	Finalize file and submit	Gain approval for clinical investigations
Process technology	Preclinical development	Identify delivery systems	Select final endpoints	Confirm target endpoints		Provide additional data if necessary

Discovery technology	Preliminary safety in humans	Technology transfer to manufacturing	Select dose ranges	Create target product profile	Gain marketing authorization
Manufacturing technology		Remove impurities		Assemble and analyze data	Gain pricing within desired band
Internal advances		Increase yield		Evaluate findings and write reports	Gain efficient reimbursement
External advances		Increase specific activity		Approve documents for regulatory purposes	Launch
Acquire expertise		Scale up		Publish findings	
		Select packaging		Pharmacoeconomic studies	
		Full scale production		Prepare market entry	
		Internal sites			
		Outsourced manufacturing			

TABLE 6.6 The Clinical Trials Process

	Biopharmaceutical Clinical Development			
	Discovery		Preclinical Development	
Stage	Early Discovery	Lead Identification	Lead Optimization	Animal Studies
Duration (Years)	2	1	1	2
Test population	Lab (in vitro) studies	Lab (in vitro) studies	Lab (in vitro) studies, animal (in vivo) studies	Animal (in vivo) studies
Stage targets	Genes... drug targets... small molecules... drug leads	Genes... drug targets... cell assays... small molecules... drug leads	Genes... drug targets... cell assays... small molecules... drug leads	Leads for human testing
Type of research	Target identification, genomics... functional genomics... proteomics...	HTS, med chem, x-ray, Gx... funx gen... proteomics... Comb chem screening...	Med chem, kinetics, metabolism, toxicology; rodent test	Various animal models, scale up, formulation, batch manufacture
Technologies in use				Positional cloning, sequencing, mass spec, structural design, cellular assays, model organisms
Objectives	Target validation		Metabolism, toxicology	Biological activity; Safety route of administration
Costs				
Success rate %	30	60	50	50
Launch probability				1:10000
Compounds tested	Thousands	Thousands	100	20
Study design				

Clinical Trials

	Phase I	Phase II	Phase III	Regulatory Review	Phase IV
	1.5	2	3	1.5	Until end of life cycle
	20–200 healthy volunteers	200–500 patient volunteers	500–5000 patient volunteers		Thousands of real-life patients
	Top leads tested in humans	Top leads tested in humans	Top leads tested in humans	New drug	Line extensions, successors
	First-in-humans safety, tolerability, pharmacokinetics, pharmacodynamic, pharmacogenomic	Safety, dose ranging, clinical proof of principle, pharmacodynamic, pharmacogenomic	Safety, efficacy, pharmacodynamic, pharmacogenomic		Long-term safety
	Genotyping, phenotyping, SNP markers	Genotyping, phenotyping, SNP markers	Genotyping, phenotyping, SNP markers		
	Safety dosage	Efficacy toxicity	Efficacy long-term safety		
	70%	50%	60%	95%	
	1:20	1:2	3:4		
	5	3.5	1.7	1.1	1
	Open label	Open label, controlled	Randomized, controlled, double-blind, multicenter		

Investigational new drug (IND) application to regulatory authorities

NDA/Biologics license application (BLA)

Commercial launch

Source: Courtesy of U.S. Food and Drug Administration, Silver Spring, MD.

THE U.S. FOOD AND DRUG ADMINISTRATION

The U.S. Food and Drug Administration (FDA; http://www.fda.gov) dates back to 1906, when the passage of the Pure Food and Drugs Act, became into a law that prohibited interstate commerce in adulterated and misbranded food and drugs. More than a century since then, the mandate of FDA has changed repetitively. Its current range of regulatory responsibilities includes biological medicines, all other drugs, as well other substances detailed in Table 6.7.

Biological Medicines under FDA

Biological products, like other drugs, are used for the treatment, prevention, or cure of disease in humans. In contrast to chemically synthesized small molecular weight drugs, which have a well-defined structure and can be thoroughly characterized, biological products are generally derived from living material—human, animal, or microorganism—are complex in structure, and thus are usually not fully characterized.

Section 351 of the U.S. Public Health Service (PHS) Act defines a biological product as a "virus, therapeutic serum, toxin, antitoxin, vaccine, blood, blood component or derivative, allergenic product, or analogous product ... applicable to the prevention, treatment, or cure of a disease or condition of human beings." FDA regulations and policies have established that biological products include blood-derived products, vaccines, in vivo diagnostic allergenic products, immunoglobulin products, products containing cells or microorganisms, and most protein products. Biological products subject to the PHS Act also meet the definition of drugs under the Federal Food, Drug and Cosmetic Act (FDC Act). Note that hormones such as insulin, glucagon, and human growth hormone are regulated as drugs under the FDC Act, not biological products under the PHS Act.

TABLE 6.7   What Does FDA Regulate?

Biologics	Drugs	Other
Product and manufacturing establishment licensing	Product approvals	Cosmetics
	OTC and prescription drug labeling	Foods
Safety of the nation's blood supply		Medical devices
Research to establish product standards and develop improved testing methods	Drug manufacturing standards	Radiation-emitting Electronic products
		Veterinary products

Source: U.S. Code of Federal Regulations, Title 21, Volume 1, Revised as of April 1, 2008. U.S. Government Printing Office via GPO Access [CITE: 21CFR3.2], Title 21-FOOD AND DRUGS, Chapter I-FOOD AND DRUG ADMINISTRATION, DEPARTMENT OF HEALTH AND HUMAN SERVICES. PART 3 PRODUCT JURISDICTION. pp. 55–56, Posted at: http://edocket.access.gpo.gov/cfr_2008/aprqtr/21cfr3.2.htm

Applications for Biologics Licenses: Procedures for Filing

Within the U.S. Code of Federal Regulations, Title 21, Volume 7, as revised on April 1, 2008, we read:

> To obtain a biologics license under section 351 of the Public Health Service Act for any biological product, the manufacturer shall submit an application to the Director, Center for Biologics Evaluation and Research or the Director, Center for Drug Evaluation and Research, on forms prescribed for such purposes, and shall submit data derived from nonclinical laboratory and clinical studies which demonstrate that the manufactured product meets prescribed requirements of safety, purity, and potency; with respect to each nonclinical laboratory study, either a statement that the study was conducted in compliance with the requirements set forth in part 58 of this chapter, or, if the study was not conducted in compliance with such regulations, a brief statement of the reason for the non-compliance; statements regarding each clinical investigation involving human subjects contained in the application, that it either was conducted in compliance with the requirements for institutional review set forth in part 56 of this chapter; or was not subject to such requirements in accordance with 56.104 or 56.105, and was conducted in compliance with requirements for informed consent set forth in part 50 of this chapter. A full description of manufacturing methods; data establishing stability of the product through the dating period; sample(s) representative of the product for introduction or delivery for introduction into interstate commerce; summaries of results of tests performed on the lot(s) represented by the submitted sample(s); specimens of the labels, enclosures, and containers, and if applicable, any Medication Guide required under part 208 of this chapter proposed to be used for the product; and the address of each location involved in the manufacture of the biological product shall be listed in the biologics license application. The applicant

shall also include a financial certification or disclosure statement(s) or both for clinical investigators as required by part 54 of this chapter. An application for a biologics license shall not be considered as filed until all pertinent information and data have been received by the Food and Drug Administration. The applicant shall also include either a claim for categorical exclusion under 25.30 or 25.31 of this chapter or an environmental assessment under 25.40 of this chapter. The applicant, or the applicant's attorney, agent, or other authorized official shall sign the application.

When clinical testing and research on a drug has been completed, the manufacturer analyzes all the data and, if the data successfully demonstrate safety and efficacy, submits a biologics license application (BLA) or a new drug application (NDA) to the FDA. The application is a compilation of the research completed during the three phases, and it includes full details of the product's formula, production, labeling, and intended use.

Investigational New Drug Application

Current federal law requires that a drug be the subject of an approved marketing application before it is transported or distributed across state lines. Because a sponsor will probably want to ship the investigational drug to clinical investigators in many states, it must seek an exemption from that legal requirement. The IND is the means by which the sponsor technically obtains this exemption from the FDA. The FDA's IND process is depicted in Figure 6.1.

The main components of an IND application are (1) introductory statement; (2) general investigational plan; (3) plans: study protocol(s); (4) plans: investigators, facilities, and institutional review board; (5) data: chemistry, manufacturing, and quality control; (6) data: pharmacology and toxicology; (7) data: previous human experience; and (8) data: investigator brochure. Recent FDA approvals of biologic products are listed in Table 6.8.

Requirements for Biologics License Application

Biological products are approved for marketing under the provisions of the Public Health Service (PHS) Act. The Act requires a firm who manufactures a biologic for sale in interstate commerce to hold a license for the product. A biologics license application is a submission that contains specific information on the manufacturing processes, chemistry, pharmacology, clinical

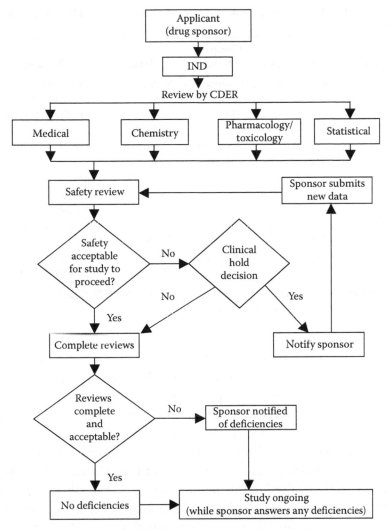

FIGURE 6.1 The IND process with the FDA. (Courtesy of U.S. Food and Drug Administration, Silver Spring, MD.)

pharmacology, and the medical affects of the biologic product. If the information provided meets FDA requirements, the application is approved, and a license is issued allowing the firm to market the product (see Figure 6.2).

42 U.S.C. §262 requires: The biological product that is subject of the application is safe, pure, and potent; the facility in which the biological product is manufactured, processed, packed, or held meets standards designed to assure that the biological product continues to be safe, pure, and potent; applicant consents to the inspection of the facility that is the

TABLE 6.8   U.S. FDA Biologic Product Approvals during 2008 and First Semester of 2009

Brand Name	Generic Name	Company Name	Date	Indication
Simponi	Golimumab	Centocor Ortho Biotech	April 24, 2009	Rheumatoid arthritis, psoriatic arthritis, and ankylosing spondylitis
Dysport	Abobotulinum toxin A	Ipsen biopharm	April 29, 2009	Cervical dystonia (spasmodic torticollis)
Ilaris	Canakinumab	Novartis	June 17, 2009	
Nplate	Romiplostim	Amgen	August 22, 2008	Immune thrombocytopenic purpura
Cimzia	Certolizumab Pegol	UCB	April 22, 2008	Crohn's disease
Arcalyst	Rilonacept	Regeneron	February 27, 2008	Cryopyrin-associated periodic syndromes

Source: Courtesy of U.S. Food and Drug Administration, Silver Spring, MD, http://www. accessdata.fda.gov/scripts/cder/drugsatfda

subject of the application. The BLA must also contain: a full description of manufacturing methods; data establishing stability of the product through the dating period; sample(s) representative of the product for introduction or delivery for introduction into interstate commerce; summaries of results of tests performed on the lot(s) represented by the submitted sample(s); specimens of the labels, enclosures, and containers; any medication guide proposed in the use of the product; and the address of each location involved in the manufacturing of the biological product. In general, for a BLA approval a biopharmaceutical manufacturer must demonstrate: no microbial or viral contamination; no endotoxin, exotoxins, pyrogens; and no nucleic acids (which were thought capable of delivering oncogenes and transforming the DNA of a potential patient). Once BLA approved, then clinical trial phases begin.

FDA Approvals in 2009

According to the Medical Marketing and Media (2009), the FDA approved 17 new molecular entities and 7 biologics license applications in 2009. That's a substantial improvement in large molecule approvals—the agency granted just three BLAs last year—and a slight downturn in new chemical compounds, from last year's 21 NMEs.

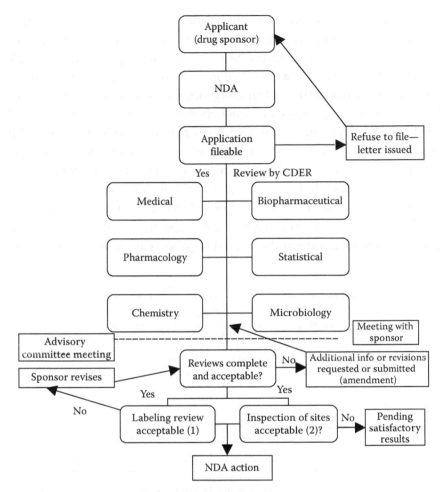

FIGURE 6.2 The NDA process with the FDA. (1) Labeling in this context means official instructions for use. (2) Manufacturing sites and sites where significant clinical trials are performed. (Courtesy of U.S. Food and Drug Administration, Silver Spring, MD.)

THE EUROPEAN MEDICINES EVALUATION AGENCY (EMEA)

In the European Union (EU), a company that wishes to bring a medicine to the market may submit a single application to the European Medicines Agency for a "marketing authorization" (license) that is valid simultaneously in all EU Member States, plus Iceland, Liechtenstein, and Norway. This is called the "centralized (or 'Community') authorization procedure," and is mandatory for certain types of medicines and optional for others (European Commission—Commission of the European Communities, 2009, pp. 118–119).

European Commission (EC) Regulation No 726/2004231 (hereafter "Regulation") lays down a centralized Community procedure for authorization of medicinal products based on a single application, a single evaluation, and a single authorization (see Figure 6.3). Pursuant to the regulation, the use of the centralized procedure is compulsory in particular for biotechnology medicinal products, orphan medicinal products, and medicinal products containing an entirely new active substance for which the therapeutic indication is the treatment of specific diseases. On the other hand, the use of the centralized procedure is optional for other medicinal products not appearing in the Annex of the Regulation and containing a new active substance not yet authorized in the Community, medicinal products which constitute a significant therapeutic, scientific, or technical innovation or which are in the interest of patients at the community level.

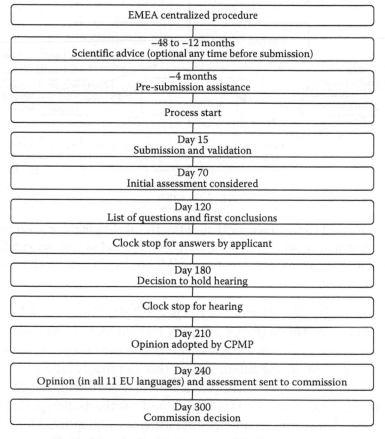

| EMEA centralized procedure |
| −48 to −12 months
Scientific advice (optional any time before submission) |
| −4 months
Pre-submission assistance |
| Process start |
| Day 15
Submission and validation |
| Day 70
Initial assessment considered |
| Day 120
List of questions and first conclusions |
| Clock stop for answers by applicant |
| Day 180
Decision to hold hearing |
| Clock stop for hearing |
| Day 210
Opinion adopted by CPMP |
| Day 240
Opinion (in all 11 EU languages) and assessment sent to commission |
| Day 300
Commission decision |

FIGURE 6.3 Overview of the EMEA centralized procedure. (Courtesy of European Medicines Evaluation Agency, London, U.K.)

Generic applications of centrally authorized medicinal products may be authorized via the centralized procedure or alternatively via the national, mutual, or decentralized procedure under certain conditions.

Procedure

According to EMEA, (European Commission—Commission of the European Communities, (2009), pp. 118–119):

Applications for Community authorisation must be submitted to the EMEA. Each application must be made in accordance with a specific format called the EU common technical document (CTD). Information that must be included in any application comprises in particular: the name and the qualitative and quantitative particulars of all the constituents of the medicinal product, the manufacturing method, therapeutic indications, contra-indications and side-effects, posology, pharmaceutical form, method and route of administration, expected shelf life, reasons for precautionary and safety measures during storage and administration of the medicinal product and disposal of waste, the risk to the environment, the results of pharmaceutical, pre-clinical tests and clinical trials, a summary of the product characteristics and a mock-up of the packaging together with a package leaflet.

Within the EMEA, the Committee for Medicinal Products for Human Use (CHMP) is responsible for drawing up the opinion of the EMEA on whether or not MA can be granted. In order to prepare its opinion, the CHMP will examine whether the product concerned meets the necessary quality, safety, and efficacy requirements. The members of the CHMP are national experts appointed by the competent national authorities. Based on the qualifications of those experts and their expression of interest in relation to a specific file, the CHMP will appoint a rapporteur and if appropriate a co-rapporteur. The scientific evaluation of the application will therefore in practice be carried out by those national experts who will prepare an assessment report with the administrative support of the EMEA. If the opinion is unfavorable, the possibility exists for the applicant to request the EMEA to re-examine the application before a final opinion is issued. All final opinions of the CHMP (positive or negative) are published on the EMEA Web site. The opinion will then be sent to the European Commission, which takes the final decision after consulting the Member States. The decision can deviate from the opinion of the CHMP, but in this case the Commission must state in detail the reasons for the deviation. A decision granting MA contains the summary of the product characteristics along with the labelling and package leaflet.

Timetable

The standard timetable for the scientific evaluation of a centralized application allows 210 days for the adoption of the CHMP opinion starting from the date of receipt of a valid application. This time limit can be suspended if the applicant is required by the CHMP to provide supplementary information. Within 15 days after receipt of the opinion, the Commission shall prepare a draft of the decision. The final decision will be taken within 15 days after the end of the consultation with the Member States. As all Commission decisions, such decisions may be challenged pursuant the rules of the Treaty.

Products Eligible for the Centralized Procedure

Community authorization via the Centralized Procedure is compulsory for products appearing in the annex to Regulation 726/2004. These include the following:

1. *Medicinal products developed via one of the following biotechnology processes*: (1) recombinant DNA technology, (2) controlled expression of gene coding for biologically active proteins in prokaryotes and eukaryotes, including transformed mammalian cells, and (3) hybridoma and monoclonal antibody methods.

2. *Advanced therapy medicinal products*: (1) gene therapy medicinal products, (2) somatic cell therapy medicinal products, (3) tissue-engineered products, and (4) combination (with medical device) advanced medicinal products.

3. *Medicinal products for human use containing a new active substance which, on the date of entry into force of this regulation, was not authorized in the Community, for which the therapeutic indication is the treatment of any of the following diseases*: (1) acquired immune deficiency syndrome, (2) cancer, (3) neurodegenerative disorder, and (4) diabetes. After May 20, 2008 any appropriate proposal to amend this list may be presented.

4. *Medicinal products designed as orphan medicinal products* pursuant to Regulation (EC) 141/2000.4.

Community authorization via the Centralized Procedure is optional for certain product types detailed in Article 3 of Regulation 726/2004: (a) Medicinal products containing new active substances not authorized in the Community at the date of entry into force of this regulation, and (b) Medicinal products for which a significant therapeutic, scientific, or technical innovation can be demonstrated in the interest of patients' health similar biological ("biosimilar") medicinal products that are developed by means of biotechnological processes must be authorized via the Centralized Procedure. Centralized Procedure is mandatory for (1) biotech products, (2) orphan drugs, (3) anticancer, diabetes drugs, HIV, neurodegenerative treatments (e.g., Alzheimer, TSE).

EMEA Marketing Authorization Application Example: Arzerra (GSK And Genmab)

Copenhagen, Denmark; February 5, 2009—"GlaxoSmithKline (GSK) and Genmab A/S (OMX: GEN) announced today the submission of a Marketing Authorisation Application (MAA) to the European Medicines Agency (EMEA) for Arzerra™ (ofatumumab) for the treatment of chronic lymphocytic leukaemia (CLL). If approved, ofatumumab would be indicated for the treatment of patients with CLL who have previously failed, or are inappropriate for, standard therapies. Ofatumumab targets a distinct binding site on the CD20 molecule of B-cells and it could become the first monoclonal antibody targeted to CD20 available for these patients. GSK and Genmab announced the submission of a Biologics License Application (BLA) to the US Food and Drug Administration (FDA) on Friday 30 January 2009.

CLL is the most common form of leukaemia in the Western world and patients have a high need for new therapy options. Currently fewer than 25 percent of patients with refractory CLL respond to current treatments resulting in much poorer clinical outcomes. "Ofatumumab is a new generation of monoclonal antibody that may provide an important new treatment for patients suffering from CLL and we plan additional studies to understand its potential in lymphomas and selected autoimmune diseases," said Carlo Russo, Senior Vice President BioPharm, GSK. "The filing of ofatumumab for refractory CLL represents the strong ongoing partnership between the GSK BioPharm and Oncology Units to developing therapies based upon novel biopharmaceutical platforms."

Source: Courtesy of Genmab Press Release, Copenhagen, Denmark, February 5, 2009, http://www.genmab.com. Copyright Genmab A/S. Used with permission.

THE JAPANESE MINISTRY OF HEALTH, LABOUR AND WELFARE

The Ministry of Health, Labour and Welfare (MHLW) (Koseirodosho in Japanese) was established by a merger of the Ministry of Health and Welfare (MHW) and the Ministry of Labour, on January 6, 2001 as part of the government program for reorganizing government ministries. The MHLW is in charge of pharmaceutical regulatory affairs in Japan, and the Pharmaceutical and Food Safety Bureau (PFSB) undertakes main duties and functions of the Ministry: it handles clinical studies, approval reviews and post-marketing safety measures, i.e., approvals and licensing. The Health Policy Bureau handles promotion of R&D, and production and distribution policies, i.e., functions related to pharmaceutical companies. The Pharmaceuticals and Medical Devices Evaluation Center (Evaluation Center) in the National Institute of Health Sciences was established to strengthen approval reviews on July 1, 1997.

As explained by the Japanese Pharmaceutical Manufacturers Association (JPMA; http://www.jpma.or.jp/english/), formal approvals and licenses are required in order to market drugs in Japan, and formal approval and/or licenses must first be obtained from the Minister of the MHLW or prefectural governor. Drug marketing approval refers to governmental permission for a drug with the quality, efficacy, and safety, or a drug that is manufactured by a method in compliance with manufacturing control and quality control standards based on an appropriate quality and safety management system to be marketed, generally distributed, and used for healthcare in Japan. Whether or not a substance under application is appropriate for human healthcare is objectively determined in light of state-of-the-art medical and pharmaceutical technology. Specifically, the Minister or prefectural governor reviews the name, ingredients, composition, dosage and administration, indications, and ADRs, of the product in an application submitted by a person with a marketing business license. A GMP compliance review is performed to assure that the plant manufacturing the product complies with the manufacturing control and quality control standards. Marketing approval is granted to products meeting these standards. This approval system is the essential basis for ensuring good quality, efficacy, and safety of drugs and related products, which is the principal objective of the Pharmaceutical Affairs Law.

Source: Japan Pharmaceutical Manufacturers Association (JPMA)— English Regulatory Information Task Force, 2009. Pharmaceutical administration and regulations in Japan, March, Posted at: http://www.jpma. or.jp/english/parj/1003.html. With permission.

Approval Review Process

Application forms for approval to market drugs are usually submitted to the PMDA. When application forms for new drugs are received by the PMDA (KIKO), a compliance review of the application data (certification from source data), GCP on-site inspection, and detailed review are undertaken by review teams of the PMDA and the team prepares a review report. The approval review process consists of expert meetings of review team members and experts to discuss important problems (see Figure 6.4). A general review conference attended by team members, experts, and representatives of the applicant is held after the expert meeting. The evaluation process followed by the PMDA is as follows: (1) interview (presentation, inquiries, and replies), (2) team review, (3) inquiries and replies, (4) review report (1), (5) expert meeting (includes at least three clinical specialists as experts), (6) general review conference (main agenda items and names of participating experts made available 2 weeks prior to meeting; presentation), (7) follow-up expert meeting, (8) review report (2), and (9) report to the evaluation and licensing division, PFSB.

For a Japanese Ministry of Health, Labour and Welfare approval example see: NEXAVAR ONYX Pharmaceuticals, Emeryville, CA, Press Release, May 20, 2009, http://www.onyxpharm.com

ACCELERATED PRODUCT AVAILABILITY

PTO Special Status

According to the U.S. PTO Manual of Patent Examining Procedures (MPEP, 2008; http://www.uspto.gov/web/offices/pac/mpep/index.htm) 708.02 Petition to Make Special [R-6]:

> In recent years revolutionary genetic research has been conducted involving recombinant deoxyribonucleic acid ('recombinant DNA'). Recombinant DNA research appears to have extraordinary potential benefit for mankind. It has been suggested, for example, that research in this field might lead to ways of controlling or treating

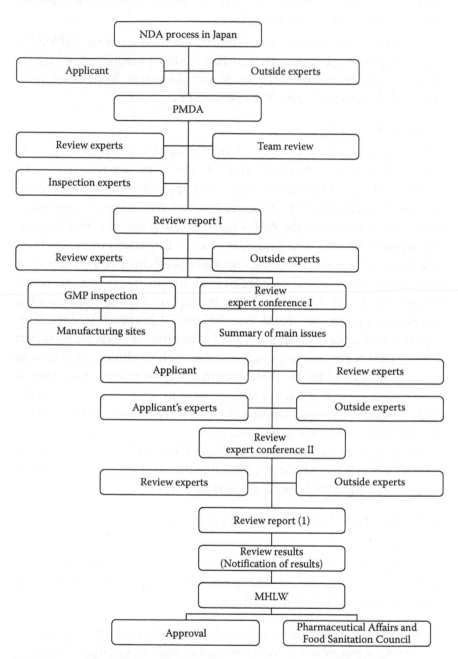

FIGURE 6.4 The NDA review process in Japan. (Courtesy of Japanese PMDA, Tokyo, Japan.)

cancer and hereditary defects. The technology also has possible applications in agriculture and industry. It has been likened in importance to the discovery of nuclear fission and fusion. At the same time, concern has been expressed over the safety of this type of research. The National Institutes of Health (NIH) has released guidelines for the conduct of research concerning recombinant DNA. These 'Guidelines for Research Involving Recombination DNA Molecules,' were published in the Federal Register of July 7, 1976, 41 FR 27902-27943. NIH is sponsoring experimental work to identify possible hazards and safety practices and procedures.

In view of the exceptional importance of recombinant DNA and the desirability of prompt disclosure of developments in the field, the U.S. Patent and Trademark Office will accord 'special' status to patent applications relating to safety of research in the field of recombinant DNA. Upon appropriate petition and payment of the fee under 37 CFR 1.17(h), the Office will make special patent applications for inventions relating to safety of research in the field of recombinant DNA. Petitions for special status should be accompanied by statements under 37 CFR 1.102 by the applicant, assignee, or statements by an attorney/agent registered to practice before the Office explaining the relationship of the invention to safety of research in the field of recombinant DNA research. The fee set forth under 37 CFR 1.17(h) must also be paid.

To qualify for a special status, the company must be a small entity (a company with fewer than 50 employees) or a nonprofit organization. The petition must state that the patent applicant's technology will be significantly impaired if a patent examination is delayed. As far as the FDA is concerned, there are essentially five ways in which companies may accelerate the introduction to market of a new drug.

FDA Well-Characterized Status

A biopharmaceutical manufacturer may petition the U.S. FDA for an immediate start of its clinical trials program, provided it can prove that its product has a "well-characterized status." Such a status indicates that the biopharmaceutical under investigation can be dependably manufactured resulting in an identical compound with given three-dimensional structure, purity, potency, and quality. For example, the manufacturer may prove that its biosynthetic growth hormone is of a well-characterized status that is identical in every shape and form to the other, already approved, commercially available growth hormones. If the FDA approves the well-characterized status, the biomanufacturer may initiate the clinical trials program, and simultaneously try to improve the manufacturing process and yield for its product.

FDA Expanded Access Exception

The FDA's expanded access exception allows a biomanufacturer to make its biopharmaceutical commercially available to patients before the product's clinical trial program is completed. This is usually done in order to allow seriously ill patients to get access to the promising drug while no other treatment alternatives are available. Once again, the biomanufacturer must apply to the FDA for the expanded access exception, providing adequate clinical data that the biopharmaceutical will be effective and safe in a certain life-threatening disease, such as terminal cancer or AIDS. These FDA regulations were put in place originally in 1987, and were recently updated in August 2009, to describe when a drug manufacturer can charge a patient for an investigational drug, in a clinical trial or expanded access program, and what costs a manufacturer can recover when charging.

FDA Accelerated Approval Process

Table 6.9 summarizes the main mechanisms for accelerated commercial availability of a biopharmaceutical accepted by the FDA, which we review further below.

According to the FDA "speeding the development and availability of drugs that treat serious diseases are in everyone's interest, especially when the drugs are the first available treatment or have advantages over existing treatments. The Food and Drug Administration (FDA) has developed three distinct and successful approaches to making such drugs available as rapidly as possible: Priority Review, Accelerated Approval, and Fast Track." (http://www.fda.gov/ForConsumers/ByAudience/ForPatientAdvocates/SpeedingAccesstoImportantNewTherapies/default.htm).

Prior to approval, each drug marketed in the United States must go through a detailed FDA review process. In 1992, under the Prescription Drug User Act (PDUFA), FDA agreed to specific goals for improving the drug review time and created a two-tiered system of review times— Standard Review and Priority Review. Standard Review is applied to a drug that offers at most, only minor improvement over existing marketed therapies. The 2002 amendments to PDUFA set a goal that a Standard Review of a NDA be accomplished within a 10 month time frame. A Priority Review

TABLE 6.9   Which Are the Main Mechanisms for Accelerated Commercial Availability of a Biopharmaceutical Accepted by the FDA?

	Accelerated Review	Priority Review	Fast Track
Statute	1992	1996	1997
Procedure	Manufacturer request	Manufacturer makes application and FDA clinical team leader recommends	Manufacturer request, approved by FDA on set criteria
Criteria	Serious or life-threatening disease, unmet medical need addressed, adequate studies supporting use of surrogate outcome, product use under restrictive prescribing	Major treatment advance No adequate therapy exists	Serious or life-threatening disease unmet medical need addressed
Benefits	Adjusted trial outcome requirements	Additional attention, expedited review	Closer interaction with FDA, possibility to submit parts of BLA as they become available (rolling review)
Requirements	Post-approval studies to extend surrogate results to clinical outcome		

designation is given to drugs that offer major advances in treatment, or provide a treatment where no adequate therapy exists. A Priority Review means that the time it takes FDA to review a NDA is reduced. The goal for completing a Priority Review is 6 months.

When studying a new drug, it can take a long time—sometimes many years—to learn whether a drug actually provides real improvement for patients such as living longer or feeling better. This real improvement is known as a "clinical outcome." Mindful of the fact that obtaining data on clinical outcomes can take a long time, in 1992 FDA instituted the Accelerated Approval regulation, allowing earlier approval of drugs to treat serious diseases, and fill an unmet medical need based on a surrogate endpoint. A surrogate endpoint is a marker—a laboratory measurement, or physical sign—that is used in clinical trials as an indirect or substitute measurement that represents a clinically meaningful outcome, such as survival or symptom improvement. The use of a surrogate endpoint can considerably shorten the time required prior to receiving FDA approval.

Approval of a drug based on such endpoints is given on the condition that post-marketing clinical trials verify the anticipated clinical benefit.

Fast track is a process designed to facilitate the development, and expedite the review of drugs to treat serious diseases and fill an unmet medical need. The purpose is to get important new drugs to the patient earlier. Fast Track addresses a broad range of serious diseases. Determining whether a disease is serious is a matter of judgment, but generally is based on whether the drug will have an impact on such factors as survival, day-to-day functioning, or the likelihood that the disease, if left untreated, will progress from a less severe condition to a more serious one. AIDS, Alzheimer's, heart failure, and cancer are obvious examples of serious diseases. However, diseases such as epilepsy, depression, and diabetes are also considered to be serious diseases. Filling an unmet medical need is defined as providing a therapy where none exists or providing a therapy that may be potentially superior to existing therapy. A drug development program (i.e., a drug plus one specific indication) can be designated as fast track anytime after submission of an IND; although sponsors potentially receive more benefits the earlier in development the designation is made. Table 6.10 lists selected FDA fast track approvals of biopharmaceuticals to date.

Fast-Track Designation Example: PEGylated Interferon Beta-1a (Biogen Idec)
Cambridge, MA, July 08, 2009 (Business Wire)—Biogen Idec (NASDAQ: BIIB) today announced the U.S. Food and Drug Administration (FDA) has granted PEGylated interferon beta-1a (BIIB017) Fast Track designation for relapsing multiple sclerosis (RMS). Biogen Idec is currently enrolling patients in a global Phase III study evaluating the efficacy and safety of either bi-weekly or once-monthly injections of PEGylated interferon beta-1a in this patient population. The FDA's Fast Track program is designed to expedite the review of new drugs that are intended to treat serious or life-threatening conditions and demonstrate the potential to address unmet medical needs. Biogen Idec plans to enrol more than 1200 patients in the Phase III, randomized, double-blind, placebo-controlled trial designed to evaluate the efficacy and safety of PEGylated interferon beta-1a in patients with RMS. The global trial, called ADVANCE, will determine the efficacy of PEGylated interferon beta-1a in reducing relapse rates in patients with RMS at one year. The study will also examine if, over time, treatment with PEGylated interferon beta-1a can slow disease progression and lead

TABLE 6.10   Selected FDA Fast Track Approvals

Proprietary Name	Applicant	Approval Date	Use
Tykerb (lapatinib ditosylate)	GlaxoSmithKline	March 13, 2007	Treatment-refractory (including Herceptin) advanced or metastatic ErbB2-overexpressing breast cancer
Cyanokit (hydroxocobalamin)	EMD	December 15, 2006	For the treatment of known or suspected cyanide poisoning
Remicade (infliximab)	Centocor	October 13, 2006	Maintenance of clinical remission and mucosal healing in the treatment of patients with moderately to severely active ulcerative colitis (UC), who have had an inadequate response to conventional therapy
Zolinza (vorinostat)	Merck	October 6, 2006	Treatment of cutaneous T-cell lymphoma
Vectibix (panitumumab)	Amgen	September 27, 2006	Treatment of metastatic carcinoma of the colon or rectum in patients who have failed standard, irinotecan- and/or oxaliplatin-containing chemotherapy regimens.
Elaprase (idursulfase)	Transkaryotic	July 24, 2006	Enzyme replacement therapy for patients with Hunter syndrome (Mucopolysaccharidosis II, MPS II)

Source: Courtesy of U.S. Food and Drug Administration, Silver Spring, MD.

to a decrease in the number of T2 hyper-intense brain lesions commonly seen in MS patients.

Source: Courtesy of Biogen Idec Press Release, Cambridge, MA, July 8, 2009, http://investor.biogenidec.com

CONTRACT RESEARCH ORGANIZATIONS

Reasons for Outsourcing

During the last 25 years, the cost of bringing a new biopharmaceutical product to the marketplace rose almost ninefold, now estimated to surpass the $1 billion mark. The reasons for escalating R&D costs will be analyzed

TABLE 6.11   Which Are the Main Reasons for Outsourcing to CROs?

1 Sponsor can convert the fixed costs of maintaining the personnel, expertise, and facilities like data management necessary for clinical trial management into variable costs

2 Nonavailability of services in-house

3 Knowledge of regulatory affairs in a particular country of interest

4 Increased complexity of clinical trials

5 Necessity for medical and clinical knowledge in specific therapeutic areas or indications

6 Increased amount of data required from clinical trials

7 Multinational and multicenter nature of current clinical trials

8 Large requirement of patient populations

9 Regionalized diseases

later in this chapter. In brief, rising costs are associated with increasing regulatory hurdles, larger patient populations, more complex medical testing required, more complex pathologies tackled, longer times, and others. Rising costs have decreased the biopharma industry's R&D productivity, eventually leading to questionable profitability. In an effort to cut costs and reduce the clinical development time, biopharmas have embarked on a process of outsourcing clinical research, through collaboration with dedicated external partners called contract research organizations (CROs).

The use of CROs allows biopharmas to control both fixed (facilities, laboratories, devices) and variable costs (reagents, bioassays, animals, patients). Furthermore, while patent protection is paramount to a biopharmaceutical's commercial profitability and return of development investments, each day of delayed R&D time may cost the biomanufacturer millions of U.S. dollars of lost commercial profits. For all these reasons (summarized in Table 6.11), the penetration of CRO services has been gradually rising over the years.

CRO Services

A contract research organization is an external partner providing critical R&D services to the biopharmaceutical industry. FDA defines a CRO (Code of Federal Regulations 21–312.3) as "Contract research organization means a person that assumes, as an independent contractor with the sponsor, one or more of the obligations of a sponsor, e.g., design of a protocol, selection or monitoring of investigations, evaluation of reports, and preparation of materials to be submitted to the Food and Drug Administration." EMEA defines a CRO as "A person or an organization (commercial, academic, or other) contracted by the sponsor to perform one or more of a sponsor's trial-related duties and functions" (see European Medicines Agency, 2002, p. 7, http://www.ema.europa.eu/docs/en_GB/document_library/Scientific_guideline/2009/09/WC500002874.pdf). According to CenterWatch, an organization providing global news, directories, proprietary market research, and analysis for clinical trials professionals and patients (http://www.centerwatch.com/), the CRO market size is estimated at $23.7 billion and growing (Zisson and Gambrill, 2010).

CROs offer a variety of services to the biopharmaceutical industry, spanning the entire R&D spectrum, from basic research all the way to product's regulatory approval and beyond. CROs range from large, full-service, global organizations to small, niche operators who specialize in isolated steps of the R&D value chain. A prominent example of the first is KENDLE, as presented in one of their press releases below.

CRO Example: Kendle

Cincinnati, OH, February 25, 2009 /PRNewswire-FirstCall via COMTEX News Network/—Kendle (Nasdaq: KNDL), a leading, global full-service clinical research organization, today reported net service revenues for the quarter ended Dec. 31, 2008, of $109.2 million, an increase of 5 percent over the same period in 2007. Excluding the impact of foreign exchange rates, revenues for the quarter increased 18 percent compared to the same period in 2007. Net service revenues for the full year were $475.1 million, an increase of 19 percent over net service revenues of $397.6 million for full year 2007. Foreign exchange rates had a negligible impact on revenue for the full year. Kendle International Inc. (Nasdaq: KNDL) is a leading global clinical research organization providing the full range of early- to late-stage clinical development services for the world's biopharmaceutical industry. Our focus is on innovative solutions that reduce cycle times for our customers and accelerate the delivery of life-enhancing drugs to market for the benefit of patients worldwide. As one of the fastest-growing global providers of Phase I–IV services, we offer experience spanning more than 100 countries, along with industry-leading patient access and retention capabilities and broad therapeutic expertise, to meet our customers' clinical development challenges.

Source: Courtesy of KENDLE Press Release, February 25, 2009, http://www.kendle.com

TABLE 6.12 How Do Biopharmaceutical Companies Select a Contract Research Organization?

1	Expertise	Environmental sustainability, molecule, regulatory validation and approval, technology base, therapeutic area, central laboratory	5	Project team	Project team (research, manufacturing, QA, regulatory, legal), clear responsibilities, responsiveness, top management
2	Deliverables	Deadlines, milestones, quality, standard operating procedures	6	Risk	Data privacy, environmental, facilities, financial, intellectual property, personnel, product, regulatory, supplier
3	Data management	Dedicated personnel, clinical trial power, data management, biostatistics, proprietary software	7	Price	Per trial phase, per trial center, per investigator, per patient, payment terms
4	Track record	Customer satisfaction, laboratory to clinical to market completions, new chemical entities, no. of customers, no. of molecules, primary investigators, clinical trial centers, no. of countries, regulatory agencies	8	Customer service	Administrative, invoicing, flexibility pre-contract and post-contract inspections, motivation, reporting, technical links (remote monitoring), willingness to change

Selection of CROs

The process by which a biopharmaceutical organization selects its CRO partner is critical for the project's success and even the biopharma's viability in the long term. Table 6.12 summarizes some of the criteria that can be used in securing the services of an ideal CRO partner. As far as the size and spectrum of services offered by the CRO are concerned, going with the largest partner may not always be in the best interest for a young biopharmaceutical start-up. Special attention needs to be allocated to the project teams on either side of the collaboration, as experience, responsibilities, responsiveness, and dedication of both teams are of crucial importance for the biopharmaceutical development.

R&D PRODUCTIVITY IN NUMBERS

We have previously mentioned that any given biopharmaceutical product needs to undergo multiple successive tests of basic research, preclinical and clinical testing before it receives marketing authorization. This long

TABLE 6.13   The Innovation Gap Is Getting Wider

Year	R&D Spending ($ Bn)	New Drug Approvals (NMEs)	Year	R&D Spending ($ Bn)	New Drug Approvals (NMEs)
1992	11.5	26	2000	26	27
1993	12.7	25	2001	29.8	24
1994	13.4	22	2002	32.1	17
1995	15.2	28	2003	33.2	21
1996	16.9	53	2004	38.8	31
1997	19	39	2005	39.4	17
1998	21	30	2006	43	18
1999	22.7	35			

Source: Pharmaceutical Research and Manufacturers of America, *Pharmaceutical Industry Profile 2009*, Annual Membership Survey, PhRMA, Washington, DC, 2009. With permission.

and arduous process may require more than 10 years and $1 billion to complete, making it seriously risky and expensive. Furthermore, it has been observed that, despite regulatory attempts to make the process more transparent and expedited, or industry attempts to make the process last shorter and cost less, the biopharmaceutical R&D productivity has been gradually reduced over the last 10 years. As indicated in Table 6.13, despite the total biotechnology R&D budget of the members of the U.S. Pharmaceutical Research and Manufacturers of America (PhRMA) rising from $11.5 billions in 1992 to $43 billion in 2006, the new molecular entity (NME) approvals dropped from 26 in 1992 to only 18 in 2006, respectively.

Biopharmaceutical companies, faced with decreased R&D productivity, are looking into new ways of shortening the times and reducing the investments required for preclinical and clinical development. Their urgency is driven by two supplemental forces, namely, an urgency to protect the remaining commercial selling time under patent protection, and also the influence of demanding investors who wish to see more pipeline compounds reaching commercial profitability, and more compounds recuperating the R&D costs it took to bring them into the marketplace at the beginning. There are various estimates of the times required to complete each clinical trial phase successfully. According to the Tufts Center for the Study of Drug Development (CSDD), the average times required to complete phase I, phase II, phase III, and the regulatory approval phase range from 16 to 33 months each, bringing the total clinical R&D time required close to 98 months (eight and one half years; see Table 6.14).

TABLE 6.14   Clinical Development and Approval Times

Times in Months	Biopharmaceutical	Pharmaceutical
Phase I	19.5	12.3
Phase II	29.3	26.0
Phase III	32.9	33.8
Regulatory approval	16.0	18.2
Total R&D	97.7	90.3

Source: Courtesy of DiMasi, J.A. and Grabowski, H.G., *Manage. Decis. Econ.*, 28, 469, 2007.

TABLE 6.15   Increasing Complexity of Clinical Trials

	1999	2005	% Change
Unique procedures per trial protocol (median)	24	35	46%
Total procedures per trial protocol (median)	96	158	65%
Clinical trial staff work burden (measured in work-effort units)	21	35	67%
Length of clinical trial (days)	460	780	70%
Clinical trial participant enrollment rate	75%	59%	−21%
Clinical trial participant retention rate	69%	48%	−30%

Source: Courtesy of Tufts Center for the Study of Drug Development, Growing protocol design complexity stresses investigators, volunteers. Impact report 10(1), 2008, January/February, Boston, MA.

The reasons behind the decrease in biopharmaceutical R&D productivity are multiple. As indicated by the Tufts CSDD in Table 6.15, some of the reasons responsible are the increasing number of required testing procedures per trial protocol, or the participants' enrollment time (increasing) or retention (decreasing) times.

According to recent industry statistics, the transition probabilities for clinical phases between biopharmaceutical and pharmaceutical drug candidates are not identical, with increased probabilities seen with biopharmaceutical inventions, as seen in Table 6.16.

TABLE 6.16   Transition Probabilities for Clinical Phases

	Biopharmaceutical (%)	Pharmaceutical (%)
Phase I–II	83.7	71
Phase II–III	56.3	44.2
Phase III—approval	64.2	68.5
Phase I—approval	30.2	21.5

Source: Courtesy of DiMasi, J.A. and Grabowski, H.G., *Managerial Dec. Econ.*, 28, 469, 2007.

TABLE 6.17   Which Are the Main Reasons for Molecule Attrition from Research to a Biopharmaceutical Product?

In vitro assay not mimic disease accurately	Disease biology incomplete
In vivo models not mimic disease accurately	Proteins, neutralizing antibodies
Acute models versus chronic human diseases	Human protein rejection in animals research
Animal–human species differences	Formulations untenable
Human population more heterogeneous	ADME problems
Toxicology only found in humans	Drug interactions
Pharmacokinetics, animal versus humans differences	Inadequate disease activity in humans
Low target affinity needs excessive dose in humans	Cannot be manufactured in commercial quantities

Source: Evens, D.P., 2005. Biotechnology and Industry research and practice: Part 1— The exploding science, the expanding products, the usage challenges and opportunities. University of Florida, College of Pharmacy Course PHA 5172. Powerpoint presentation posted at: http://www.cop.ufl.edu/safezone/pat/pha5172/evens-powerpoint-0.5.htm. With permission.

It therefore becomes apparent that reasons for molecule attrition (compounds being progressively rejected throughout the R&D phase) during the biopharmaceutical industry's R&D efforts are not only multiple and critical, but that they should all be individually challenged and improved on the way to a productivity increase so critical for the industry. The main reasons for such an attrition are listed in Table 6.17.

Efforts to increase the biopharmaceutical R&D productivity have focused, among other parameters, to the industry-specific success factors, the most important of which are focused around people, processes, pipeline, profits, organization, and performance, as summarized in Table 6.18.

As an indication of the massive effort involved in biopharmaceutical R&D, we need only to quote Genentech, according to which "the research department at Genentech houses approximately 1100 researchers, scientists and post-docs and covers a wide range of groundbreaking scientific activity—from molecular biology and protein chemistry to bioinformatics and small molecule drug discovery" (http://www.gene.com/gene/research/).

For various examples of approaches to lower biopharmaceutical drug development costs and time see: National Institute of Standards and Technology (NIST), Planning Report 07-1, Economic Analysis of the Technology Infrastructure Needs of the U.S. Biopharmaceutical Industry, Prepared by: RTI International for National Institute of

TABLE 6.18   What Are the Most Important Biopharmaceutical R&D Success Factors?

People	Process	Pipeline
Build expertise	Use life cycle management	Pursue multiple indications
Recruit and retain talent	Use portfolio management	Maximize product options
Define roles and responsibilities	Share knowledge and info	Use novel technologies
Have and support Investigators	Operate globally	Use enabling technologies
	Work in product teams	Create full pipeline at all research stages
	Kill compounds early	
Profits	**Biopharm organization**	**Perform**
Meet unmet medical needs	Recognize R&D excellence	Maintain accountability
Develop best in class	R&D, true integration	Perform consistent
Focus resources	Common objectives X organ	Use efficient data capture and analysis and reporting
Support optimal product pricing and reimbursement	Freedom to operate (patents)	Use innovative technology
	Reward speed and quality	Have internal champions
	Create research alliances	

Source: Evens, D. P., 2005. Biotechnology and Industry research and Practice: Part 1—The Exploding science, the expanding products, the usage challenges and opportunities. University of Florida, College of Pharmacy Course PHA 5172. Powerpoint presentation posted at: http://www.cop.ufl.edu/safezone/pdt/pha5172/evens-powerpoint-0.5.htm. With permission.

Standards & Technology, November 2007, available at: http://www.nist.gov/director/planning/upload/report07-1.pdf.

BUSINESS APPROACHES TO IMPROVING R&D PRODUCTIVITY

We have previously mentioned the intense pressures on biopharmaceutical R&D to perform faster and better. A large variety of methods have been previously proposed, and most of them have been tested already, with varying degrees of success. All the efforts proposed focus around four major techniques of improving R&D productivity; (1) increasing the future sales potential of the drug candidates, in other words, choosing drug projects more carefully; (2) decreasing the time required, in other words, doing things faster, or turning successive processes into parallel, or decreasing decision time delays; (3) increasing the probability of success, in other words, attracting better minds to research more promising candidates, using better assays or tests; (4) reducing the costs required, in other words reducing the number and duration of tests, going for higher product efficacy that gives higher statistical significance, which in turn, reduces the number of subjects and tests required. In the following sections, we focus on some of the ideas already proposed and/or implemented by biopharmas.

In-Licensing

In the previous chapter, we have presented the role of in-licensing in biopharmaceutical development. Several biopharmas, faced with expiring pipelines, reduced in-house R&D productivity, increased failures, and ongoing risks of development, have turned to in-licensing for quickly securing new product candidates in support of their internal research efforts. While in-licensing offers new product candidates with reduced cost and faster than internal efforts, it requires significant business development resources, it may reduce the resources available for other internal projects, and is not devoid of future risks.

As reported by Hall (2004), its significance for the biopharmaceutical industry is constantly rising, and it is estimated that in 2003, licensed products accounted for more than $70 billion in revenue for the top 20 global pharmaceutical companies. According to research by Wood Mackenzie, licensed products will account for $100 billion by 2008 and will represent a third of the industry's total projected revenue. Furthermore, according to a 2009 European Commission Pharmaceutical Sector Inquiry Report, 25% of molecules in clinical development during 2007 were previously acquired or in-licensed (see Table 6.19).

TABLE 6.19   Percentages of Molecules Acquired or In-Licensed by Originator Companies during Preclinical Research, Clinical Development, or Pending Marketing Authorization (2007)

Phase	% of Company's Own Molecules	% of Molecules Acquired or In-Licensed
Preclinical research	88	12
Clinical development	75	25
MA pending	65	35

Source: European Commission—Commission of the European Communities, Pharmaceutical sector inquiry final report. EC, Brussels, SEC(2009) 952, July 8, 2009, Posted at: http://ec.europa.eu/competition/sectors/pharmaceuticals/inquiry/communication_en.pdf. With permission.

Merger and Acquisition

Biopharmaceutical M&A activity with the aim of improving R&D productivity is one of the most common methods used by biopharmaceutical companies. As mentioned in the previous chapter, various synergies, economies of scale, enhanced credibility, access to new products and markets, knowledge transfer, vertical integration and diversification, or replacement of products under expiring patents have been some of the major reasons driving the M&A trend. However, biopharmaceutical M&A is not always easy to accomplish successfully. For example, internal resistance to change, completely opposite corporate cultures, lost brain capital due to restructuring, new operational models that have not been tried before, or problems in reducing the number of research sites often turn the M&A irrelevant to an R&D productivity increase.

Strategic Alliances and Partnerships

Strategic alliance is an alternative to a product in-licensing or company M&A mentioned above. Under an R&D strategic alliance agreement, the two parties agree to share intellectual property, know-how, bioassays, tools, reagents, laboratories, facilities, and scientists in order to pursue a common R&D goal. Although a partnership needs to be constantly monitored and ideally managed in order to bear fruits, the biopharmaceutical industry has been steadily relying on an increasing number of alliances aimed at increasing R&D productivity.

New Organizational Structure and Decision-Making Process

In any given biopharmaceutical company, especially the most established and commercially successful, it is often unavoidable to implement several organizational levels and numerous cross-functional responsibilities. For example, the R&D function needs to effectively and efficiently control the company's pipeline, while, at the same time liaising or even competing for resources with other in-house functions, such as manufacturing, sales and marketing, or logistics. As far as the R&D department per se is concerned, the traditional functional unit is a project team, staffed with various skills (e.g., molecular biologists, biochemists, pharmacologists, physicians, pharmaceutical technologists, and others) and aiming at achieving certain milestones within any given period of time.

Alternative organizational structures and decision-making models have been proposed for biopharmaceutical R&D. First, organizing independent

R&D teams capable of bringing a molecule from start to finish (vertical structures). Second, organizing teams responsible for any given process step, e.g., basic research for all in-house candidate molecules. Third, organizing R&D across therapeutic areas, e.g., neurology. Fourth, organizing R&D across indication areas, e.g., Parkinson's versus Alzheimer's disease. Fifth, setting up centers of excellence, for example, independent facilities working on a specific technology (e.g., DNA chips) or a bioassay (e.g., autoimmune models in primates). Sixth, R&D teams coming up with approved indications (top-down development), or seventh, commercial teams directing research toward profitable segments (bottom-up). It is imperative that individual biopharmas have to carefully select their mode of R&D organization, according to their internal characteristics and resources.

Strategic Alternative #1: Focus on Therapeutic Areas
By focusing on select therapeutic areas, a biopharma may achieve the following: (1) thorough understanding of the disease mechanisms involved, (2) more resources targeted on the same indication, (3) more molecules being researched and approved on the indication, (4) better scientific specialization, (5) molecules approved for treating various stages of any given disease (complete therapeutic portfolio), or (6) better regulatory and opinion leader contacts and insights. For example, Amgen has assembled a multidisciplinary group of chemists and biologists who together approach the challenge of drug discovery using multiple potential therapeutic modalities. This novel approach allows them to choose the best target for attacking a disease and to use the modality most likely to affect that target. The research program has grown spectacularly, yielding a heightened understanding of human disease, and innovative new approaches to improving human health (http://www.amgen.com/science/overview.html).

Strategic Alternative #2: Focus on Targets (Treatment Platforms)
Instead of focusing on specific disease indications, biopharmas may focus on certain molecular targets, often implicated for various disease pathologies. Therefore, by gaining thorough expertise on these targets, a biopharma may even discover therapies for multiple indications, all associated with the same underlying mechanism. The advantage of super specialization is increased awareness, expertise, and focus, while the disadvantages include the selection of a molecular target that does not yield a therapeutic product candidate easily (often called a non-druggable target). Other disadvantages include going after various

indications simultaneously, or switching among target mechanisms necessitating a complete renewal of all skills needed in-house.

Strategic Alternative #3: Spin-Off Research
A biopharmaceutical company with a product candidate just entering preclinical development is faced with successive preclinical and clinical trial phases, each involving different sets of skills, assays, tools, and finances. It is obvious that, in order to reach regulatory approval and commercial availability, the company must master all involved tasks of R&D, and also find the significant resources to finance them. What if the biopharma, still in preclinical target discovery and validation, assigned the whole stage to an external, knowledgeable partner, such as a CRO, with a remit to reduce a potentially large number of thousands of drug hits down to 20 drug leads? If this outsourced step was successful, could the biopharma outsource the whole preclinical phase? OK, you guessed it. How about spinning off research completely? This idea is just beginning to appear in biopharmaceutical R&D. The so-called virtual biopharmas (see Chapter 13) manage a network of external partners from afar. The future will tell.

For a research spin-off example see: EISAI & QUINTILES, Quintiles, Quintiles Press Release, Research Triangle Park, NC, October 30, 2009, http://www.quintiles.com

R&D Reorganization Examples

During the past few years, AstraZeneca aligned its discovery research along therapeutic units of 600-800 people each. GlaxoSmithKline divided the company's discovery component from lead molecule selection to Phase I trials into Centers of Excellence for Drug Discovery (CEDDs). Each CEDD is therapeutically aligned or devoted to a technology platform, with 240-400 people per therapeutically defined CEDD and 60-150 people per technology defined CEDD.

J&J split pharma activities into three business units: biologics group focused on haematology, oncology and immunology; virology group focused on HIV and HCV; and CNS IM, which focuses on CNS, infection and metabolic diseases and cardiology. Roche created research units focused on specific disease biology areas (DBAs). Each DBA has 300-500 people.

TECHNOLOGY APPROACHES TO IMPROVING R&D PRODUCTIVITY

In addition to the business approaches to improving R&D productivity, a huge effort is underway to increase the productivity through the use of new, cutting-edge technologies. Most of these new technologies did not even exist 10 years ago, while today a growing number of biopharmas is trying to gain the know-how, install, and apply them in their R&D departments. Let's review some of these approaches.

Platform Technology Contributions

The use of a platform technology allows a biopharmaceutical researcher to automate a certain step of R&D so that a large number of alternatives can be tested reliably, effectively, and efficiently, saving time and money, and thus improving ultimate productivity. There is a wide variety of biotechnology platform technologies in use today. For example, the polymerase chain reaction, micro-RNA chips, DNA chips, combinatorial drug discovery, biomarkers, or monoclonal antibodies are some of the most widely used technologies today.

Biomarkers are biological properties that can be measured in tissue samples. These can vary in their nature, for example, they can be specific molecules, cells, genes, hormones, enzymes, and others. Their function can be predictive, diagnostic, or prognostic. They serve a hugely positive role in biopharmaceutical research, since they can be used as "surrogate endpoints" in preclinical and clinical research. In other words, when a chronic and severe disease is being studied, instead of expecting actual clinical symptoms to appear in the test subjects after years of disease progression, a biomarker (e.g., an enzyme alteration) may be easily measured and serve as a predictive endpoint (risk indicator) for this disease.

Monoclonal antibodies are also another significant platform technology. Let's hypothesize that a certain disease is associated with a given receptor. The receptor is subsequently isolated, sequenced, and cloned. By the use of a monoclonal antibody platform technology, specific antibody molecules can be constructed to bind and attack the receptor. Having this platform (vehicle) of specifically attacking the receptor, a multitude of drug candidates can be constructed to attach onto the antibody and thus be transported to attack and destroy the target.

Cooperative Platform Technology Development

As described above, a platform technology can significantly increase the productivity and efficiency of biopharmaceutical drug development. Nevertheless, the creation of any such platform may prove resource- and time-consuming, and also risky on its own. Biopharmas faced with such a possibility, have one of three options: (1) develop it in-house, (2) outsource it, or (3) develop it in collaboration with other interested biopharmas, by way of an R&D consortium. The latter process saves the participating company's time and money, reduces risk, and also allows them to specifically target R&D challenges by designing a custom-built platform technology around them.

Form Biopharma Consortium

If two biopharmaceutical enterprises can combine their forces in commonly developing a platform technology, then they can also form much closer relationships, aimed at commonly solving their overall R&D challenges. For example, biopharmas may form a consortium in the form of a joint venture (see Chapter 5) that is aimed at taking a certain family of products all the way through the R&D continuum to regulatory approval. Alternatively, the joint venture may be created to specifically develop a new bioassay, a new animal model of research, a new manufacturing process, a new research tool, a new biomarker, etc.

Share Open Source Innovation

The advent of the World Wide Web of interconnected computers gave a significant boost to humanity's collective intellectual capacity. This was achieved by interconnectivity, the free and fast exchange of ideas, better communication, and a degree of newly found virtual "camaraderie." Enlightened thinkers then took this exchange of ideas one step further. What if globally dispersed virtual thinkers worked collectively on a given project, each adding his or her knowledge, experience, ideas, and suggestions to the common project? The movement was first called *open-source*, whereas all contributors had access to the creation of a project, all had the power to comment upon and improve on the others' suggestions, while the final product was available to all free of charge. *Web 2.0* was starting to form.

The first products of open-source innovation were collective software-engineering efforts (Linux), as well as collective knowledge repositories, called wikis. Open source later entered even the world of healthcare biotechnology. If global, virtual, anonymous users were able to form a collective encyclopedia, what if global, virtual, anonymous researchers combined their intellectual capacity to solve biotechnology-related R&D challenges. This can either be achieved on a free basis, or even posting a research challenge on a Web site and offering a monetary reward for the solver. Examples of such efforts can be seen in Innocentive (http://www. innocentive.com).

STRATEGIES FOR CONSERVING THE MONEY

As previously described, the biopharmaceutical R&D process is both time- and resource-consuming. Starting from basic research and progressing a biopharmaceutical drug candidate all the way to regulatory approval may require in excess of 12 years. In addition, according to the Tufts Center for the Study of Drug Development the average cost to develop a new prescription drug stood at $802 million (DiMasi, 2001). These figures include costs related to drug target discovery, preclinical studies, and also include drug development failures. It goes without saying that the biopharmaceutical industry is keen on conserving the money of R&D, bringing new biopharmaceuticals to the marketplace shorter, and with less money consumed during the process.

R&D Cost Estimates

The cost of a study depends on many factors, especially the number of sites that are conducting the study, the number of patients required, and whether the study treatment is already approved for medical use. Clinical trials follow a standardized process. Table 6.20 indicates the major factors driving R&D costs at each stage of the process.

TABLE 6.20   What Are the Factors Driving R&D Costs at Each Stage of the Process?

	Research					Development				
	Basic Research	Target ID	Target Validation	Screening	Optimization	Preclinical Development	Phase I	Phase II	Phase III	Registration
Unit cost x										
Stage duration x										
# Candidates x										
# Patients x										
Stage total										

TABLE 6.21 Distribution of Costs in Clinical and Preclinical Phases at Global Level (2007)

Costs	In % of Total R&D
Preclinical (including basic research)	8
Phase I	12
Phase II	20
Phase III	60

Source: European Commission—Commission of the European Communities, Pharmaceutical sector inquiry final report. EC, Brussels, SEC(2009) 952, July 8, 2009, Posted at: http:// ec.europa.eu/competition/sectors/pharmaceuticals/inquiry/ communication_en.pdf. With permission.

TABLE 6.22 What Are the Estimated Costs of Pharmaceutical Clinical Trials per Phase?

	Phase I	Phase II	Phase III	FDA Approval
Likelihood of eventual FDA approval	20%	30%	67%	81%
Average years to completion	0.5–1	1.5	3.5	0.5–2
Supporting animal studies	$500,000	$1 million	$1.5 million	N/A
Average number of clinical trial subjects	50	200	300	N/A
Average per subject cost	$12,000	$12,000	$6,000	N/A
Approval costs	N/A	N/A	N/A	$1.3 million

Source: Stewart, J.J., Biotechnology valuations for the 21st century. MILKEN Institute Policy Brief 27, Santa Monica, CA, 2002. With permission.

Taking things one step further, The European Commission 2007 Pharmaceutical Sector Inquiry (Table 6.21) and the MILKEN Institute (Table 6.22) have previously published the distribution of costs in preclinical and clinical phases and the estimated costs per clinical trial phase, respectively.

Do Biopharma Costs Differ?

The Tufts Center for the Study of Drug Development (CSDD) has even compared biopharmaceutical versus pharmaceutical R&D costs. Using compound-specific costs for a sample of 17 investigational biopharmaceuticals from 4 firms, a time series of annual preclinical and clinical expenditures for a biotech firm, estimated average development times and phase transition probabilities for over 500 therapeutic recombinant proteins and mAbs, they estimated average preclinical period, clinical period, and total costs per approved new biopharmaceutical (DiMasi and Grabowski, 2007). They found out-of-pocket (cash outlay) cost estimates of $198 million, $361 million, and

TABLE 6.23   How Do Capitalized Costs per Approved Biotech
Product Compare with Those of Time-Adjusted Pharmaceutical
Products (in 2005 $ Million)?

	Nonclinical Costs	Clinical Costs	Total Costs
Biotech	615	626	1241
Pharma	439	879	1318

Source: DiMasi, J.A. and Grabowski, H.G., *Manage. Decis. Econ.*,
        28, 469, 2007.

$559 million per approved new biopharmaceutical for the preclinical period, the clinical period, and in total, respectively (in year 2005 dollars). These figures include the costs of compound failures. Adding time costs to cash outlays, they found cost estimates of $615 million, $626 million, and $1241 million per approved new biopharmaceutical for the preclinical period, the clinical period, and in total, respectively (in year 2005 dollars).

If past growth rates in R&D costs for traditional pharmaceutical firms are applied to the results in DiMasi et al. (2007), then total capitalized biopharmaceutical cost per approved new molecule appears to be essentially the same as estimated total capitalized per approved new drug for traditional pharmaceutical firms (see Table 6.23).

Cost-Mitigating Strategies

Two strategic options exist for improving biopharmaceutical R&D productivity: (1) Reduce the costs/risks/timescales of the current system through buying or collaborating with biotech companies, or outsourcing to/collaborating with Asia, (2) Reengineer the system: upgrading regulatory science to level of discovery science requires global consensus from industry, legislators, and regulators. One of the major innovations of the last two decades for R&D business process is the emergence of outsourcing to complement the traditional vertical integration model of the pharmaceutical companies. The outsourcing partners help the pharmaceutical companies to mitigate risk, reduce cost, and more importantly, focus on investing and developing unique in-house expertise that will sustain their competitive advantages.

QUESTIONS

1. What are the key steps in the R&D process of biological drugs?
2. What does the U.S. FDA regulate? Provide one example per category.
3. What is the investigational IND process with the FDA?

4. What is the NDA process with the FDA?

5. What is the centralized NDA process with the European EMEA?

6. What is the NDA process with the Japanese MHLW?

7. Which are the main mechanisms for accelerated commercial availability of a biopharmaceutical accepted by the FDA?

8. Which are the main reasons for outsourcing biopharmaceutical R&D to contract research organizations (CROs)?

9. Which are the main reasons for molecule attrition from research to a biopharmaceutical product?

10. Which are the main business and technology approaches to improving R&D productivity?

EXERCISES

1. Visit the web pages of the FDA and the EMEA. Then name all the biopharmaceuticals that were approved by the two agencies over the last two full years.

2. The biopharmaceutical R&D process is comprised of several distinct steps. By visiting biopharma web pages, name one biopharmaceutical in development at each of the different steps. Use different company examples per step.

3. You are the chief scientific officer (CSO) of a biopharma presenting to the Board of Directors the company's clinical trial results. What tools and parameters are you going to use, and how are you addressing your department's shortfalls?

4. Both FDA and EMEA are not known for easy to navigate web pages. By surfing through their maze of pages, collect information on all of your company's competitors presently active in the field of rheumatoid arthritis.

5. The FDA NDA process may stumble upon several obstacles (see relevant figure). By accessing publicly available web resources, provide actual examples of how biopharmaceutical companies are addressing such blocks.

6. Provide five examples of biopharmaceuticals approved by either of the mechanisms available for accelerated commercial availability with the FDA.

7. You are the CSO of a top 10 biopharma. Present to the Board of Directors why you are recommending the outsourcing of a certain R&D project, and why you are proposing one of the top-10 CROs. Which criteria have you based your two proposals on?

8. The clinical development and approval times, as well as the costs involved for new biopharmaceuticals remain a contested issue between proponents and critics of the biopharmaceutical industry. By choosing two opposing views, attempt to objectively identify realistic estimates for the times and costs involved.

9. Which R&D parameters may be responsible for potential differences in approval times and costs involved for pharmaceuticals or biopharmaceuticals with the FDA?

10. By using their corporate web pages, attempt to describe how 10 prominent biopharmas are addressing their R&D productivity problems over the last 5 years.

REFERENCES

Arnold, M., 2009. FDA BLA approvals rose in 2009 while NMEs stumbled. Medical Marketing and Media, December 31, 2009. Posted at: http://www.mmm-online.com/fda-bla-approvals-rose-in-2009-while-nmes-stumbled/article/160496/

Biogen Idec Press Release, Cambridge, MA, July 8, 2009, http://investor.biogenidec.com

Burrill & Company Press Release, San Francisco, CA, March 10, 2009, http://www.burillandco.com

COVANCE, 2009. Corporate presentation at the *UBS Global Life Sciences Conference*, September 21, 2009. PowerPoint presentation posted at: http://ir.covance.com/phoenix.zhtml?c=105891&p=irol-presentations

DiMasi, J., 2001. Risks in new drug development: Approval success rates for investigational drugs. *Clinical Pharmacology & Therapeutics* May, 69, 297–307.

DiMasi, J.A. and Grabowski, H.G., 2007. The cost of biopharmaceutical R&D: Is biotech different? *Managerial and Decision Economics* 28, 469–479.

European Commission—Commission of the European Communities, 2009. Pharmaceutical sector inquiry final report. EC: Brussels, SEC(2009) 952, July 8, 2009. pp. 118–119. Posted at: http://ec.europa.eu/competition/sectors/pharmaceuticals/inquiry/communication_en.pdf

European Medicines Agency, CPMP/ICH/135/95 ICH Topic E6 (R1)—Guideline for Good Clinical Practice, Step 5 Note for Guidance on Good Clinical Practice (CPMP/ICH/135/95), p. 7, London, U.K., July 2002. Posted at: http://www.ema.europa.eu/does/en_GB/document_library/Scientific_guideline/2009/09/WC500002874.pdf

Evens, D.P., 2005. Biotechnology and industry research and practice: Part 1—The exploding science, the expanding products, the usage challenges and opportunities. University of Florida, College of Pharmacy Course PHA 5172. PowerPoint presentation posted at: http://www.cop.ufl.edu/safezone/pat/pha5172/evens-powerpoint-0.5.htm

Genmab Press Release, Copenhagen, Denmark, February 5, 2009, http://www.genmab.com

Hall, J., 2004. A decade (and ½) of deals. BioPartnerships—A Pharmaceutical Executive and Biopharm International Supplement, October, pp. 18–24.

Japan Pharmaceutical Manufacturers Association (JPMA)—English Regulatory Information Task Force, 2009. Pharmaceutical administration and regulations in Japan, March 2009. Posted at: http://www.jpma.or.jp/english/parj/1003.html

KENDLE Press Release, Cincinnati, OH, February 25, 2009, http://www.kendle.com

National Institute of Standards and Technology (NIST), Economic analysis of the technology infrastructure needs of the U.S. Biopharmaceutical Industry, Boulder, CL, Available at: http://www.nist.gov/director/prog-ofc/report07-1.pdf

ONYX Pharmaceuticals Press Release, Emeryville, CA, May 20, 2009, http://www.onyxpharm.com

Pharmaceutical Research and Manufacturers of America, 2009. *Pharmaceutical Industry Profile 2009*. Washington, DC: PhRMA.

Quintiles Press Release, Research Triangle Park, NC, October 30, 2009, http://www.quintiles.com

Stewart, J.J., 2002. Biotechnology valuations for the 21st century. MILKEN Institute Policy Brief 27, April, Santa Monica, CA.

Tufts Center for the Study of Drug Development, 2008. Growing protocol design complexity stresses investigators, volunteers. Impact report 10(1), January/February, Boston, MA.

Tufts Center for the Study of Drug Development, 2009. *Outlook 2009*. Boston, MA: Tufts CSDD, 2009.

U.S. Code of Federal Regulations, Title 21, Volume 1, Revised as of April 1, 2008. U.S. Government Printing Office Via GPO Access [CITE: 21CFR3.2], Title 21-FOOD AND DRUGS, Chapter I-FOOD AND DRUG ADMINISTRATION, DEPARTMENT OF HEALTH AND HUMAN SERVICES. PART 3 PRODUCT JURISDICTION. pp. 55–56. Posted at: http://edocket.access.gpo.gov/cfr_2008/aprqtr/21cfr3.2.htm

U.S. Patent and Trademark Office (USPTO), 2008. *The Manual of Patent Examining Procedure* (*MPEP*), Chapter 2100 on Patentability. Eighth Edition, August 2001, Latest Revision July 2008. Posted at: http://www.uspto.gov/web/offices/pac/mpep/mpep_e8r6_2100.pdf

Zisson, S. and Gambrill, S., 2010. 2009: Light at the end of a tough year. CenterWatch Monthly. Posted at: http://www.centerwatch.com/cwmonthly-complimentary/00x00x00x00_ThisMonthPDF.pdf (accessed on January 31, 2010).

## CHAPTER 7

Biomanufacturing

Despite the nation's economic slowdown, America's pharmaceutical research and biotechnology companies invested a record $65.2 billion in 2008 in the research and development of new life-changing medicines and vaccines—an increase of roughly $2 billion from 2007, according to analyses by the Pharmaceutical Research and Manufacturers of America (PhRMA), Washington, District of Columbia and Burrill & Company, San Francisco, CA (2009).

B IOPHARMACEUTICALS ARE MEDICINES PRODUCED through the use of biotechnology techniques. Biopharmaceuticals may belong to different classifications. According to their biochemical structure, they can be nucleic acids (RNA, DNA) or proteins (interferons). According to their physiological function, they can be distinguished in hormones, growth factors, thrombolytic agents, interferons, interleukins, and more. As far as their healthcare application is concerned, they can have therapeutic applications (recombinant insulin), preventive applications (vaccines), or diagnostic ones.

In Chapter 6, we studied in detail the biopharmaceuticals' research and development process. In this chapter, we will move into their manufacturing method, with its unique applications and challenges. Overall, biologics are produced by modifying a gene of a host organism to specifically encode for the production of a biopharmaceutical. Various host organisms have been used to date, for example, microbial cells (*Escherichia coli*), mammalian cells (Chinese hamster ovary [CHO] cells), or plant cells in culture. Furthermore, instead of isolated cells in culture, whole living organisms have been genetically altered in order to produce biologicals, including whole plants and animals. Biopharmaceuticals are produced in special, clean room environments, under the strictest good manufacturing practices (GMPs), and their manufacturing is closely monitored by the relevant regulatory authorities (such as the FDA, EMEA, J.MHLW) we have described previously.

CHEMICAL VERSUS BIOPHARMACEUTICAL PRODUCTION

The manufacturing of biopharmaceuticals (large molecular weight entities) bears unique differences from the respective manufacturing of low molecular weight medicines. Let us compare the two processes at the beginning.

Manufacturing Low Molecular Weight Drugs

Low molecular weight medicines (e.g., aspirin) are usually organic compounds. Their manufacturing is achieved with the help of organic chemistry, i.e., the successive steps of adding chemical atoms and side chains to a molecular frame. Organic chemistry requires the use of pure chemical compounds under closely monitored reaction conditions (i.e., air, temperature, humidity, light, or the presence of catalysts). The resulting pharmacologically active compounds are then purified, isolated, characterized, and sterilized before mixing them with inactive excipients and additives in order to make them into a pharmaceutical dosage form (e.g., pill, capsule, granules) than can easily be administered to the patient.

Production of rDNA Products

Biologics are complex, organic compounds of high molecular weight, comprised of sugars, nucleic acids, and proteins. In nature, they are produced by microorganisms, animals, or humans. Before the advent of the modern biotechnology techniques, biologics had been isolated from their original sources, for example, urinary gonadotrophins, or cadaver insulin. Those early methods were of questionable ethics, of low yield, of low efficacy, and highly contaminated with other physiological or pathological substances, later manifesting themselves as pathogens or side-effect-causing contaminants.

Modern biotechnology techniques have allowed the safe, effective, efficient, and fast production of large quantities of high molecular weight biologics under the strictest manufacturing practices. The basic technology is the genetic alteration of a host organism in order to produce the required biologic, and the subsequent purification and isolation of this biologic product. The whole process therefore involves the genetic engineering of the host genetic material, which is far more complex and conditions-sensitive than organic chemistry. Because of this fundamental

TABLE 7.1   What Are the Main Classes of Biopharmaceuticals?

Months	Weeks
Large and complex proteins or assemblies, e.g., erythropoietin, interferons, therapeutic vaccines, interleukins, monoclonal antibodies, clotting factors, plasminogen activators, colony stimulating factors	Small and simple Peptides Naked DNA Small molecule chemicals

difference in the manufacturing procedure, the manufacture of biologicals (from now on biomanufacturing) is closely associated with the process used, resulting in different purity, efficacy, and safety for the biological even after small modifications in the manufacturing process. This fact has led to the seminal characterization, that when it comes to biologicals "the process is the product." Table 7.1 summarizes the main classes of biopharmaceuticals, either belonging to large and complex proteins, or small and simple biomolecules. Their respective manufacturing processes can last for months, or weeks, respectively.

As far as the host organisms used in the production of biopharmaceuticals, Table 7.2 lists the main expression hosts used today, as well as representative biologicals produced from these hosts.

TABLE 7.2   Production and Purification of rDNA Products

Expression Hosts			
E. coli	CHO Cells	BHK Cells	*S. cerevisiae*
Therapeutic hormones	Therapeutic hormones	Haemopoietic growth factors	Therapeutic hormones
Human insulin, insulin glargine	Human choriogonadotrophin, follicle-stimulating hormone	Erythropoietin omega	Insulin aspart
Haemopoietic growth factors	Haemopoietic growth factors	Coagulation factors	Haemopoietic growth factors
Filgrastim	Erythropoetin alpha, erythropoetin beta, darbopoetin	Factor VII A	Surgramostim
Thrombolytic agents	Coagulation factors		Anticoagulants
Reteplase, saruplase	Factor VIII, factor IX		Lapirudin
Interferons	Thrombolytic agents		
Interferon alpha 2b, interferon beta 1a	Alteplase, tenecteplase		
Interleukins	Therapeutic enzymes		
Interleukin-2, Interleukin-11	Dornase alpha, glucocerebrosicase		

Source: Adapted from Bhopale, G.M. and Nanda, R.K., *Curr. Sci.*, 89, 4, August 25, 2005.

BIOMANUFACTURING PLATFORMS

Platform Systems Widely Used

We have previously mentioned that there are various host organisms (or production platforms) used in biomanufacturing. The selection of one versus the other platform for any given biological depends on the molecular complexity of the biologic, its physicochemical properties, as well as the required production yield (see below). The major platforms used rely on either microbes or mammalian cells. The first category includes bacteria (mainly *E. coli*) or yeast. The second category includes mainly CHO cells in culture. Almost 90% of all the currently marketed biopharmaceuticals (including the biggest selling blockbusters among them) rely on the use of three systems, mainly bacteria, yeast, and CHO cells. Lately, mainly due to the significant production capacities required, alternative platform systems have been introduced, such as whole, living plants or animals, a process requiring the production of a genetically modified plant or animal strain, called a transgenic organism. The major biomanufacturing platform systems used today and their respective advantages are summarized in Table 7.3.

Expression System Decision Framework

We have previously mentioned that the selection of a biomanufacturing platform for any given biological depends on the molecular characteristics, as well as the required production yield. In Figure 7.1, Arthur D. Little has suggested an expression-system decision framework, where the main determinants of the platform to be used are molecular glycosylation (adding to molecular complexity), and overall protein complexity of the produced biologic. Let us now review the major

TABLE 7.3 Which Are Some of the Alternative Biomanufacturing Modes?

Conventional mammalian cells in bioreactor	Regulators are comfortable, manufacturing routine, product has high efficacy, very expensive
Yeast expression	High yield, protein product dissimilar to mammalian derived. Cheap, fast
Bacterial expression	High yield, useful only for smaller proteins. Cheap, fast
Transgenic plants— seeds or moss	High yields, cheap, great potential
Transgenic animals—goats	Longer lead times, high product yield, similar to cell-derived product, cheaper

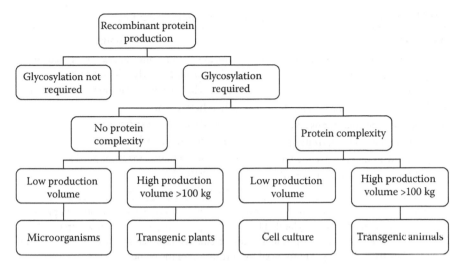

FIGURE 7.1 Expression system decision framework. (From Andersson, R. and Mynahan, R., The protein production challenge, In Vivo: The Business and Medicine Report, 2001. With permission.)

biomanufacturing platforms in more detail, starting from the lower complexity platforms.

Bacteria

Bacteria are a very large and diverse group of unicellular organisms. These organisms belong to the genus *Bacillus*, are few micrometers in length, do not possess a nucleus (so-called prokaryotes), and are found in every habitat on Earth, even inside (gut) or on the outside surface (skin) of humans in the millions. There are two specific bacteria that have been utilized as biomanufacturing platforms, mainly for their simple structures and their detailed characterization to-date, namely, *E. coli* and *Bacillus subtillus*. The advantages and disadvantages of using bacteria as production platforms for biopharmaceuticals are summarized in Table 7.4.

Yeast

Yeasts are another group of microorganisms belonging to the kingdom *Fungi*. Compared to bacteria, they are also unicellular, a few micrometers in length, but possessing a nucleus (so-called eukaryotes). A specific yeast species, namely, *Saccharomyces cerevisiae* has been used since the antiquity in making bread or beer. Other yeasts that have been chosen as biomanufacturing platforms include *Pichia pastoris* or *Hansenula*

TABLE 7.4   Bacteria as Production Platform for Biopharmaceuticals

Advantages	Disadvantages
Well understood molecular biology	Protein refolding and separation of incorrectly folded from properly folded product
Simple vector construction	
Rapid cell growth	Proteins lack posttranslational modifications
High intracellular expression levels	Micro-heterogeneity
Secretion into periplasm possible	Poor extracellular expression
Simple cell bank characterization	Fusion partner may be required
Easy to grow in inexpensive media	Removal of endotoxins from product (Gram-negative)
Established regulatory track record	
	N-terminal methionine

Source: Courtesy of GE Healthcare, Bioprocess—Target molecules—Recombinant proteins, Buckinghamshire, England, http://www4.gelifesciences.com/aptrix/upp01077.nsf/ Content/bioprocess~target±molecules~recombinant±proteins#, 2010. © 2010 General Electric Company–Reproduced by permission of the owner.

TABLE 7.5   Yeast as Production Platform for Biopharmaceuticals

Advantages	Disadvantages
Lack endotoxins; GRAS	Heterologous proteins may be incorrectly glycosylated and folded
Established large-scale fermentation technology	
Low media costs	Recombinant proteins are generally overglycosylated
Genetics well understood	
Proteins properly folded	Complex vector construction
High expression levels and rapid growth	Low intracellular expression
Natural secretor	Difficult to lyse

Source: Courtesy of GE Healthcare, Bioprocess—Target Molecules—Recombinant Proteins, Buckinghamshire, England, http://www4.gelifesciences.com/aptrix/upp01077. nsf/Content/bioprocess~target±molecules~recombinant±proteins#, 2010. © 2010 General Electric Company–Reproduced by permission of the owner.

polymorpha. The respective advantages and disadvantages of using yeasts in biomanufacturing are listed in Table 7.5.

Mammalian Cells

Mammals are vertebrate animals whose females possess mammary glands. They are large, complex, multicellular and multitissue animals, they breathe air, and they range in size 1000-fold from 30 mm to 30 m in length! Certain mammalian cells have been successfully used as biomanufacturing platforms, including the CHO, baby hamster kidney (BHK), murine hybridoma cells, or human cell lines. Their advantages and disadvantages as biologic production platforms are seen in Table 7.6.

TABLE 7.6   Mammalian Cells as Production Platform for Biopharmaceuticals

Advantages	Disadvantages
Correct posttranslational modifications	Expensive
Properly folded proteins	Require expensive media
Easily secreted	Slow growth and low production levels
Good regulatory track record	Potential oncogene contamination
	Extensive cell bank characterization

Source: Courtesy of GE Healthcare, Bioprocess—Target Molecules—Recombinant Proteins, Buckinghamshire, England, http://www4.gelifesciences.com/ aptrix/upp01077.nsf/Content/bioprocess~target±molecules~recombinant± proteins#, 2010. © 2010 General Electric Company–Reproduced by permission of the owner.

BOEHRINGER INGELHEIM Proposal: Example for Mammalian Cell Culture and Microbial Production (*Yeast, E. Coli, pDNA, CHO and Others*)

Optional: The Boehringer Ingelheim group is one of the world's 15 leading pharmaceutical companies. Headquartered in Ingelheim, Germany, it operates globally with 142 affiliates in 50 countries and more than 41,500 employees. Since it was founded in 1885, the family-owned company has been committed to researching, developing, manufacturing and marketing novel products of high therapeutic value for human and veterinary medicine.

Boehringer Ingelheim can be regarded as a pioneer in industrial biotechnology. With a workforce of more than 2,000 employees at their sites in Austria and Germany they have world leading facilities dedicated to the development and production of biopharmaceuticals using mammalian cells, microorganisms and yeast as host organisms. In microbial fermentation, they use the most modern technologies for production, coupled with state-of-the-art extraction and purification procedures in fermentation scales up to 6,000 litres and with a total capacity of about 12,000 L. Besides interferons, various proteins, scaffolds and antibody fragments, they also manufacture plasmid DNA for gene therapy on a commercial scale. In mammalian cell culture they are Europe's leading manufacturer for therapeutic proteins and monoclonal antibodies with a total capacity of 180,000 L. In addition they have state-of-the-art development facilities including a 2,000 L pilot plant for production of clinical trial material. They offer the entire process chain from genetic engineering to the therapeutic drug product including fill & finish and worldwide registration. All of their manufacturing processes are conducted according to GMP standards. To date they have registered biopharmaceuticals with the European, Canadian and US regulatory authorities. They have generated many successful long-term partnerships in biopharmaceutical production with the world's leading pharmaceutical and biopharmaceutical companies.

Source: Courtesy of Boehringer Ingelheim, *Our Expertise in World-Class Contract Manufacturing for Your Success Brochure,* http://www.boehringer-ingelheim.com/biopharm. With permission.

Benefits of Newer Systems

The need for the development of newer and improved biomanufacturing expression systems originated from the following necessities: (1) increased yield, (2) production stability, (3) simplicity, (4) batch contamination improvement, (5) higher protein complexity, (6) more human-like characteristics, (7) increased production volumes, (8) reduced costs, (9) increased production portability, and (10) increased production scalability. There is presently a plethora of newer systems, although their commercial and/or research use remains under 10% of the global biological production.

According to Rader (2008), some of the novel expression systems (in terms of human biopharmaceuticals) include those based on bacteria other than *E. coli* (e.g., *Pseudomonas* fluorescents and *Caulobacter crescentus*); fungi (e.g., *Chrysosporium lucknowense*); improved human cell lines (e.g., PER.C6); yeasts culturable in glucose, ethanol, or other simple media and/or that provide human-like glycosylation; algae ranging from single cells through whole plants (e.g., Lemna); various insect cells and whole insects; a wide variety of terrestrial plants (e.g., safflower and tobacco); and various transgenic animals. Completely cell-free systems are also becoming available.

TRANSGENICS

General Applications of Transgenic Organisms

As described above, a transgenic organism has had its genome (gene sequence) altered with biotechnology techniques, so that it now contains a new gene specifically encoding for the production of a new protein. Because the resulting organism does not contain the original genome, it is called a transgenic organism, one that contains a mixture of gene sequences coming from different organisms.

The addition of a new gene into an organism may be achieved with either natural or artificial methods. For example, natural methods are based on the use of special bacteria or viruses that can transfer new genetic material to another species. Artificial methods range from the genetic engineering of a virus into containing a new gene and then infecting the host organism, or injecting pure DNA sequences into the nucleus of an embryo to be artificially implanted, or utilizing special "gene guns," etc. The resulting transgenic organism can be either a plant or an animal that can reproduce the desired protein in mass quantities, later collected and purified from its leaves, or milk, respectively. The potential use of transgenic organisms is just emerging. For example, they can be used to produce hard-to-make proteins. Alternatively, animals may be created as disease models, or others that may recognize and exhibit a foreign pathogen, thus acting as living diagnostics. The use of transgenic plants or animals for the production of biopharmaceuticals is collectively called "pharming."

Transgenic Plants

Transgenic plants have been around for centuries. These new species were either created by chance (cross hybridization) or by purposeful farmers, attempting to primitively alter the characteristics of their plants, seeking a better color, appearance, height, yield, or resistance to disease and lack of water. By the use of modern biotechnology techniques, plants can now be directed to produce specific biologics to be used in human disease diagnosis, prevention, or treatment. In the case of phytopharming recombinant proteins—as for example, EPO—they are usually expressed in the seeds or leaf of the recombinant plant. The use of plant transgenics presents the advantages and disadvantages listed in Table 7.7.

According to KKY Partners (2010), biopharmas are turning to mass cultivation of row crops (e.g., tobacco and corn) that can be transgenically modified in order to produce biologicals with diverse functions. Additional advantages of plant transgenics is the avoidance of large, initial biomanufacturing-related capital expenses, as well as the easy scalability of

TABLE 7.7   Transgenic Plants as Production Platform for Biopharmaceuticals

Advantages	Disadvantages
Low initial investment, medium timescale (months), unlimited scale-up potential, faster than transgenic animals, very low costs <5$/g, safe, no risk of pathogen contamination, edible crops can be used, active complex proteins (sIgA)	Some crops cannot be regenerated, vulnerable to weather, not 100% biologically contained unless via chloroplast transformation

Source: Courtesy of GE Healthcare, Bioprocess—Target Molecules—Recombinant Proteins, Buckinghamshire, England, http://www4.gelifesciences.com/aptrix/upp01077.nsf/Content/bioprocess~target±molecules~recombinant±proteins#, 2010. © 2010 General Electric Company–Reproduced by permission of the owner.

production by just adding additional acreage to the cultivated transgenic plant. The "first wave" of clinical applications includes edible vaccines, antibiotics, anti-HIV drugs, and anticlotting agents, among others. Edible vaccines have already been developed for Hepatitis-B, bacterial Lt-B toxin that causes "Traveller's Disease" and TGVE (transmissible gastro-enteritis virus), while pipeline products include albumin, aprotinin, trypsin, lacto-ferrin, and various monoclonal antibodies.

Some of the plant-derived pharmaceuticals currently in the pipeline for the treatment of human disease are listed in Table 7.8.

Some of the high-profile players in plant-based transgenics include the following companies: BASF Plant Science, Bayer CropScience, Biolex, Dow AgroSciences, Dupont, EdenSpace, Icon Genetics, Ventria Bioscience, Mendel Biotechnology, Metabolix, Pioneer Hi-Bred, Phytomedics, and Syngenta Biotechnology.

Transgenic Animals

As in the case of transgenic plants, genetically altering the genome of animals in order to produce a new protein is a novel biomanufacturing

TABLE 7.8 Plant-Derived Pharmaceuticals for the Treatment of Human Diseases That Are in the Pipeline for Commercialization

Product	Class	Indication	Crop
Various single-chain Fv antibody fragments	Antibody	Non-Hodgkin's lymphoma	Viral vectors in tobacco
E. coli heat-labile toxin	Vaccine	Diarrhea	Transgenic maize Transgenic potato
Gastric lipase	Therapeutic enzyme	Cystic fibrosis, pancreatitis	Transgenic maize
Hepatitis B virus surface antigen	Vaccine	Hepatitis B	Transgenic potato Transgenic lettuce
Human intrinsic factor	Dietary	Vitamin B12 deficiency	Transgenic Arabidopsis
Lactoferrin	Dietary	Gastrointestinal infection	Transgenic maize
Norwalk virus capsid protein	Vaccine	Norwalk virus infection	Transgenic potato
Cyanoverin-N	Microbicide	HIV	Transgenic tobacco
Insulin	Hormone	Diabetes	Transgenic safflower
Lysozyme, lactoferrin, human serum albumin	Dietary	Diarrhea	Transgenic rice

Source: International Service for the Acquisition of Agri-Biotech Applications (ISAAA), Pocket K No. 26 Molecular Pharming and Biopharmaceuticals, ISAAA, Manila, May 2007, http://www.isaaa.org. With permission.

platform that can address the following production issues. First, there is a growing number of approved biopharmaceuticals that are commercially approved for the treatment of human disease. Second, because of their superior efficacy and safety characteristics, biopharmaceuticals are slowly gaining market share from traditional pharmaceuticals in a number of indications. Third, better diagnostic tools allow the diagnosis of more patients suffering from severe and chronic diseases that could potentially be treated by biopharmaceuticals. Fourth, the traditional biomanufacturing platforms are very hard to scale, and often require the buildup of additional new facilities, requiring significant delays, very high capital expenses, and often resulting in temporary product shortages in the marketplace. In conclusion, pharming can offer quick, scalable, economic, and safe production opportunities for the growing needs of modern therapeutics in biopharmaceutical molecules. The advantages and disadvantages of using transgenic animals as biomanufacturing platforms are listed in Table 7.9.

Transgenic Animal Applications
Pharming technology has been applied to goats, cattle, pigs, sheep, rabbits, and chickens. Sheep and cattle, for example, have been transformed for the expression of human factor VIII and IX, which are needed for the treatment of haemophilia or fibrinogen that is used for the treatment of wound healing. Transgenic chicken, cows, and goats are utilized for the production of monoclonal antibodies. Mostly, the recombinant protein is expressed in the milk of the transgenic mammals but it could also be directed to the blood, urine, or to the eggs (of transgenic chicken). Currently, an increasing number of field and clinical trials are running and the first protein that is produced by pharming has gained market approval: In August 2006, the European Commission granted market authorization to ATryn®. The U.S.-based biotech company GTC Biotherapeutics produces ATryn® in the milk of female goats carrying a transgene for human antithrombin.

According to Engelhard et al. (2007), antithrombin is an important anticoagulant in human serum and is applied for the prophylaxis of venous thromboembolism in surgery of patients with congenital antithrombin

TABLE 7.9   Transgenic Animals as Biopharmaceutical Production Platforms

Advantages	Disadvantages
Active complex proteins, accurate glycosylation, yields up to 40 g/L milk, herds can be bred	Very slow (years for cloning), upscale slow (breeding), BSE and other pathogens, cloning very labor-intensive and yet to be optimized, host protein contamination, expensive: 100 K–300 K$/animal, public ethical concerns

deficiency. Antithrombin products were previously derived from human plasma. The complex structure of antithrombin precludes its efficient production in traditional bioreactors. Thus, recombinant human antithrombin can only be produced in higher organisms as expression platform.

Transgenic Animal Model Development

According to Brusick (1998), the first step in developing a transgenic organism is to identify, prepare, and purify the DNA coding of the particular trait desired. The transgene contains not only the gene of interest, but a promoter sequence which controls the gene's function. The purity of the DNA construct is extremely important in order to avoid any toxic effect on the embryo. Purification is accomplished via electroelution or glass bead adsorption. The goal is to provide DNA that is free of salts, organic solvents, or traces of agarose, in a correct and sterile buffer, and not sheared or nicked. In addition, the DNA must be at the proper concentration. Although several methods of genetic transfer have been developed, three techniques are used in the production of most transgenic animals: microinjection, viral transfer, and genetic manipulation of the embryonic stem cell culture.

For a pharming example see: GTC Biotherapeutics, Framingham, MA, GTC Biotheropeutics Corporate Profile, http://www.gtc-bio.com

BIOMANUFACTURING PROCESS DEVELOPMENT

Biopharmaceutical production is a complex and demanding operation. It has four critical objectives. First, product quality needs to be guaranteed, for example, the resulting product needs to be primarily safe and effective, it needs to have a minimum specific activity, it needs to abide to strict standards (GMP), and it needs to be reproducible in its nature, quality, and quantity in every facility it may be created. Second, the production process needs to produce the desired quantity, so that it meets all required commercial and research needs, and it also needs to be scalable, so that it quickly meets any unforeseen spikes in demand. Third, bioproduction needs to meet strict time requirements, for example, quickly supply all research demand, later be scaled-up in order to meet the commercial launch demands, and obviously support the product throughout its life cycle, especially under the critical patent protection period. Finally, it needs to be cost-efficient, so that it produces the required yields; it meets the planned cost-of-goods requirements, and also offers a profitable commercial alternative that is compatible with the existing private market, government reimbursement, or formulary limitations.

Fermentation versus Cell Culture

Biopharmaceutical products can be produced by two distinct methods, namely, fermentation or cell culture, both called bioreactions. In the fermentation process, the production platform (bacteria or yeast) is based on living organisms that are allowed to grow under special, carefully monitored conditions in a bioreactor. This is a relatively expeditious and simple process, the microorganisms are kept healthy, vigorous, and well producing, and the whole process may require 2–3 days for a given batch to be produced. Biopharmaceutical molecules produced in this way are relatively simpler and less sensitive to the complex bioreactor conditions (e.g., biosynthetic penicillin).

Alternatively, the cell culture is a process of growing and multiplying isolated cells (e.g., CHO cells) in a culture, in a more complex and time-consuming process. This process may require up to 8 weeks to complete, and may require the frequent relocation of the growing tissue culture in bigger containers, often called roller-bottles for they have to be constantly rotated so that the cells do now grow asymmetrically over a single spot. This process is also resource-consuming, since a large bioreactor is not always usable, and it may require special robots for the rolling operation. In the end, the resulting biopharmaceutical products are usually complex molecules (e.g., biosynthetic FSH; Gonal-F). The final product may be found intracellularly or may be secreted extracellularly.

Key Steps in Process Development

Biomanufacturing can be subdivided into three distinct activities: (1) bioprocess development, (2) scale-up for manufacture of clinical test materials, and (3) large-scale, commercial manufacturing. Living cells serve as mini-factories that can manufacture the appropriate proteins. Because biotechnology companies make complex molecules for human use, we need to monitor, control, and document all aspects of the complicated process—the raw materials, environment, utilities, equipment, and procedures—to ensure we make safe, active, and consistent product.

Development of Production Strain

The development of a biopharmaceutical production strain starts with the insertion of a specific gene into the host cell, using either a transfection vector or direct injection, in a process described earlier.

Cell Bank Creation and Characterization

After a single cell has been transfected, it is allowed to multiply in a controlled medium, and under every other possible condition closely controlled (temperature, humidity, oxygen, light, etc). When the single cell has grown to a cell culture (with thousands of cells), this is called the *research cell bank (RCB)*. Using an aliquot of the RCB, the first tests are done: (1) cells are checked for homogeneity, (2) cells are checked for similarity with original cell, (3) the cellular genome is checked for containing the exact gene sequence inserted, (4) the cells are lysed, the biopharmaceutical is collected, purified, and analyzed, and its exact characteristics are checked versus the desired, and previously declared and approved characteristics, and (5) different methods of isolation are checked for their resulting yields. If all is found according to specifications, the cell is called the *master cell bank (MCB)* and is frozen in aliquots, ready to be used in future production runs. When the production apparatus is ready, a single aliquot from the master cell line is selected, thus becoming the *working cell line (WCB)*. The cell line is then thawed and allowed to grow in small containers under set conditions. After another round of tests following the primary multiplication, the cell line is transferred into larger containers (roller bottles, flasks, or bioreactors) and allowed to multiply under strict specifications.

Only a handful of highly specialized professionals are allowed to handle the master and working cell lines, which are then stored under surveillance, or are used in production under constant computer monitoring of multiple parameters. MCB and WCB aliquots are also stored outside the main biomanufacturing facilities in remote and secure locations.

Scale-Up Process

The scale-up of a cell culture process can be very difficult and time-consuming, taking as long as several months before researchers can obtain a product. The entire process of producing a biotech product from start to finish is often called a campaign and is usually divided into two main parts: upstream and downstream. Upstream processes involve production of the protein product, most often by using cells (microbial, insect, or mammalian) growing in culture. Downstream processes include the recovery, purification, formulation, and packaging of the protein product.

Upstream Phase

According to Amgen Scholars (2010), upstream processing begins with the cells that scientists create or engineer to make the protein product.

To begin a campaign, scientists remove and thaw a vial of cells from the cell bank and initiate a cell culture in a flask containing a small volume of growth media. The initial volume of media can be as little as 5 mL. The media provides the nutrients and the optimum environment for cells to survive. Scale-up is done by gradually transferring the growing cells into successively larger growth vessels containing larger media volumes. The cells are constantly dividing as long as the growth environment remains favorable. Therefore, more and more cells are present with each step. The greater the number of cells, the more protein product is generated.

Downstream Phase

In the downstream phase of manufacturing, the protein product is isolated from the cells that produced it. Proteins found inside the cell (intracellular proteins) require special protocols to extract them for purification. Usually, this involves bursting the cells open to release the protein product, which then has to be purified away from the other components that were inside the cell. Proteins found outside of the cell (extracellular proteins) can be easier to isolate. After harvesting the protein product, the next step is clarification. This is where scientists separate the protein from cellular debris. Then, they apply the protein solution to a series of chromatography columns to obtain a pure protein product. Purification of protein mixtures by column chromatography separates proteins based on physical and chemical properties such as size, shape, or electrical charge. Additional purification steps remove any residual DNA and deactivate any viral particles that may be present. Researchers verify the isolation and purification of the protein product through confirmed testing protocols. The protein product is then formulated according to the R&D specifications and packaged for use by physicians and patients.

Primary Recovery Unit Operations

Genentech provides a brief overview of biologics manufacturing at its company Web site (http://www.gene.com/gene/news/kits/corporate/manufacturing.html). In summary, when the cells grow to sufficient numbers, they are transferred to large-scale production tanks and grown for about another 2 weeks. At this point in the process, the protein or antibody can be harvested. The cells are engineered to secrete the protein or antibody into the cell culture media, so the first step in the purification process is to separate the cells from the media. The media is then subjected to several additional purification steps that remove any cellular debris, unwanted proteins, salts, minerals, or other undesirable elements. At the end of the purification process, the product is suitable for human use.

Analytical Development

The analytical development is taking place during the process development and is of critical importance to the final product. It involves two complementary functions. First, through quality control, it needs to constantly monitor the quality of the manufactured product on conformity with the internally developed specifications that have also been declared and approved by the regulatory authorities. Second, it needs to verify that these specifications are followed identically and dependably after every production batch, so that no unforeseen manufacturing problems may cause deviation from the acceptable specifications. In other words, the process needs to stay on course, and the identical destination needs to be reached each and every time in biomanufacturing.

Formulation and Fill/Finish

After the analytical assays described above deliver a dependably safe, effective, and pure biological, the product needs to be made into a formulation, i.e., the final dosage form administered to the patient. The formulation chosen is dependent on its physicochemical properties (soluble, solid, acidic, heat-sensitive), its pharmacodynamic properties (where does the product go into the body and what does it cause), and its pharmacokinetic properties (how long does it stay in the body and how does it get deactivated or excreted).

The basic consideration here is the following: capitalize on its properties in order to make the active substance remain within the target tissue above a minimum effective concentration and below a minimum toxic concentration until the next dose is conveniently administered. When these considerations are made, the proper formulation is chosen, and the bulk, final product needs to be safely modified into becoming its final formulation form, e.g., turned into a capsule, which surrounds it with an inactive cellulose layer that delivers it safely past the stomach's acidic content. It is imperative that all inactive additives and excipients chosen are to be declared to the regulatory authorities and remain constant throughout the manufacturing process, or until an improvement becomes available.

Biomanufacturing Regulation

The FDA, the EMEA, and other regulatory agencies regulate and inspect equipment, facilities, and processes used in the manufacturing of pharmaceutical and biologic products prior to approving a product. If, after receiving clearance from regulatory agencies, a company makes a material change in manufacturing equipment, location, or process, additional regulatory review and approval may be required. Biomanufacturers must also adhere to current Good Manufacturing Practices, or cGMP, and product-specific regulations enforced by the FDA following product approval. The FDA, the EMEA, and other regulatory agencies also conduct regular, periodic visits to reinspect equipment, facilities, and processes following the initial approval of a product. If, as a result of these inspections, it is determined that the equipment, facilities, or processes do not comply with applicable regulations and conditions of product approval, regulatory agencies may seek civil, criminal, or administrative sanctions and/or remedies against biomanufacturers, including the suspension of their manufacturing operations.

For a biomanufacturer example see: DSM Pharma, DSM Annual Report 2008, Heerlen, the Netherlands, http://www.dsm.com

GLOBAL BIOMANUFACTURING IN NUMBERS

According to BioProcess Technology Consultants, a specialized consultancy in biologic process and product development (Levine, 2009; http://www.bioprocessconsultants.com/index.php; With permission), in 2007, 27 biopharmaceutical products had worldwide sales in excess of $1 billion. Nine manufactured by microbial fermentation, including Lucentis, an antibody fragment. Eighteen manufactured in mammalian cell culture. Nine antibody-based products, including Lucentis. Monoclonal antibodies represent the fastest growing segment of the pharmaceutical industry. Monoclonal antibodies remain 85%–90% of the biologics product pipeline. Approximately 70% of all biopharmaceutical products in development are produced in mammalian cell culture. For 2007, total biologics sales exceeded $75 billion. This represented 11% of total pharmaceutical market, showing a 16% annual growth rate, and equivalent to approximately 23 metric tons total product. Of this quantity, insulin accounts for >50% of total product.

In addition, according to Ransohoff et al. BPTC Cell Culture Capacity Report (2007; With permission), the global biopharmaceutical demand for 2007 was as follows:

- Mammalian recombinant products   95 kg

- Mammalian MAb products   5,753 kg

- Microbial recombinant products   17,183 kg

- Microbial MAb products   0.4 kg

The State of Mammalian Cell Culture Capacity

According to Levine (2009; With permission) there is currently sufficient capacity worldwide to meet annual production needs for all biopharmaceutical products and new capacity is under construction in several regions. There is adequate but slightly tightening mammalian cell culture capacity through 2013. Contract manufacturing organization (CMO) capacity will remain an option for companies. Probability of sufficient capacity through the end of the decade is very high with relatively few new volume driver products being approved and growth of the existing large volume commercial products slowing during this period. Its capacity is set to increase from approximately 2.5 million liters in 2008 to approximately 4.1 million liters in 2013. In 2008, approximately 52% total installed capacity was fully utilized, growing to approximately 73% by 2013.

For a biomanufacturing facility example see: GENENTECH's Vacaville Product Operations, GENENTECH, San Francisco, CA, http://www.gene.com/gene/news/kits/corporate/vacaville-backgrounder.html

BIOMANUFACTURING STRATEGY

We have previously described the process steps involved in biopharmaceutical development. Table 7.10 summarizes these steps and their respective time requirements, spanning the entire biopharmaceutical development and manufacturing value chain.

Contract or Build?

Having completed the process development phase during clinical development, a biopharmaceutical organization is faced with a critical strategic dilemma, that is, assigning a large capital expense toward the building

TABLE 7.10 What Is the Biopharmaceutical Development and Manufacturing Value Chain?

Year	-2	-1	0	1	2	3	4	5
Cell line development	▓							
Cell line banking		▓						
Process development		▓						
Process optimization			▓	▓				
Process validation					▓			
Manufacturing	TOX	Phase I	Phase II		Phase III			
Output		<50 g	<100 g		<3 kg			
Clinical phase plant		▓	▓	▓				
Commercial plant					▓	▓	▓	▓
Clinical trials			Phase I	Phase II			Phase III	

Note: Shaded areas indicate biopharmaceutical development stages during which the listed processes (in rows) take place.

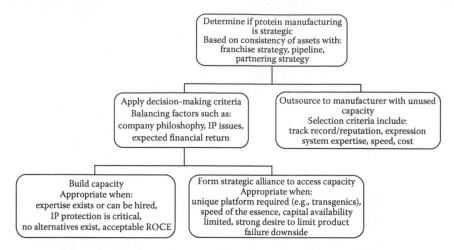

FIGURE 7.2   Make/collaborate/buy decision framework. (From Andersson, R. and Mynahan, R., The protein production challenge, In Vivo: The Business and Medicine Report, 2001, Arthur D. Little Analysis, 2001. With permission.)

of a new full-scale manufacturing facility, or collaborating with an external manufacturing expert, or even buying a completed facility from another organization that no longer needs it. This dilemma is nicely depicted in Figure 7.2 by Arthur D. Little. The major considerations to be made along this strategic framework are overall corporate strategy, protection of intellectual property, speed, cost, financial returns, and risks involved.

Building Capacity

By studying the annual financial reports of major biopharmaceutical companies, it can easily be estimated that constructing a new biopharmaceutical commercial facility requires up to 5 years and burns capital expenses of up to $500 million. Commercial facility construction thus needs to be initiated during preclinical development, so that it provides both the clinical research material and the commercial material needed after launch.

As described above, process development needs to come first and be declared, inspected, and eventually validated by the regulatory authorities. When this is achieved, facility development also needs to be validated by the same authorities, who are closely involved in facility design approval, GMP manufacturing adherence, and final product specifications' validation. Facility development is planned incrementally, so that initial process development is achieved and sufficient material is produced for phase I and II trials, while final process development, optimization, scalability, and validation are achieved in time for phase III trials.

In order to complete the validation process, biomanufacturers need to run through repetitive test production runs, and submit their respective manufacturing samples to the regulatory authorities for specification adherence and reproducibility testing. Having achieved the regulatory validation, the whole biopharmaceutical manufacturing process needs to be fully implemented and remain unchanged throughout the product's commercial life cycle, unless manufacturing improvements are planned and are approved by the authorities in advance of implementation. Building a biomanufacturing plant in-house offers several advantages, but is not devoid of disadvantages. For example, critical know-how is obtained, incremental improvements are easier, and there is better control on GMP, quality, and costs, while scalability can easily be added later. The in-house biomanufacturing is often done in international locations that offer ample access to intellectual capital, easy access to raw materials, manufacturing safety, political stability, and tax incentives. Puerto Rico and Ireland are some of the most prominent examples.

On the other hand, in-house manufacturing may be plagued by large capital expenses, long lead times (e.g., making capacity decisions more than 5 years before a product's commercial introduction), and also difficulties in switching manufacturing technologies or products or sites, not previously foreseen.

Manufacturing Strategy Timeline
As previously described, a complete manufacturing strategy blueprint needs to be in place in advance of phase III trials. However, building or not the manufacturing facility is not the only major concern. For example: How much capacity is planned? Can capacity be scaled up later? What products are to be produced, and are they compatible? Where are the products going to be sold, and have the respective regulatory agencies validated it? Who are the ideal facility designer and constructor? Are raw material providers identified, selected, and validated? Has the specialized personnel been recruited? Have we secured the proper electrical, water, and waste management? How about clean-room and cold-chain requirements? Is the plant secure from malicious acts of vandalism? Does the plant have easy access to transportation routes (ports, airports, highways)? Can we attract the maximum investment incentives? The list goes on.

If the above prerequisites are not met, critical problems may arise, for example, product over- or under-capacity. Either of these negative scenarios carries huge financial consequences for the biopharma. For example, in the case of excess capacity, the biomanufacturing facility would

TABLE 7.11   Differences in Biotech versus Pharma Capacity Planning

Protein Production	Active Pharmaceutical Ingredients (API)
5–6 year lead time to build new facilities	Shorter lead time to build new facility
Rate of technology change high	Technology not changing rapidly
Processes require fit with facility—modifications required to fit	Less complicated processes allow for easier plan changes
No robust CMO market	Excess capacity in industry

be forced to scale back its production capacity for a certain period of time. This is accompanied by carrying over inflexible fixed costs, such as manufacturing facility leasing, equipment leasing, utility bills, water and air treatment bills, property taxes, and more. In addition, fixed costs will include those originating from a large manufacturing organization, that is highly specialized and specifically trained, making their downsizing a difficult task.

Due to the critical nature of biomanufacturing, capacity planning is far more difficult than that performed in small molecule (traditional) pharmaceutical manufacturing, as summarized in Table 7.11.

Biomanufacturing Challenges

Unfortunately, in-house biomanufacturing is not for the faint-hearted biopharma executive. One of the most critical issues faced is capacity exceeding or trailing demand. This challenge is inherently related to the quality of sales forecasting, which can never be ideal, especially in the commercial introduction of new biological entities (NBE), meaning new biopharmaceuticals that work with a completely different mechanism of action than the existing, "reference" treatment alternatives. Despite ongoing efforts to improve the industry's forecasting accuracy, however, subjective input from medical opinion leaders, changing consumer demands, economical recessions that bring additional product, reimbursement constraints, and unexpected side effects can always play a negative role in the quality of biomanufacturing forecasting.

An additional factor to make the problem worse is the extremely long lead time required for biomanufacturing changes in technologies used, specifications followed, products produced, or capacities employed. This is due to the fact that manufacturing process alterations are dependent on long process development. To state this fact in a different way, biomanufacturing depends on living organisms, and they have their way! For example, changing technologies may result in contaminations, or loss of yield. A change in specifications required may necessitate a new bioreactor. A change in products produced may necessitate a different microorganism, different containers, and conditions. Finally, an unexpected scale-up may require leasing new land, adding new bioreactors, and time-consuming regulatory validations.

A frequent example used to showcase the critical effects of biopharmaceutical production shortages is the one relating to Enbrel (etanercept) originally launched by Immunex in 1998, which faced severe shortages and lost sales during 2001, later acquired by Amgen which significantly increased its production capacity with time. Faced with such problems, proactive biomanufacturers need to constantly monitor the market evolution for their products, and gradually add capacity, long before any shortages may occur. An illustrative example of such a strategy is shown in Table 7.12, describing GENZYME's increasing manufacturing capacity.

Another challenge facing biomanufacturing is the rare, but devastating receipt of a warning letter by the relevant regulatory agency. For example, a final product may have been found contaminated, a new batch may have been found outside the approved specifications, a batch may be causing unexpected local site injection reactions, or a plant catastrophe (e.g., failure of clean-room generators) may have occurred. The above unexpected events may eventually bring a regulatory letter demanding the immediate discontinuation of all production operations, and the required corrections to be started immediately, such as decontamination, new generators and monitors, new tests, and obviously a completely new process development, validation, and approval. Faced with such unforeseen events, small biopharmas often decide to completely outsource production, until a later stage in the company's life cycle.

TABLE 7.12   Biomanufacturing Example: GENZYME's Increasing Manufacturing Capacity

2006	2009	2011
Total = 8,000 L	Total = 20,000 L	Total = 32,000 L
		Myozyme 3 × 4 kL
		Fabrazyme 2 × 2 kL
	Myozyme 2 × 4 kL	Fabrazyme 2 × 2 kL
	Fabrazyme 2 × 2 kL	Cerezyme 2 × 2 kL
Cerezyme 4 × 2 kL	Cerezyme 4 × 2 kL	Cerezyme 4 × 2 kL

Source: Courtesy of Genzyme Corporation, Genzyme Annual Report 2008, Cambridge, MA, 2008, 2009.

BIOMANUFACTURING FORECASTING

We have previously mentioned the critical nature of forecasting in planning and building biomanufacturing facilities. In principle, future biopharmaceutical use is based on total population, disease prevalence and incidence, diagnosis rate, treatment rate, existence of alternatives, pricing and reimbursement, and patient adherence to therapy.

Let us take these parameters in consideration. First, disease incidence may be changed by a pandemic (e.g., H1N1 flu-virus). Second, diagnosis rate may change with better tools (e.g., pharmacogenomics) or physician and public education. Third, treatment rates may change due to the issuance of new therapeutic guideline. Fourth, treatment alternatives may appear, either pharmacologic (from biopharmaceutical competitors) or non-pharmacologic (e.g., radiations or hyperthermia). Fifth, pricing may change due to competition or government-imposed reductions. Sixth, reimbursement rates may change due to state fiscal problems, or changing laws, or opinion leader recommendations. Finally, patient adherence may improve after education or additional services, such as nurse and psychologic support at home.

And forecasting problems do not end there. For example, new molecular entities require certain strategic assumptions to be made. In addition, forecasting input may carry subjectivity (similar to the placebo effect) or bias. A product's regulatory approvability may prove a difficult target to achieve. Unexpected side effects may necessitate forecasting changes. And long-term toxicity, new technologies, better prevention, or primary healthcare can all play a significant role in changing important forecasting parameters.

Problems encountered above may necessitate changes in excipients, additives, formulations, specifications, and more. These changes will, in turn, necessitate new process or facility development delays, ranging from 6 months (new process), 1 year (new regulatory validation), 2 years (new formulation), 3 years (new production platform), and even 5 years (new biomanufacturing facility). It becomes apparent that, first, the forecasting process is an art by itself, and second, that in-house scalability needs to be available, or manufacturing outsourcing should be considered.

Factors That Will Impact Future Capacity

We have previously mentioned the basic future usage considerations, namely, population, prevalence, incidence, diagnosis rate, treatment rate, alternatives, pricing, reimbursement, and adherence to therapy. All these factors will lead to a basic capacity forecasting. Let us see what additional factors may impact future biopharmaceutical capacity, in chronological order: (1) platform technologies for anticipated products, (2) product in-licensing, (3) approvability of pipeline by regulatory authorities, (4) funding sources (secondary offering, borrowing) for capital expenses, (5) outsourcing manufacturing, (6) product number entering the market place, (6) sales and marketing success (or failure), (7) peak sales potential, impacting the economies of scale, (8) competitive product launches, (9) process development improvements, (10) production problems and warning letters, (11) product withdrawals (own and competitive), (12) pricing changes (proactive or reactive), (13) reimbursement/Formulary changes (e.g., negative opinion by U.K.'s NICE), (14) government healthcare reform, (15) merger or acquisition, (16) contract manufacturing for third parties by the biopharma itself, (17) lifecycle management (see Chapter 12), and (18) patent protection expirations.

As far as the process of forecasting is concerned, there are two major issues to be considered. First, forecasting the size of the global market, and second, forecasting the penetration of own and competitive products, based on their respective competitive advantages. Table 7.13 presents a method of forecasting biomanufacturing demand for a given biopharmaceutical. Armed with this information, biomanufacturing executives then proceed in estimating the tissue cell culture volume required for the estimated demand, either for a clinical phase product (Table 7.14) or a commercial product (Table 7.15).

Furthermore, Table 7.16 summarizes a method for estimating biomanufacturing supply, either on a global scale for any given indication, or comparing the capacities of industry or contract manufacturers (see below).

TABLE 7.13   How Do You Estimate Biomanufacturing Demand?

1	Market differentiation	Microbial and mammalian cell culture markets
		Clinical and commercial markets
2	Probability weighing factors	Accounting for multiple products targeting same indication
		Assumptions for probability of success and time to market
3	Estimate existing and future requirements	Estimated dose and dosing regimen
		Probability and time of launch
		Competition in indication area

TABLE 7.14   How Do You Estimate Global Cell Culture Volume Required for a Given Commercial Biopharmaceutical Product?

	Parameter	Units	Informational Sources	Formula
1	Global annual product sales	USD	Company financial reports, industry reports	
2	Product pricing	USD/mg		
3	Product amount annually required	kg		1×2
4	Per patient annual dosing	g/patient	Prescribing information, regulatory documents	
5	Treatment population	Patients		3×4
6	Expression level/overall yield	g/L	Published data	
7	Technology for manufacture		Literature	
8	Cell culture volume annually required	L		$3 \times 6 \times 7$

TABLE 7.15   How Do You Estimate Global Cell Culture Volume Required for a Given Clinical Phase Biopharmaceutical Product?

	Parameter	Units	Informational Sources	Formula
1	Per patient annual dosing	g/patient	Prescribing information, regulatory documents	
2	Indication prevalence	Patients per year	Disease prevalence databases	
3	Market penetration	% of prevalence	Indication, number of products in indication	
4	Product amount annually required	kg		$1 \times 2 \times 3$
5	Expression level/overall yield	g/L	Published data	
6	Technology for manufacture		Literature	
7	Cell culture volume annually required	L		$4 \times 5 \times 6$

TABLE 7.16   How Do You Estimate Biomanufacturing Supply?

1	Current supply	Bioreactor number
		Bioreactor volume
		Production platform
		Intended facility use (non-GMP, clinical, or commercial)
2	Future supply	Planned bioreactor number
		Planned bioreactor volume
		Production platform
		Forecast years "on-line"
		Intended facility use (non-GMP, clinical, or commercial)

Biomanufacturing Supply Forecasting Example: Cerezyme and Fabrazyme (Genzyme)

Genzyme Provides Update on Cerezyme and Fabrazyme Supply— Date: September 23, 2009. Genzyme Corporation (NASDAQ: GENZ) today provided an update on its progress to restore supplies of Cerezyme® (imiglucerase for injection) and Fabrazyme® (agalsidase beta) for patients worldwide and revised its 2009 revenue guidance for these products. The company is now approximately half-way through the anticipated shortage period for Cerezyme and Fabrazyme, the restart of the Allston Landing manufacturing facility is complete, and if production continues to proceed as planned, Genzyme expects that it can begin meeting anticipated patient demand for both products during the first quarter of 2010.

All six bioreactors at the Allston plant are fully operational and have reached the point in their production cycles when their anticipated output and the timing of product release can be predicted with more certainty. Cerezyme production is proceeding on track, with four bioreactors producing bulk material at levels in the higher range of Genzyme's historical experience for the product. The company anticipates that newly produced Cerezyme will be available for shipment beginning in November and December as planned. The first shipments of newly produced Fabrazyme are now expected to occur in mid-December, and the volume of finished product initially available for release will be lower than anticipated. There are several factors that have contributed to the production delay and lower product volume. Fabrazyme bioreactors were re-started later than planned in order to perform preventative maintenance and sanitization procedures related to the decontamination of the facility. In addition, output from the two Fabrazyme bioreactors is expected to be in the lower range of Genzyme's historical experience for the product. Also, to ensure global access to Fabrazyme as quickly as possible, Genzyme has been processing bulk material in smaller batches, which leads to faster availability of final product but also leads to losses in process efficiency and lower overall volume. As a result, additional product conservation measures are now needed to help ensure that the limited remaining Fabrazyme inventory can be made available to as many patients as possible until new material is available.

In June, Genzyme determined that its Fabrazyme inventory was sufficient to support approximately 80 percent of global patient demand through October. Dose conservation guidelines were implemented by the Fabry physician and patient community to help ensure that the reduced product supply was distributed according to clinical guidelines. To date, these conservation measures have been successful. Today, Genzyme has enough Fabrazyme inventory to cover 80 percent of forecasted demand through October, the last remaining month of the original dose conservation plan. However, to help ensure the global availability of the remaining Fabrazyme inventory until new product is available, Genzyme will begin shipping enough products to meet approximately 30 percent of forecasted global patient demand starting October 1st, until the end of 2009. Revised clinical guidelines are expected to be formulated by stakeholder working groups and regulatory authorities to establish the basis for use of this material. Individual treatment decisions will need to be made by patients and physicians, as locally appropriate, with the aid of these guidelines.

Source: Courtesy of Genzyme Press Release, Cambridge, MA, September 23, 2009, http://www.genzyme.com. © Genzyme Corporation 2008, 2009. With permission.

BIOMANUFACTURING COSTS AND TIMELINES
Manufacturing Cost Estimation

In the early years of healthcare biotechnology, producing and launching a new biotherapeutic was all about bringing a new molecular entity to the world, and creating a therapeutic history along the way. As things progressed, more biopharmas were incorporated, and more companies imitated the success of the history-making Genentech–Eli Lilly alliance. Today, there are more than 200 biotherapeutics in commercial use, and hundreds more are in pipeline. As expected, the name of the game has since changed.

Today's biopharmas are engaged in fierce competition, either with big pharma and generics manufacturers of traditional pharmaceuticals, or with other biopharmas and big pharma competing with their own biotherapeutics. Dwindling R&D productivities, increasing sales and marketing expenses, and rising manufacturing expenses (both capital and variable), are necessitating a change in the biomanufacturing model toward "leaner, and meaner" manufacturing. The result is a significantly increased emphasis on process development, facility development, raw material sourcing, and cost-of-goods visibility. The latter is one of today's biomanufacturing priorities. A variety of models and modeling tools are in use, each with its own advantages and disadvantages. Let us review some of the most commonly applied COGS estimate methodologies.

Calculation-Based Modeling

The simplest method for estimating biomanufacturing COGS is by using calculation-based models. Let us see how they work. The whole manufacturing process is broken down to individual steps, for example, cell bank creation and characterization, scale-up process, upstream phase, downstream phase, and formulation fill and finish. Every single step is then divided into smaller components, for example, the addition of raw materials, mixing, fermenting, separating, isolating, and filling. Every individual component requires certain raw materials (reagents, culture media, water, ammonia, oxygen), various tools (chromatography columns, centrifugation devices), supplementary processes (e.g., bioreactor cleaning), energy, etc. The whole process (usually run in production batches) gives the final product, exhibiting a certain yield.

We have just outlined the biomanufacturing variable costs, that is costs that change by the number of product units produced (move quantities of raw materials are needed for more biopharmaceutical injection vials produced). Superimposed to the variable costs are fixed manufacturing costs, that is costs that do not change by the number of product units produced, for example, capital costs to build the facility, the cost of money borrowed in order to cover capital expenses, as well as various facility-related taxes (state, city, municipal, environmental), temperature control, clean-room conditions, cold chain, water and sewage treatment, insurance, fire safety, security, and remote monitoring. When all the above costs, both variable and fixed, are entered into a detailed software program (starting from the proverbial spreadsheet to a highly complicated, custom-made database), the final cost of goods can be estimated. It then becomes apparent that, for example, producing a single batch of 10,000 prefilled syringes of the biopharmaceutical has cost the biopharma $250,000, bringing the syringe unit COGS to $25. If every single process step, its individual inputs (chemicals, water, and energy) and its outputs (liters of diluents, weight of bulk product isolate and number of final production vials) are monitored, then an initial COGS estimate becomes easily, timely, and economically available. Care needs to be allocated to the assumptions and approximations needed along the process, for example, chromatography column specificity when binding the active substance, or the effect of centrifugation or freeze-drying on the actual production yield.

By going through the calculation-based modeling, a biomanufacturer ends up with a COGS estimate, but no actual insight into where exactly along the process resources were consumed the most. In other words, within the $250,000 production batch cost used above, the total amino-acid tab was $13,000, while chromatography costs $3,000. Apparently, it would be ideal if amino acids were preserved in a subsequent production run.

Activity-based costing (ABC) brings a new dimension in biomanufacturing COGS estimation. Here, individual raw materials and procedural costs are grouped in order to provide cost estimates per activity, for example, chromatographic separation of microorganism cellular material. Here, chromatography becomes an individual "cost center" and is further scrutinized. It may eventually turn out that the addition of nutritional amino acids could not be reduced in cost, but instead, alternative separation methods could reduce the chromatography tab down by 60%, to $1200. An issue with ABC becomes the allocation of fixed costs across cost centers, for example, the payment of taxes or executive salaries per cost center that requires certain assumptions on its own.

Monte Carlo Simulations   In the costing processes described above, all costs were recorded as individual and factual parameters. For example, amino acid costs and water treatment costs were recorded as such, and a total cost was devised. To take a calculation-based model to the next level of sophistication and to extend a simple cost analysis, Monte Carlo simulations can be useful.

Let us hypothesize that instead of purchasing and adding individual amino acids, a biomanufacturer obtained access to a raw protein source, combining several of the amino acids previously bought separately. Or, by adding oxygen at a final bioreactor concentration of X, a better production yield was achieved than by adding oxygen at a concentration of Y. A Monte Carlo simulation, named for the casinos of Monte Carlo, Monaco, uses statistical simulation of a process or model to analyze a multitude of outputs and scenarios. By the use of statistical models, a biomanufacturer can input alternative scenarios and compare the final costs estimated for each scenario. It is exactly this possibility of mixing and matching materials, devices, processes, and durations that can significantly improve cost visibility and lead to significant production yield increases and cost decreases.

A new parameter entering the COGS estimate through statistical modeling is the statistical dimension of each scenario evaluated, often called a "probability density function (PDF)." After the PDF of oxygen dilution is estimated, alternative scenarios of replacing raw materials or altering conditions can be tried and compared.

Discrete Event Modeling   Now let us go back to the previous cost models, for a moment. We have either added raw material and process costs, or estimated both individually, and then mixed and matched them in alternative scenarios. Have we missed anything? The answer is yes. There are still more parameters we should not have ignored in our cost estimates. Let us hypothesize that after each raw material is received at the manufacturing facility, it is sterilized in a dedicated facility by a team of three production workers. The team is well trained, experienced, and conscientious. However, they have been told by their predecessors that in-between sterilization runs the device needs to be kept open to cool at room temperature, for about 8 h. And later down the production process, another team is laboring on the chromatography columns by eluting them with ethanol in-between runs for 14 h. Is there a new parameter emerging that we have never taken into consideration in our previous models? Yes! Time lost in-between processes, processes run successively, while they could have run concurrently. Devices replaced every four production batches, instead of six. Errors acceptable by personnel up to 0.5% of yield. Replacement times, cooling times, downtimes, instrument sensitivities, wastage, absenteeism, and more.

The process of taking all these new parameters into consideration is achieved by discrete event modeling. In other words, another software tool is implemented, encompassing materials, processes, tools, costs, errors, delays, designs, specifications, and variations that all play a role in biomanufacturing COGS. Here everything is brought under the sun. The resulting insight is far superior to previous models. For example, if scale-up is done on a facility's ground floor, and downstream purification is done on the first floor of an adjacent facility, transportation of the unfinished product between facilities leads to time delays, resulting in two production batches per month, instead of three! Voila! Biopharmaceutical manufacturing costs have been estimated by experts, for either low-dosage or high-dosage biopharmaceuticals. Figure 7.3, indicates the respective costs involved, while Table 7.17 provides selected biomanufacturing cost examples of protein therapeutics.

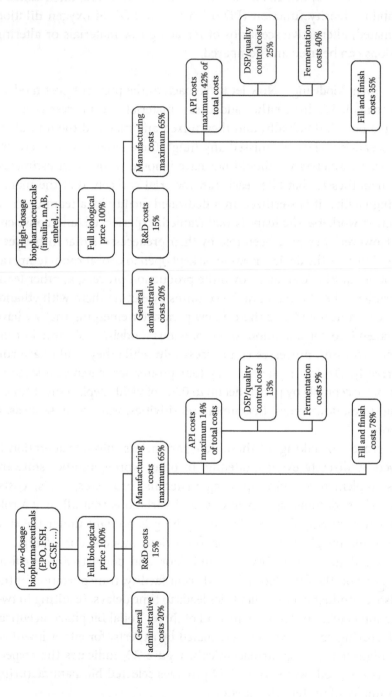

FIGURE 7.3 Biopharmaceutical manufacturing costs (CoGS).

TABLE 7.17   Biomanufacturing Cost Examples of Protein
Therapeutics

	Biomanufacturing Cost
Insulin	$375/kg
Tissue plasminogen activator	$23,000/kg
Human growth hormone	$35,000/kg
Erythropoetin (Epogen)	$840,000/kg

Source: Courtesy of Committee on Bioprocess Engineering, National Research Council, *Putting Biotechnology to Work: Bioprocess Engineering*, Washington, DC, 132 pp, 1992. Reprinted by permission from the National Academics Press, © 1992, National Academy of Sciences.

Manufacturing Capital Cost Estimation

We have previously briefly mentioned some of the biomanufacturing costs belonging to the fixed cost category. A major proportion of these belong to capital costs, namely, the significant expenses required to build a new biomanufacturing facility. Table 7.18 describes how a biomanufacturer can estimate its fixed capital costs for a new facility.

CONTRACT BIOMANUFACTURING

We have previously described the complexities, cost requirements, and risks involved with biomanufacturing. We have also reviewed several factors that may lead to unexpected biopharmaceutical over- or under-capacities. Faced with these challenges, biomanufacturers have chosen alternative pathways for manufacturing their products.

For established biopharmas, such as Amgen, Genentech, and Genzyme, significant cash flows, multiple commercial and pipeline products, and gradually growing market shares driving demand have led them to completely internalize biomanufacturing in an effort to control their own destinies. On the other side of the bioindustry spectrum, young, biotechnology start-ups that have never reached commercialization yet have avoided undertaking the huge capital expenses, risks, and capacity constraints associated with in-house manufacturing, opting to outsource their operations to external contract manufacturing organizations, so-called CMOs. In recent years, the latter model has even taken a more extreme turn, with various biopharmas deciding to operate with a small handful of experienced executives leading most of their operations on an outsourced basis. For example, by in-licensing compounds from academia, later giving them to CROs for further development, CMOs for manufacturing, and even contract sales

TABLE 7.18 How Does a Biopharmaceutical Company Estimate Its Fixed Capital Costs Required for a Biopharmaceutical Plant?

Item	Description	Cost	Formula
A	Total plant direct cost		$1 + 2 + 3 + 4 + 5 + 6 + 7 + 8 + 9 + 10 + 11 + 12 + 13 + 14$
1	Land		
2	Equipment		
3	Installation		
4	Process piping		
5	Instrumentation		
6	Insulation		
7	Fire safety		
8	Security		
9	Electrical		
10	Manufacturing vehicles		
11	Manufacturing facilities		
12	Office facilities		
13	Auxiliary facilities		
14	Surrounding space		
B	Total plant indirect cost		$15 + 16 + 17$
15	Engineering		
16	Construction		
17	Inspection and validation		
C	Total plant cost		$A + B$
D	Other plant costs		$18 + 19 + 20$
18	Building permit		
19	Contractor's fee		
20	Contingency		
E	Direct fixed capital		$C + D$

organizations (CSOs) for sales and marketing they have created the virtual biopharma model, which will be further discussed in Chapter 13.

Can We Avoid Outsourcing Our Biomanufacturing?

There are several major factors that induce biopharmaceutical companies to consider bio-outsourcing. These include avoidance of capital expenditures and investment in biomanufacturing; flexibility to meet changing volume requirements; lack of internal biomanufacturing expertise, experience, and personnel; a need to reduce time-to-market for their product(s). According to Ransohoff (2007), based on current industry success rates, the probability of approval for a phase II product is approximately 26%. Therefore, if a company decides to build a manufacturing facility for a phase II product, it faces a 74% chance that the facility will not be needed upon its completion. Not surprisingly, the vast majority of biopharmaceutical companies do not want to assume this level of risk, nor can they afford the cost and time required to build their own biomanufacturing facilities. Instead, many companies choose to outsource manufacturing to CBMOs.

Most industry experts estimate that it costs between $350 and $900 million (depending upon the product) to build, equip, and validate a biomanufacturing facility. Furthermore, it may take as long as 5 years before a dedicated production facility can be built and made operational. Finally, most regulatory experts agree that the decision to build a commercial manufacturing facility should be made around the time a product is in phase II clinical testing. Table 7.19 summarizes the main advantages of building one's own biomanufacturing capacity versus outsourcing.

Key biomanufacturers include the following organizations: Amgen, Wyeth, GSK, Genentech, Novo Nordisk, Intermune, Ligand, Baxter, Genzyme, Biogen, DSM, Diosynth, Lonza Biologics, Merck Serono, Boehringer Ingelheim, Celltrion, Cora Biomanufacturing, Xcellerex, Avecia, GTC Biotherapeutics, Pharming, Eden Biodesign, and Genopole Biomanufacturing Center.

Table 7.20 describes the results of a biomanufacturing outsourcing survey for the period 2006–2011, published by BioProcess Consultants in 2007.

Bio-Outsourcing Disadvantages

Despite its benefits, bio-outsourcing is not without potential drawbacks. For example, Mintz (2005) has listed the following: First, many companies feel that they must maintain manufacturing control over a product to ensure regulatory compliance and product quality. Second, patent and proprietary information concerns can arise. Third, some companies are not willing to invest the time, effort, or costs required to identify, qualify, and transfer technology to a CBMO. Finally, there are considerable tax incentives and benefits for companies that build their own biomanufacturing facilities.

As far as the selection process for a contract biopharmaceutical manufacturer is concerned, Table 7.21 identifies the most commonly used criteria by major biopharmas.

Contract Biomanufacturing Agreement Example: Morphotek®, Inc. and Lonza Group Ltd.

> Exton, PA/Basel, Switzerland, May 19, 2009—Morphotek®, Inc., a subsidiary of Eisai Corporation of North America, and Lonza Group Ltd. jointly announced today that they have executed a manufacturing services agreement to support the development and manufacturing

TABLE 7.19 What Are the Advantages of Building Own Capacity versus Outsourcing Biopharmaceutical Production?

#	Own Capacity	Outsourcing
1	Design/build to optimize process	Need to make decision long before capacity needs are finalized
2	Expertise in manufacturing leads to capacity and improvements for future products	Large capital investment is avoided
3	Control over quality and regulatory issues	New technologies/process improvements may create obsolete or idle internal capacity
4	Enables flexibility in developing long-term strategy for clinical and commercial production	Large companies have leveraged in-house resources with specialized, competent partners
5	Maintain lower cost of goods	Smaller companies cannot master the entire skill range within the industry
6	Possible off-shore manufacturing to decrease tax burden	Even well-established companies may lack the flexibility to implement and perform critical projects in a timely fashion
7	Focus on drug discovery (the science) and leave manufacturing (risk, expertise, investment) to others	Moving multiple projects forward simultaneously
8	Integrate all operations under control of the operating company	Rationalizing manufacturing facilities
9		Reduce and control operating costs
10		Function difficult to manage/out of control
11		Share risks
12		Search for efficiencies in the drug development cycle
13		Extending pharmaceutical company capacity
14		Pharmaceutical industry consolidation
15		Augmenting small sponsor resources and experience
16		Access to specific therapeutic expertise
17		Globalization

of a subset of antibodies in Morphotek's therapeutic antibody pipeline. The agreement will reserve capacity for commercial manufacturing of Morphotek's lead compound farletuzumab (also known as MORAb-003), which recently entered Phase III clinical trials for ovarian cancer under a Special Protocol Assessment (SPA) agreement with the U.S. Food and Drug Administration (FDA). The collaboration between both parties already encompasses several other monoclonal antibodies currently in clinical or preclinical development.

Source: Courtesy of LONZA Press Release, Basel, Switzerland, May 19, 2009, http://www.lonza.com

TABLE 7.20   PCO Outsourcing Strategy 2006 and 2011

% PCO Outsourcing	2006 (%)	2011 (%)
Mammalian cell culture	45	60
Microbial	38	60
Fermentation	15	40
Yeast plant cells	15	35

Source: Ransohoff, T.C., *The Ever-Changing Landscape of Biopharmaceutical API Outsourcing*, DCAT/ISM/ICIS Strategic Sourcing Summit & Showcase, New Brunswick, NJ, October 24, 2007, Posted at: http://bioprocessconsultants.org/PDFs/RansohoffDCAT.pdf. With permission.

TABLE 7.21   How Do Biopharmaceutical Companies Select a Contract Manufacturing Organization?

1	Capacity	Batch size, lead time, location, volume availability
2	Expertise	Production platform, technology base, processes (upstream and downstream), therapeutic area, molecule, environmental sustainability, regulatory validation and approval
3	Deliverables	Deadlines, yields, quality, standard operating procedures
4	Track record	New chemical entities, laboratory to clinical to market completions, number of customers, number of molecules, production lines, customer satisfaction, regulatory agencies
5	Project team	Top management, project team (research, manufacturing, QA, regulatory, legal), responsiveness
6	Risk	Intellectual property, platform, product, facilities, supplier, financial, environmental, regulatory, personnel
7	Price	Per batch, per kilogram, per vial, laboratory versus clinical versus commercial, extra production runs, payment terms
8	Customer service	Technical links (remote monitoring), reporting, motivation, flexibility, willingness to change, inspections, administrative

CONTRACT BIOMANUFACTURING IN NUMBERS

Recent surveys conducted by the American Society for Microbiology and BioPlan Associates, Inc. indicated that in 2004 approximately 35% of biopharmaceutical companies outsourced some of their biomanufacturing activities (ranging from bioprocess development through commercial manufacturing). This number is expected to grow to 47%–50% by 2008. The survey data also showed that a higher percentage of companies involved in microbial fermentation outsourced biomanufacturing activities compared with companies that use mammalian cell culture, since manufacturing using microbial fermentations is considered to be a more "mature" technology than mammalian cell culture.

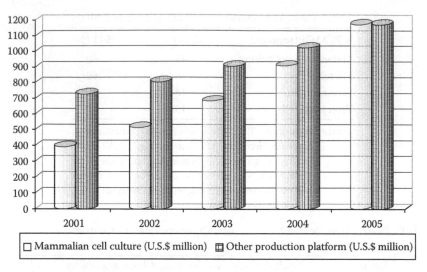

FIGURE 7.4   CMO market revenue evolution.

Figure 7.4 depicts the CMO market revenue evolution, in terms of mammalian cell culture between 2001 and 2005.

According to CBDMT (2008), contract biomanufacturing is a significant market estimated at €2.3 billion this year with an annual growth of about 10%–15%. Pharmaceutical biomanufacturing could account for more than 20% of the global contract manufacturing market in 2012. For both mammalian cell culture and microbial fermentation capacities, product development companies currently control 70%–80% of the industry capacity. But we know that the outsourcing of biomanufacturing will increase in the next 5 years.

Furthermore, according to *Business Insights*, "the global PCM market was worth $26 billion in 2007 and is expected to grow at a CAGR of 11.4% to reach $40 billion by 2011. Catalent is the largest CMO in the world, with revenues of $1.8 billion in 2007. The PCM market is highly fragmented, with the top 10 players in the market holding less than 30% of total market share. Contract manufacturing in India and China is forecast to expand at a CAGR of 20% through to 2011. Biopharmaceutical manufacturing is forecast to have increased by 15% in 2008, driven by sales growth of biologics."

Source: Courtesy of *Business Insights*, Key players in pharmaceutical contract manufacturing: Market developments, outsourcing hotspots and growth strategies, London, U.K., March 23, 2009.

QUESTIONS

1. Which are the main differences in the manufacturing of low molecular weight versus those with high molecular weight pharmaceuticals? Provide examples of molecules and manufacturing methods.
2. Which are some of the alternative biomanufacturing platforms? Provide examples of molecules and platforms.
3. What are the main advantages and disadvantages of the alternative biomanufacturing platforms?
4. Describe the process of either transgenic plant or animal model development. Provide examples of molecules and their manufacturers.
5. Which are the key steps in biomanufacturing process development?
6. Which are the major deciding factors in biomanufacturing's make/collaborate/buy decision framework?
7. How can you forecast future biomanufacturing capacity and demand for any given biopharmaceutical?
8. Which are the main methods used in biomanufacturing cost estimation?
9. What are the advantages of building own capacity versus outsourcing biopharmaceutical production?
10. How do biopharmaceutical companies select a contract manufacturing organization?

EXERCISES

1. Choose one of the top biopharmaceutical companies in the world, according to sales. Then, by using publicly available web resources, describe in detail their biomanufacturing platforms and their respective locations.
2. You are the global head of biomanufacturing at a biopharmaceutical start-up. Their first molecule is approaching clinical trials, and you are in charge of its clinical supplies program. Pick on of the available platforms and defend its merits versus alternative platforms. Use a commercial biopharmaceutical as an example.
3. Transgenic plants and animals have faced significant scepticism concerning their safety. Choose either side of the debate and defend your arguments as best you can.
4. Several commercially available biopharmaceuticals are produced in large-scale bioreactors. Select any given molecule and describe its manufacturing specifics. A good place to start is the companies' own SEC fillings in the United States.

5. You are the global head of manufacturing facilities with a European biomanufacturer. You need FDA approval for your new U.S.-based facility. Find what it takes for such an approval, and summarize the relevant steps and timelines involved.

6. Choose one of the top contract biomanufacturers. Then, study their capabilities and resources, and describe them to your classmates. What do you believe are their unique competitive advantages?

7. The biopharmaceutical industry is full of biomanufacturing incidences, where either product shortages, production contaminations, or production oversupplies have been reported. By using publicly available web resources, select any case study and present what happened.

8. Choose one of the top-selling recombinant beta-interferons in the marketplace. Then, estimate the global cell culture volume required to cover its annual demand. Explain any assumptions you used to reach your estimate.

9. Your biopharmaceutical employer is planning to commercially launch a new recombinant follicle-stimulating hormone (FSH) in the future. Find out which biomanufacturers are producing it anywhere in the world today. Present 10 manufacturing locations as examples.

10. Identify 10 biomanufacturers located in either China or India. What are their manufacturing capabilities and capacities today?

REFERENCES

Amgen Scholars, 2010. Scale-up and manufacturing. Posted at: http://www. amgenscholars.eu/c/document_library/get_file?uuid=8e1f5edd-77e1–48f7– 8b14–1fddde015b27&groupId=14 (accessed on April 7, 2010).

Andersson, R. and Mynahan, R., 2001. The protein production challenge. In Vivo: The Business and Medicine Report, May 2001.

Bhopale, G.M. and Nanda, R.K., 2005. Recombinant DNA expression products for human therapeutic use. *Current Science* 89(4): 614–622.

Boehringer Ingelheim, *Our Expertise in World-Class Contract Manufacturing for Your Success Brochure*, Ingelheim am Rhein, Germany, http://www. boehringer-ingelheim.com/biopharm

Brusick, D., 1998. Transgenics in pharmaceutical development: An evolving role. *Biopharmaceutical Focus* 3(1), August 1998.

Business Insights, Key players in pharmaceutical contract manufacturing: Market developments, outsourcing hotspots and growth strategies, London, U.K., March 23, 2009.

CBDM.T®, The market and business intelligence company reviews. The biomanufacturing market, Press Release, September 15, 2008. Posted at: http://cbdmt. com/index.php?id=5&did=11

Committee on Bioprocess Engineering, National Research Council, 1992. *Putting Biotechnology to Work: Bioprocess Engineering*, Committee on Bioprocess Engineering, National Research Council. National Academy of Sciences: Washington, DC, 1992. http://www.nap.edu/catalog/2052.html

DSM Annual Report 2008, Heerlen, the Netherlands, http://www.dsm.com

Engelhard, M., Hagen, K., and Thiele, F. (eds.), 2007. *Pharming: A New Branch of Biotechnology*. Europaische Akademie, Graue Reihe, 43: Bad Neuenahr-Ahrweiler, Germany, November 2007.

GE Healthcare, 2010. Bioprocess—Target molecules—Recombinant Proteins, Buckinghamshire, England, http://www4.gelifesciences.com/aptrix/upp01077. nsf/Content/bioprocess~target±molecules~recombinant±proteins#

Genentech, San Francisco, CA, http://www.gene.com/gene/news/kits/corporate/vacaville-backgrounder.html

Genzyme Press Release, Cambridge, MA, September 23, 2009, http://www.genzyme.com

GTC Biotherapeutics, Framingham, MA, http://www.gtc-bio.com

International Service for the Acquisition of Agribiotech Applications (ISAAA), 2007. Pocket K No. 26 Molecular pharming and biopharmaceuticals. ISAAA: Manila, May 2007.

KKY Partners, LLC, 2010. Biopharming. PowerPoint presentation posted at: http://www.kkypartners.com/Bio Pharming 8–30.ppt (accessed on April 7, 2010).

Levine, II.L., 2009. Challenges and solutions for biopharmaceutical manufacturing. BioProcess Technology Consultants, Inc., Cambridge HealthTech PepTalk Conference, San Diego, CA, January 15, 2009. Posted at: http://www.bioprocessconsultants.com/PDFs/Levine_Challenges_and_Solutions2009.01.15.pdf

LONZA Press Release, Basel, Switzerland, May 19, 2009, http://www.lonza.com

Mallik, A., Pinkus, G.S., and Sheffer, S., 2002. Biopharma's capacity crunch. *The McKinsey Quarterly*, Special Edition—Risk and Resilience: 9–11, August 06, 2002.

Mintz, C.S., 2005. Outsourcing biomanufacturing. Contract Services Europe, Feb/March 2005, pp. 26–31. Posted at: http://www.biojobblog.com/Outsourcing %20Biomanufacturing.pdf

Rader, R.A., 2008. Chapter one—Expression systems for process and product improvement. *BioProcess International*, Supplement: 4–9, June 2008.

Ransohoff, T.C., 2007. The ever-changing landscape of biopharmaceutical API outsourcing. DCAT/ISM/ICIS Strategic Sourcing Summit & Showcase, New Brunswick, NJ, October 24, 2007. Posted at: http://bioprocessconsultants.org/PDFs/RansohoffDCAT.pdf

V

Marketing

V

gottshatr

## CHAPTER 8

Biomarketing Planning

Expanded development of monoclonal antibodies worldwide supports projected global sales growth of 14% per year through 2012. While the number of new mAb approvals has remained essentially flat in recent years, annual approvals are set to increase—one mAb has been approved in 2008 and four are undergoing FDA review.

Source: Tufts Center for the Study of Drug Development, Outlook 2009, Tufts CSDD, Boston, MA, 2009.

The American Marketing Association (AMA) defines marketing as "the activity, set of institutions, and processes for creating, communicating, delivering, and exchanging offerings that have value for customers, clients, partners, and society at large" (http://www.marketingpower.com/AboutAMA/Pages/DefinitionofMarketing.aspx). According to the Pharmaceutical Research and Manufacturers of America (PhRMA, 2008) "appropriate marketing of medicines ensures that patients have access to the products they need and that the products are used correctly for maximum patient benefit" (p. 12). They go on to proclaim that "our relationships with healthcare professionals are critical to achieving these goals because they enable us to: a) inform healthcare professionals about the benefits and risks of our products to help advance appropriate patient use, b) provide scientific and educational information, c) support medical research and education, and d) obtain feedback and advice about our products through consultation with medical experts" (pp. 3–5).

In general, the most important promotional tools for biopharmaceutical firms are (1) personal selling, (2) advertising, (3) public relations and publicity, and (4) web promotion. Before we delve into these activities in Chapter 9, in the present chapter we focus on the nature of the biopharmaceutical marketing's four Ps, the conduct of environmental analysis, the activities of segmentation, targeting and positioning, as well as planning and budgeting.

THE FOUR Ps OF BIOPHARMACEUTICAL MARKETING

Professors Neil Borden and Jerome McMarthy of the Harvard Business School identified in the mid-1960s a set of company actions influencing the consumer decision to buy the company's goods or services (Borden, 1965). This set of actions was coined "marketing mix," and was comprised of the now famous four Ps, namely, product, place, price, and promotion. In our study of biopharmaceutical marketing, we analyze the importance of the four Ps for biopharmaceuticals, and also explain its similarities and differences from the consumer goods marketing.

Product in the healthcare biotechnology industry is defined as a mass-produced good (or tangible object), in the form of a biopharmaceutical therapeutic medicine (e.g., a pill, capsule, granules, spray, or injection), or a biosynthetic preventive vaccine (usually an injection), or a biotechnological diagnostic test (e.g., home pregnancy test) that is sold to the public. Price is the amount of money a customer pays when buying a product. However, due to the universally precious nature of people's health and the role nations play in preserving their citizens' health, the price of biopharmaceutical medicines, vaccines, or diagnostics is often supplemented by state/private health coverage, or is so-called reimbursed by the states at various percentages of their original selling price. Place is the location where these biotechnology products can be purchased by the customer (at retail locations) or a patient can have them administered (at an outpatient clinic, a hospital, etc.) under medical supervision.

Promotion in the healthcare biotechnology industry is every means of communication used by the biotechnology industry in making its products known to the public, either the physicians who prescribe them, or the patients who use them, or even patients and families considering their use. The promotional activities used by biotechnology companies are usually advertising, public relations, word of mouth, web activities, and personal selling. Figure 8.1 depicts the four Ps of a biopharmaceutical product. Each and every aspect of the four Ps, as well as all promotional activities used by the healthcare biotechnology industry, will be discussed in detail in Chapters 8 and 9. We start our study by presenting how the industry marketing professionals go about their marketing strategies and tactics.

MARKETING STRATEGY

In our previous chapters, we have dreamt of a biotechnology start-up named Advanced Therapies, which was incorporated by a few ex-academic researchers, who patented their invention and later went about attracting the finances to take their drug candidate molecules through vigorous testing and hopefully all the way to commercialization. As the clinical trial phase was approaching, they all realized that they were gradually faced with the enormous task of interacting with various external audiences (e.g., financial analysts, financiers, physicians, regulators, patients, and the media) who not only had their own views and expectations, but also needed to be informed and become interested in the upcoming company product portfolio. It soon became apparent that their pharmacological and molecular biology backgrounds were not sufficient to interact with all their audiences, and decided to hire an experienced biotechnology company marketer who would gradually assist them in setting up a new and critical in-house function. As soon as the marketer was in place, she requested an immediate board meeting at which to make a presentation about how she perceived the company's ideals, vision, mission, and core values. Let us see what these entities mean.

Biopharma Vision, Mission, and Core Values

A company's vision is the ideal future state of the company, as desired by the company's top management. In the healthcare biotechnology industry, a company's vision may take the form of any of these examples below:

- We strive to become the top biotechnology company in the world.

- We wish to be among the top 10 largest pharmaceutical companies in the world by global sales.

- We want to be the worldwide leaders in neurological biotherapeutics.

The company's vision needs to be powerful, visionary, and challenging. In doing so, it seeks to motivate its employees, entice its customers, thrill its stakeholders, and align all its resources behind a common goal. Its time horizon is more than 10 years ahead, so that it does not realign too often, and it gives ample time to all employees to focus all their energy and dedication to the achievement of this audacious long-term goal. Table 8.1 outlines the components of a company's vision statement. Having set the long-term goal, the company's employees then proceed in a top-down approach in setting functional, divisional, therapeutic area, and territory

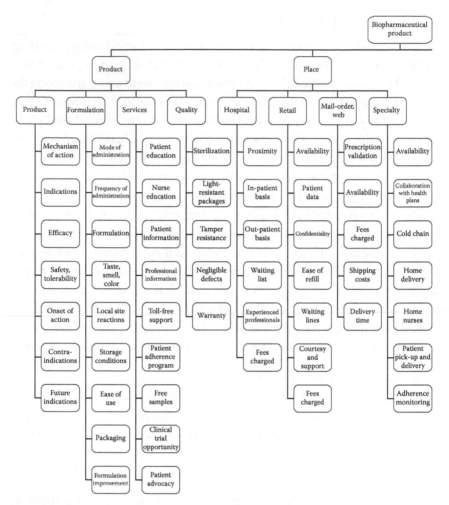

FIGURE 8.1　The four Ps of a biopharmaceutical product.

plans that cover every single company function, from the worldwide to a regional, country, and finally local territory scale. As the table indicates, the company's vision is gradually transformed to an overall strategic plan, and then respective business plans, therapeutic area strategic plans, and global and local marketing plans.

The company's vision is also related to the company's mission and values, which we review and compare below. A company's mission is a set of business objectives and goals that attempt to bring the company closer to its desired vision. The company's mission has thus been also called its reason for existence, credo, or creed. A typical

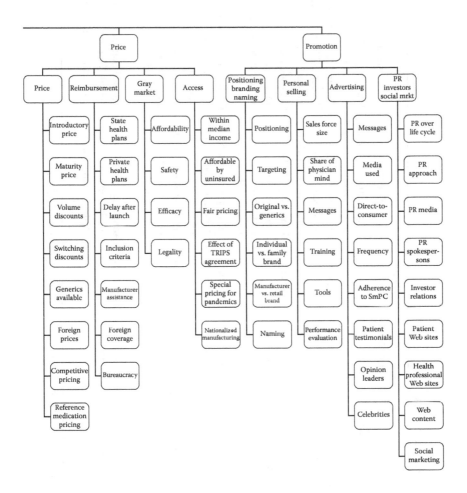

biopharmaceutical mission statement would be the following statement: "We wish to become a market leader in human immunology therapeutics, growing our global volume sales by 10%, by the year 2015, harnessing biotechnology in the fields of rheumatoid arthritis, ulcerative colitis, and psoriasis, in order to provide our prescribers and their patients the best in anti-TNF therapies, and thus becoming their partner-of-choice." Table 8.2 indicates how a biopharmaceutical company can come up with its mission statement.

We have just mentioned how a company's mission statement is progressively transformed into functional, global, and local plans. The whole

TABLE 8.1 What Is the Biopharmaceutical Strategy Framework?

Strategy Level	Content	Area	Responsibility	Time Frame	Objectives	Example
Vision	Desired future company state	Company in the future	Board of directors	Long term	Long-term profitability and survival	Top five global companies
Strategic plan	Which therapeutic areas, which regional markets	Company therapeutic/regional priorities	Executive Committee	5 years	Focus on core competencies and core national markets	CNS and cardiovascular leader in United States, Europe, Asia
Business plan	Portfolio selection Resource allocation	Allocation of resources across company departments	Executive Committee	3 years	Balanced portfolio selection and strategy-driven resource allocation	Sales and R&D investments equally in three therapeutic areas
Therapeutic area strategy plan	Which products, which customers, which claims	Therapeutic area worldwide	Headquarters therapeutic area team	3 years	Building a sustainable competitive advantage for every product	Product X the leading antiasthma choice by respiratory doctors
Global marketing plan	Product, distribution, pricing, and promotional strategies	Therapeutic area marketing mix	Headquarters therapeutic area marketing team	Next year	Designing the elements of each product's marketing mix on a global scale	Intensive distribution, premium pricing, heavy advertising
Local marketing plan	Implementation of marketing mix in national market	SBU within a national market	National SBU marketing team	Next year	Adjusting the global marketing mix strategy to individual national markets	Detailed marketing mix activity plan for product X in market Y

Source: Dogramatzis, D, *Pharmaceutical Marketing: A Practical Guide*, CRC Press, Boca Raton, FL, 2001. With permission.

TABLE 8.2 How Do You Come Up with a Biopharma Mission Statement?

Alternative Names	Role	Contents	Example
Mission	Set the starting points	Core products	To become market leader in …
Corporate objectives	Give directions	Target customers	By yearly growing by …
Reason for existence	Unite the people	Geographic areas	By the year …
Credo	Define product mix	Core technologies	Harnessing biotechnology …
Creed	Define markets	Company values	To provide our partners with …
Corporate belief	Describe organizations	Survival, profit, and growth goals	And becoming the preferred partner
Corporate goals and values	Set geographical areas		
Corporate philosophy	Define market ranking		
Management statement	Identify core technologies		
Reason d'être	Define desired growth		
Guiding principles	Identify the self concept		
Foundations	Set desired public image		
Value statement			
Business purpose			

Source: Dogramatzis, D., *Pharmaceutical Marketing: A Practical Guide*, CRC Press, Boca Raton, FL, 2001. With permission.

strategy cascade is further assisted by declaring the company's guiding values, a valuable tool set of ethical principles, business orientations, and aspirations that help guide the whole organization in its everyday performance. As a stellar example of biopharmaceutical company values, let us review those of Amgen listed below.

For a biopharma values example see: Amgen Values, AMGEN Annual Report 2008, Thousand Oaks, CA, http://www.amgen.com

ENVIRONMENTAL ANALYSIS

Having defined their vision, mission, and values, Advanced Therapies' founders, together with their newly hired chief marketing officer (CMO), are now well into the process of galvanizing their 5 year global strategic plan. Their strategic retreat will take them through four grand steps: (1) environmental analysis (external and internal); (2) market segmentation, targeting, and positioning; (3) choosing a segment strategy; and (4) marketing planning and budgeting. As always, we start from step #1, external analysis. A thorough external analysis focuses on three main views: (1) the macroenvironment, (2) stakeholders and trends, and (3) the competitors.

The Macroenvironment

The macroenvironment comprises of all societal forces that may affect the company's operations today or into the future. Biopharmaceutical marketers often focus on five or six major societal forces, namely, demography, politics, economy, natural forces, technology, and culture.

Demography is the study of human population characteristics, for example, size, location, density, age, gender, race, and occupation. These important parameters are closely monitored in the developed world, and one of the most useful monitoring tools is the periodic conduct of a population-wide census. A census attempts to account for every single person in a given country and may record numerous population parameters, such as birth rate, fertility rate, death rate, life expectancy, education, language, nationality, religion, ethnicity, marital status, and employment. The study of demographic parameters is significant for biopharmaceutical marketing for two critical reasons: (1) They give an estimate of market segment size for the products to be marketed and (2) they describe important characteristics of each segment identified that are interrelated to the product characteristics, and thus give an indication of the importance of each segment on the product's marketing. For example, a common demographic segmentation of the population is groups of people born over certain periods of time, such as the baby boomers, or people born en masse following the Second World War between the years 1946 and 1964. This generation will be turning into senior citizens following 2010, a very significant statistic for biopharmas active in neurological diseases often manifesting among seniors.

The political environment is of paramount importance to the biopharmaceutical industry. This includes the national, federal, state, city, and municipal authorities who set all health-related laws, regulations, and decrees, and thus influence almost every aspect of biopharmaceutical marketing. For example, the political environment is critical in approving a patent, a clinical trial, a product to be commercially launched, the ongoing pharmacovigilance process, the product's pricing, reimbursement, inclusion into formularies, etc. Aspects of the political regulation processes affecting the industry have been studied in Chapter 6 and will also be further studied in Chapters 9 and 10.

The economic environment plays another important role for the biopharma industry. First, the relative strength of national economies plays a direct role in stock market valuations and financings, a make-or-break process important for biopharmaceutical research and development. Second, national currency fluctuations play a role in imports and exports, as well as global profitability of biopharmaceutical multinational corporations. Third, the economic power of national governments dictates their healthcare policies, including the pricing of new treatments, the reimbursement of hospital treatments, medicines, and diagnostics, as well as the life-long insurance coverage and pension schemes of their countries' citizens. Fourth, the economic power (purchasing power) of a country's citizens plays a significant role in seeking diagnosis and treatment, paying for new medicines, or covering the required co-payment for healthcare products and services they receive.

As far as the natural environment is concerned, a biopharma is dependent on the availability of natural resources, such as raw materials, water, air, energy, and more. In addition, it requires protection and safety from natural disasters, such as hurricanes, floods, earthquakes, tsunamis, etc. Furthermore, it needs to abide to strict regulation concerning the natural environment, for example, air pollution, sewage management, crop contamination, accidental cross-breeding from transgenic species, etc.

The technological environment refers to a biopharma's access to high-technology academic institutions, highly educated personnel, technology incubators and incentives, IP protection, available IP, new ideas, tools, devices, platforms, and technologies, venture capital and mature stock markets, and more. The biopharmaceutical industry is especially technology-hungry due to the very nature of genetic manipulations needed to produce new therapeutics, vaccines, or diagnostics. It is an explained phenomenon, therefore, that countries possessing highly advanced technological environments have been the effective beacons for biotechnology advancement, and are also associated with biotechnology IP production and commercialization.

Another aspect of the macroenvironment is the cultural environment, not so much related with fine arts and humanities, but instead the one referring to the common attitudes, values, beliefs, and behavior that defines a country's existence. For example, the attitudes and beliefs toward age and gender, and health and disease, are some of the important factors defining a country's attitudes versus the life-saving products and services of a biopharmaceutical company. Furthermore, the citizens' beliefs on genetic manipulation of the DNA, monoclonal antibodies, diagnostic DNA testing, stem cell research, and transgenic organisms also play a critical role in defining their responses toward healthcare biotechnology. A biopharma's future, therefore, is inextricably related to each market's culture, and huge and continuous efforts need to be allocated toward public education, public relations, and web communications for the company's messages to become known and accepted.

Professor Porter's Five Forces Model

Following the analysis of their external macroenvironment, Advanced Therapies' core team is now ready to study their more closely related, and interactive microenvironment. On the proposal of their energetic CMO, they have all decided to use a very practical, and by now famous, external analysis tool based on the five forces' model, originally proposed by Professor Michael Porter (http://www.isc.hbs.edu/) of Harvard Business School in 1979. According to this model, the five forces affecting the industry are (1) industry competitors, (2) new entrants, (3) suppliers, (4) buyers, and (5) substitutes. Let us analyze them one by one.

Industry Competitors

This force is described by the number of existing competitors, their respective products, their competitive advantages (product differentiation or lower cost), their market shares, the total market and competitor growth, the maturity of the market and the competitors, the competitor strategies, their alliances, etc. It is also associated with reduced competition (due to competitors falling into bankruptcy or diversifying into other markets), as well as the barriers to exit (e.g., stock market conditions, government limitations, or patient outcry) when a competitor wishes to exit the marketplace.

New Entrants

This force refers to the number of competitors who are attempting to enter the specific market. For a biopharmaceutical company with commercialized products fighting Alzheimer's disease, new entrants could become potential competitors in Alzheimer's per se, or in the greater therapeutic area of neurology. The rate and number of new entrants is related to the existing "barriers to entry." These barriers exist either due to governmental regulations, or specific market conditions, or characteristics and strengths of the incumbents themselves. For example, governmental regulations impose clinical trial, marketing approval, pharmacovigilance, pricing, reimbursement, formulary, and custom duties and taxation barriers. Industry incumbents impose economies of scale, lower cost base, preferential relationships with regulators, prescribers and the media, access to distribution channels, competitive advantages, intellectual property, internal know-how, and therapeutic area expertise. Furthermore, market conditions posing an entry barrier may be an access to financing and incentives, exit opportunities through robust stock market exchanges, "buy local" campaigns, or historic barriers.

Suppliers

This is an important force for the biopharmaceutical industry, referring to the bargaining power of industry's suppliers. For biopharmas, important suppliers are those providing raw chemicals, or facility constructors, lab tool and reagent providers, contract research organizations (CRO), contract manufacturers, formulation specialists, syringe manufacturers, and others. These suppliers exert a bargaining pressure on biopharmas, which is related to the availability of alternative manufacturers, their costs charged, the importance of uninterrupted supply, their desire to forward-integrate (e.g., a CRO planning to commercialize biopharmaceuticals of its own), and the quality of products and services provided.

Buyers

Biopharmas are faced with three different classes of buyers. First, their immediate targets, i.e., physicians prescribing their products. Second, individual diagnosed patients suffering from diseases treated by biopharmaceuticals, often called individual buyers. Third, biopharmas often have to convince hospitals, state insurance funds, private insurance companies, or pharmacy benefit organizations (PBOs) to include their products in their critical reimbursement or formulary lists. These buyers are called institutional buyers and also possess a significant bargaining power versus the biopharmaceutical industry.

Substitutes

This force refers to the availability of therapeutic alternatives to the biopharmaceuticals themselves. Substitution may arise from (1) other branded biopharmaceuticals, (2) branded chemical (traditional) medicines, (3) generic substitutes, (4) diet and exercise, (5) occasionally psychological (non-pharmacologic) support, and (6) alternative treatments (e.g., homeopathy, yoga, ancient Chinese medicines, ancient Indian medicines, herbal remedies, meditation, acupuncture). Although the highly sophisticated technology of biopharmaceuticals, as well as the chronic and severe characteristics of certain indications are not easily substituted or treated by alternatives, the significant level of patients discontinuing their biopharmaceutical therapies due to low tolerance and adherence makes these patients candidates for alternative (and more "natural") treatments.

STAKEHOLDER AND TREND ANALYSIS

The Corporate Stakeholder Concept

The analysis of Advanced Therapies' five forces took the core team a full morning, and they all decided to continue into the afternoon with the stakeholder and trend analysis. As the CMO proclaimed, corporate stakeholders are all those groups of individuals who may affect, or be affected by, the biopharmaceutical company's actions. Stakeholder theory was first popularized by Edward Freeman (http://www.darden.virginia.edu/corporate-ethics/video_stakeholder_theory/index.html) in 1983, and today is a critical component of a company's strategic management process.

The existence of distinct stakeholder groups, their individual needs and wants, their influence on the organization, as well as the means by which a biopharmaceutical enterprise may interact with and manage this relationship for the benefit of both sides is of paramount importance for its long-term success and sustainability. Before the core team, however, could begin the strategic management process, they set out to identify and describe them in detail.

Who Are Biopharma's Stakeholders?

A biopharmaceutical company stakeholder is any individual or group that can be influenced by, or exert an influence on the biopharma, whether a positive or a negative one. Stakeholders have often been distinguished into (1) *primary*, that is individuals who are directly affected by an organization's actions, (2) *secondary*, that is those who are indirectly affected, and (3) *key*, that is primary/secondary stakeholders who play a significant role for the organization, either directly or indirectly. Looking into the biopharmaceutical industry, one would quickly identify three major stakeholders, namely, prescribers, regulators, and patients.

However, a quick look into Table 8.3 would reveal a long list of important stakeholders. For example, patient families and advocates, primary care physicians, health management organizations (HMOs), nursing

TABLE 8.3 Which Are the Pharmaceutical Environment's Major Stakeholder Characteristics?

	Patients	Prescribers	Hospitals	Influencers	Financers	Regulators
Who are they	Patient	Physicians	Hospitals (state, private, military)	Opinion leaders	Reimbursement funds	Ministry of Health
	Patient advocates	Non-specialists/ specialists	Clinics	Pharmacists	Insurance companies	Registration Author
	Patient families		HMOs	Wholesalers	Employers	Pricing Authority
			Ambulatory care	Nurses	MCOs	Patent Office
			Nursing homes	Social workers		Drug Organization
				Consultants		Ethics Committees
				Suppliers		Formulary Comm.
Needs	Best possible health care	Medical rationale	Increase clientele	OLs need professional recognition and advancement	Protect patient benefits	Preserve public health
	Lowest cost	Efficacy	Increase market share		Contain costs	Provide coverage
	Information	Safety	Contain costs	Healthcare professionals need access to choice		Ensure efficacy and safety
	Choice	Tolerability				Ensure fair pricing
	Privacy	Quality of life		Pharmacists need information and protection of profit margin		
	Humane treatment	Credibility				
	Efficacy	Practice expansion				
	Safety	Information				
Issues	Rx vs. OTC choice	Up-to-date info	Discounts			
	Compliance		Long payment terms			
	Health organizations	Insurance funds	Thought leaders	Physicians	Dispensers	Patients

(continued)

TABLE 8.3 (continued)   Which Are the Pharmaceutical Environment's Major Stakeholder Characteristics?

	Patients	Prescribers	Hospitals	Influencers	Financers	Regulators
Role	Create diagnosis and treatment algorithms and recommendations	Set reimbursement for diagnosis and treatments May create diagnosis and treatment algorithms	Conduct clinical trials Present trial results Write articles Develop Rx guidelines Early adopters	Diagnose and treat most patients	Chain pharmacies may offer patients screening, patient reminder programs May suggest different but equivalent product options	Seek diagnosis and treatment Increasingly knowledgeable about treatment options
Influence on Rx	High	High	Medium	High	Low	Medium
Ability for biopharma to change behavior	Low	Low	High	High	Low	Medium

Source: Dogramatzis, D., *Pharmaceutical Marketing: A Practical Guide*, CRC Press, Boca Raton, FL, 2001. With permission.

homes, pharmacists, social workers, reimbursement funds, national registration and drug organizations, as well as formulary committees, all play an active and critical role in biopharmaceutical industry's regulation, profitability, and sustainability. A thorough identification, characterization, and plan of action for each individual stakeholder category are therefore an integral part of a biopharma's strategic planning cascade.

Stakeholder Analysis

Stakeholder analysis is the process of identifying each individual stakeholder group, describing their respective role, defining their needs and wants, predicting their attitude and potential response to a specific action by the biopharma organization, and managing that response to the benefit of the biopharma organization. For example, if a biopharma plans to launch an innovative and expensive new biopharmaceutical, it needs to identify the potentially positive reaction from patient advocates and assist in having their voice heard by the regulators, while at the same time predicting the objections of a formulary committee and trying to identify ways for potential inclusion and reimbursement. Table 8.3 identifies the industry's key stakeholders, and describes their respective roles, needs, and critical issues for the industry to manage.

When conducting a stakeholder analysis, the biopharma executives need to identify the groups involved, what is their reason for existence, what matters, why, and when, and what are the potential consequences for the biopharma. Furthermore, as far as the biopharma is concerned, what is their potential sales impact (upside or downside), how can they be managed, who needs to do what, by when, and at what cost for the organization so that all potential upsides are maximized and downsides are minimized or eliminated, if possible.

Trend Analysis

Completing the first part of their external environment analysis, Advanced Therapies' team then becomes occupied with what are the expected major trends (societal, governmental, prescriber, patient, public) that may affect their strategic planning horizon, and what is their respective expected impact. Having defined these trends, the team then sets about defining internal responsibilities in managing the impact of all major trends, as well as deadlines involved, and resources required to

TABLE 8.4   How Do You Identify Important Emerging Trends for Our
Biopharmaceutical Brand?

Potential Trend	Probability	Impact	Key Trends	Type of Impact	(Volume, Price, Cost)	Size of Impact (Upside/Downside)	Effect on Segments	Planned Action	Action Metrics	Responsible	Deadline

Source: Dogramatzis, D., *Pharmaceutical Marketing: A Practical Guide*, CRC Press, Boca
Raton, FL, 2001. With permission.

effectively responding and/or adapting to potential marketing environment changes. Table 8.4 describes a trend analysis template that may be
used by biopharmaceutical industry marketers.

COMPETITIVE ANALYSIS

Competitive analysis is an integral part of a biopharmaceutical strategic cascade. It belongs to the external analysis process, and is the
major theme of many strategic frameworks (see Porter's five forces
above), tools, and templates. The competitive analysis process is comprised of knowledge gathering and analysis, competitor identification, strategic rationale analysis (the way each competitor competes),
competitive advantage analysis (what makes them unique), and SWOT
analysis (their strengths, weaknesses, opportunities, and threats—see
below). In addition, product portfolio analysis (their products, price,
place, promotion), attribute analysis (customer needs satisfaction),
market share and growth analysis, as well as organizational analysis
(how big they are, where they are based, functional division, organizational graphs, and subsidiaries). The expected outcome of a thorough
competitive analysis is the formulation of a robust internal competitive
strategy, its implementation, constant monitoring, and its adjustment
over the planning horizon.

Strategic Rationale

A biopharmaceutical competitor's strategic rationale is comprised of their corporate mission (see above), their competitive stance (offensive, defensive, imitator, niche player), their competitive advantages used in the battlefield (product characteristics, price, or cost-base), as well as their chosen image (positioning) in the minds of their customers (see below), and their strategic responses (observed or anticipated) to industry moves (e.g., how would they react if Advanced Therapies reduced the prices of their future portfolio?).

Thorough analysis of a competitor's strategic rationale gives critical insights into every competing biopharma. For instance, it reveals their strengths and weaknesses, it predicts their future moves, and it counters their attacks, or maximizes the effectiveness of the strategies chosen to fight them. Table 8.5 describes how the core team opted to analyze their competitors, by rating their organizational and product parameters on a scale of 1 = lowest to 10 = highest competitive advantages versus their own profile. Furthermore, as the strategic brainstorming continued into the late night hours, the core team came up with a detailed product head-to-head analysis for their therapeutic area planned for commercial launch (see Table 8.6).

Competitive Analysis Example: Biogen Idec

Competition among products approved for sale may be based, among other things, on patent position, product efficacy, safety, convenience, reliability, availability and price. In addition, early entry of a new pharmaceutical product into the market may have important advantages in gaining product acceptance and market share. Accordingly, the relative speed with which we can develop products, complete the testing and approval process and supply commercial quantities of the product to the market will have an important impact on our competitive position. We may face increased competitive pressures as a result of the emergence of biosimilars. Most of our marketed products, including AVONEX, RITUXAN and TYSABRI, are licensed under the Public Health Service Act as biological products. Unlike small molecule drugs, which are subject to the generic drug provisions (Hatch-Waxman Act) of the U.S. Food, Drug, and Cosmetic Act, there currently is no process in the United States for the submission or approval of biological products based upon abbreviated data packages or a showing of sameness to another approved product. There is

TABLE 8.5   How Do You Perform a Biopharmaceutical Competitor Analysis?

Date

Analyst

Grading	1 = Lowest, 5 = Average, 10 = Highest		
Aspect	**Parameters**	**Product A**	**Product B**	**Product C**
Competitor assumptions	New products			
	New formulations			
	New pricing			
Positioning	Current			
	Future			
SWOT analysis	Strengths			
	Weaknesses			
	Opportunities			
	Threats			
Customer need	Efficacy	5	7	9
	Safety	8	8	7
	Price	6	8	10
Industry competition	Sales volume	5	5	8
	Sales revenue	8	8	9
	Profit	9	6	8
	Market share	6	6	8
Product line competition	Strategy	7	7	5
	Differentiation	8	5	9
	Customer image	7	7	8
	Product price	8	8	7
	Promotion strategy	8	6	7
	Distribution strategy	6	7	5
Organization competition	Marketing structure	7	8	6
	Marketing strengths	8	8	9
	Sales force structure	8	7	7
	Sales force strengths	6	8	8

Source: Dogramatzis, D., *Pharmaceutical Marketing: A Practical Guide*, CRC Press, Boca Raton, FL, 2001. With permission.

public dialogue at FDA and in the Congress, however, regarding the scientific and statutory basis upon which such products, known as biosimilars or follow-on biologics, could be approved and marketed in the United States. We cannot be certain when, or if, Congress will create a statutory pathway for the approval of biosimilars. In Europe, the European Medicines Agency, or EMEA, has issued guidelines for approval of biological products through an abbreviated pathway, and

TABLE 8.6   How Do You Perform a Biopharmaceutical Head-to-Head Product Analysis?

	Product A	Product B	Product C	Product D
Product comparison				
International nonproprietary name				
Cell origin				
Amino acids				
Glycoprotein				
Specific activity				
Dosage form				
Route of administration				
Indication				
Treatment				
Clinical data comparison				
Side effects				
Marketing				
Positioning				
Targeting				
Profiling				
Pricing				
Distribution models				
Promotional activities				
Promotional share of voice				
Main messages				
Sales force size and characteristics				

Source: Dogramatzis, D., *Pharmaceutical Marketing: A Practical Guide*, CRC Press, Boca Raton, FL, 2001. With permission.

the first biosimilars have been approved. If a biosimilar version of one of our products were approved, it could have a negative effect on sales of that product.

Source: Courtesy of Biogen Idec Annual Report 2008, Cambridge, MA, http://www.biogenidec.com

INTERNAL ANALYSIS

Having completed a detailed external analysis over the first day of their marketing retreat, Advanced Therapies' team is now well into the second day facing the critical task of internal analysis. Being new to the biopharmaceutical marketing arena, they continue to be led by their experienced

CMO, who asks them to focus on two supplemental analyses, namely, their resources and situational ones.

Resource Analysis

In Chapter 2, we studied the critical importance of intellectual property management, and in the process we compared some of the characteristics of tangible versus intangible assets. While they are both seen as valuable resources, a biopharma's resource analysis would not be complete if it did not focus on all three types of resources available, namely, tangible assets, intangible ones, and organizational capabilities. A biopharma's tangible assets include their land properties, office and laboratory facilities, equipment, reagents and chemicals, raw materials on hand, tissue cultures and test animals, office furniture and supplies, informational technology, communication infrastructure, and more. For a young biopharma start-up, very few of these tangible resources are fully paid for, while most are leased on a short- or long-term basis.

The respective intangible assets include, first and foremost, its patents, upon which their future product portfolio will be based. In addition to internally created patents, additional patents will have been in-licensed and now belong to the biopharma's patent portfolio. Furthermore, several trademarks will by now have been registered, its scientific personnel will definitely be responsible for dozens of trade secrets, while freedom to operate will also have been purchased for those missing technologies that are needed for product commercialization.

In addition to tangibles and intangibles, Advanced Therapies will also possess certain organizational capabilities that are difficult to match by their future competitors. For example, the companies' founders are all trained molecular biologists and pharmacologists who have a direct in-depth knowledge of the entire R&D process. They also have preferential access to their alma mater's IP portfolio, as well as an impressive scientific publication track record and personal knowledge of the national neurology and immunology medical associations' boards. These are famed opinion leaders with whom they liaise almost daily and plan to use them as future advisors and spokespersons. Furthermore, the company is located at an incubator with superb facilities and shared resources, they have secured exclusivity contracts for their raw materials, they have devised a bioreactor concept that is unique in the industry, and also share a dedication, open communication, camaraderie, and academic atmosphere that makes Advanced Therapies an ideal place to work for bright industry scientists and marketers.

Taken together, their tangible and intangible assets, as well as their unique organizational capabilities make them an empowered organization that is poised to quickly capitalize on their impressive IP portfolio.

Situational Analysis

The second component of their internal analysis focuses around the characteristics of the overall healthcare market, their targeted therapeutic area, their unique competitive advantages, as well as every other organizational aspect, and how these characteristics compare with those of the major industry competitors. By identifying and analyzing several of these parameters and comparing them with the competition, a biopharma can not only describe their market segment attractiveness, but also their company's position vis-à-vis the competition. Table 8.7 provides a detailed example of a biopharmaceutical situational analysis.

Internal Analysis Example: Neulasta (Amgen)

We market Neulasta® and NEUPOGEN® primarily in the United States and Europe. Filgrastim is also marketed under the brand name GRANULOKINE® in Italy. Neulasta® was initially launched in the United States and Europe in 2002 and is indicated for reducing the incidence of infection associated with chemotherapy-induced neutropenia in cancer patients with non-myeloid malignancies. Administration of Neulasta® in all cycles of chemotherapy is approved for patients receiving myelosuppressive chemotherapy associated with at least a 17% risk of febrile neutropenia. NEUPOGEN® was initially launched in the United States and Europe in 1991. Our principal European patent relating to G-CSF expired on August 22, 2006. Upon expiration of this patent, some companies have and other companies may receive approval for and market biosimilar products and other products to compete with Neulasta® and NEUPOGEN® in Europe, presenting additional competition, as further discussed below.

Neulasta® and NEUPOGEN® could face competition in some circumstances from companies marketing or developing treatments for neutropenia associated with chemotherapy, for bone marrow and PBPC transplant patients, and AML. NEUPOGEN® competes with Neulasta® in the United States and Europe. U.S. and international NEUPOGEN® sales have been adversely impacted by conversion to Neulasta®. However, we believe that the conversion in the United States is substantially complete and

TABLE 8.7 How Do You Perform a Biopharmaceutical Situational Analysis?

Factor	Market Attractiveness	S	M	W	Company Position	S	M	W
Market								
Extent								
Growth								
Customers								
Potential								
Product								
PLC stage								
Complexity								
Added value								
Patents								
Differentiation								
Competition								
Concentration								
Capacity								
Vertical integration								
Price sensitivity								
Profitability								
Profit								
Cost structure								
Gross margin								
Personnel								
Structure								
Working Condition								
Quality								
Other factors								
Team spirit								
Government support								

Source: Dogramatzis, D., *Pharmaceutical Marketing: A Practical Guide*, CRC Press, Boca Raton, FL, 2001. With permission.

that a significant amount of the conversion in Europe had already occurred. The following table reflects companies and their currently marketed products that primarily compete with Neulasta® and NEUPOGEN® in the United States and Europe in the supportive cancer care segment.

Source: Courtesy of AMGEN Annual Report 2008, Thousand Oaks, CA, http://www.amgen.com

SWOT ANALYSIS

Continuing on with the internal analysis, countless models and tools have been proposed to assist marketers in their marketing planning quest. One of the most widely used is the SWOT analysis (stands for strengths, weaknesses, opportunities, and threats), originally proposed by Albert Humphrey at Stanford University. This analytic process is focused on a given business objective or venture, and analyzes both internal (strengths and weaknesses) and external characteristics (opportunities and threats) that define its probabilities for achievement. For example, a biopharmaceutical SWOT analysis may be associated with the commercial viability of Advanced Therapies, or the eventual marketing launch of its leading drug candidate in the U.S. market. SWOT analysis is a useful strategic analysis tool in biopharmaceutical marketing. It is imperative that should a SWOT analysis indicate that a given project is not achievable, in a well-thought, objective manner which is validated by all participating organizational functions (R&D, regulatory, marketing, legal), then a different business objective should be pursued instead.

In order for a biopharmaceutical SWOT analysis to be performed, four essential steps need to be completed. First, a set of pertinent business parameters need to be selected as indicators of strengths, weaknesses, opportunities, and threats. Second the parameters need to be weighted, in order for a final score to be derived. Third, the relevant business segments need to be chosen for analysis. Finally, all business segments are scored and are compared with each other for viability, and a priority rating is derived. Table 8.8 describes a basic SWOT model that can be used for a biopharmaceutical SWOT analysis.

TABLE 8.8   How Do You Perform a Biopharmaceutical SWOT Analysis?

Strengths and Weaknesses (SW)	Weight	Segment A		Segment B		Segment C	
		Rating	Score	Rating	Score	Rating	Score
Parameter A							
Parameter B							
Total	100						
Opportunities and Threats (OT)	Weight	Segment A		Segment B		Segment C	
		Rating	Score	Rating	Score	Rating	Score
Parameter C							
Parameter D							
Total	100						

Source: Dogramatzis, D., *Pharmaceutical Marketing: A Practical Guide*, CRC Press, Boca Raton, FL, 2001. With permission.

TABLE 8.9   Which Are Some of the Most Common Examples of Factors Used in a Biopharmaceutical SWOT Analysis?

S (Internal)	W (Internal)	O (External)	T (External)
Best clinical trial program	Complex dosage scheme	Changing epidemiology	Aggressive compet campaign
Contact with authorities	Lack of disease expertise	Changing politics	Comp tech breakthroughs
Cost-effective	Lack of financial resources	Changing world climate	Competitive clin. trial program
Crosses bodily barriers	Lack of human resources	Chronic treatment possibilities	Competitive mergers
Disease management program	Lack of technology know-how	Co-marketing with others	Entry of generics
Efficacy	Limited clinical data	Competitor withdrawals	Eroding market share
Fast onset of action	Limited premarketing effort	Discovery of new diagnostic	Government bias to competitor
Global reach	Low acceptance of new drug	Disease treatment guidelines	Increased regulation
Good company image	Low prescriber awareness	Globalization	Industry rivalry
Good contact with prescribers	Multiple product priorities	Govern. anti-generic barriers	Late market entry
Good patient compliance	Old manufacturing technology	High pricing environment	Loss of tender business
High gross margin	Weak R&D portfolio	Higher disease awareness	Low patient compliance
Innovative class		Low market fragmentation	Low physician compliance
Large patient experience		Many new products vs. old one	Negative publicity
Large prescriber experience		Market growth	New product launches
Large therapeutic category portfolio		Market size	Patent expiration
Long half-time		Patient advocacy groups	Price reductions
Long patent protection		Patient education	Price wars
Mixing during administration		Population aging	Regulatory delays
No impurities		Positive clinical results	
No interactions		Positive publicity	
Patient-friendly dosage		Pricing received	
Patient-friendly formulation		Reduction of trade barriers	
Pharmacoeconomic expertise		Reimbursement received	
Room-temperature storage		Research/Quality award	

TABLE 8.9 (continued)   Which Are Some of the Most Common Examples of Factors Used in a Biopharmaceutical SWOT Analysis?

S (Internal)	W (Internal)	O (External)	T (External)
Safety		Sales seasonality	
Specialized sales force		Societal changes vs.	
Superior segment		disease	
knowledge		Tender business	
Therapeutic category		Unmet therapeutic	
leadership		need	
Tolerability			

Source: Dogramatzis, D., *Pharmaceutical Marketing: A Practical Guide*, CRC Press, Boca Raton, FL, 2001. With permission.

Note: Always choose the 10 most important factors to list. A larger SWOT list defeats its purpose.

As far as the biopharmaceutical strategic parameters to be used as indicators, Table 8.9 lists a large number of the most commonly used indicators for S-W-O-T analysis in the industry.

MARKET SEGMENTATION

What Is a Market Segment

Advanced Therapies' core team is now well into their second day of their marketing retreat, deep into the beautiful countryside in the north of San Francisco. It is time to enter their second phase of strategic analysis, namely, the phase including their market segmentation, profiling, targeting, and positioning. Before they can start, their CMO gives them a brief definition of a market segment. A market segment is a group of individuals or organizations (individual or institutional consumers) that have similar characteristics making them have similar needs for products or services.

Let us think of some potential market segments in the biopharmaceutical industry. First, patients suffering from rheumatoid arthritis in need for a new safe and effective medicine that will improve their quality of life. Second, private medical specialists in rheumatology who are in need for a new medicine to prescribe to their chronic patients. Third, the state health insurance fund covering all state employees, which is in need of a new safe and effective RA medicine that will be not only financially beneficial in the long term, but will also reduce morbidity and absenteeism among the state employee patients.

Unfortunately, the board of directors becomes originally confused. Their basic confusion comes from the definition of a biopharmaceutical market segment, that, is how big or how small can a segment be practically studied and targeted by marketers. Here's some defining criteria that will reduce their confusion from the outset: (1) a market segment is distinguishable from other segments; (2) a segment is homogeneous; (3) a segment responds similarly to a market action, e.g., a medicine's commercial launch; (4) a segment is reachable by a given market action, e.g., a promotional campaign; (5) a segment is commercially meaningful, e.g., a single global patient with limited adherence to prescribed medicines cannot be a viable commercial segment, (6) a segment may appear, change characteristics, or disappear, making market segmentation a continuous and evolving process.

What Is Market Segmentation

Market segmentation is the process of dividing a biopharmaceutical market into distinct market segments. As mentioned above, crude market segmentation would suggest the existence of three groups, namely, physicians, patients, and institutional buyers. However, by following the segment criteria described above, the patient group could be further subdivided into the following segments: (1) never diagnosed, (2) seeking the advice of a physician, (3) newly diagnosed, (4) placed on a diet, (5) prescribed a medication for the first time ("pharmacologically naive"), (6) prescribed a new medication ("switching patients"), (7) patients not responding to therapy ("non-responders"), and (8) patients not adhering to therapy ("non-compliant"), and more.

There are multiple variables used for biopharmaceutical market segmentation. The most commonly used are (1) geographical (e.g., country characteristics, population, climate), (2) demographic (e.g., age, gender, education, income, standard of living), (3) psychographic (e.g., personality, lifestyle, values, attitudes), (4) behavioral (e.g., needs, usage, loyalty, adherence), (5) technological (motivation, attitudes versus biotechnology), (6) pathological (e.g., signs and symptoms, years after diagnosis, relapsing, morbidity, mortality, quality of life), (7) pharmacological (e.g., previously untreated, on treatment, nontolerated, nonadherent, switching), and others.

It is imperative that these patient segments are all important to a biopharma, and special marketing plans may be created for each one in the future. In general, a biopharma marketer is faced with four market segmentation steps: (1) segment identification, (2) segment analysis (profiling), (3) segment evaluation (market attractiveness analysis), and (4) segment selection (targeting). We study these four steps in detail. First, we focus on segment identification and profiling, especially among physicians and patients. Figure 8.2 indicates the significance of segmentation in biopharmaceutical marketing.

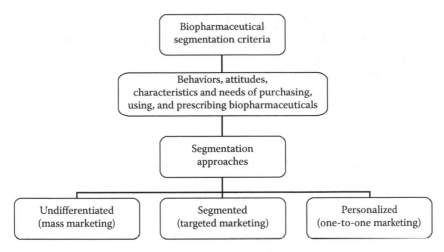

FIGURE 8.2   Why segment in biopharmaceutical marketing?

SEGMENT ANALYSIS (PROFILING)

Having identified a series of distinct market segments, industry marketers are faced with the task of analyzing these segments in detail, a process called segment profiling. The goal of profiling is threefold: (1) identify segment characteristics that are pertinent to a given biopharmaceutical product and rate them for importance (e.g., volume market potential), (2) identify product characteristics that are pertinent to the given segment's needs and rate them (e.g., safety, efficacy), and (3) based on steps 1 and 2, rate the market attractiveness of the chosen segment for the given biopharmaceutical product (e.g., primary, secondary, etc.). Table 8.10 provides a template for performing a biopharmaceutical segment analysis (Step 1), while Table 8.11 gives an example of a biopharmaceutical product attribute analysis (Step 2).

Based on the above two templates, the case is made for the primary market segments to be targeted. A more detailed segment profiling is then performed, where industry marketers attempt to closely monitor today's market characteristics, and further extrapolate these into the future in an attempt to forecast the market segment evolution over the planning period (usually 3, 5, or 10 years ahead). Table 8.12 provides a global biopharmaceutical market data template.

Based on the above primary segment profiling, marketers can then derive the biopharmaceutical product's global market potential over the planning period, by incorporating even more prescriber, patient, and product attributes and assumptions, as seen in Table 8.13.

TABLE 8.10   How Do You Perform a Biopharmaceutical Segment Analysis?

Market Potential	Ther Area A	Ther Area B	Ther Area C
Potential market size			
Available market size			
Served market size			
Average prescription value			
Value market potential			
Volume market potential			

Opportunity	Ther Area A	Ther Area B	Ther Area C
Market growth			
Number of competitors			
Patient satisfaction			
Price sensitivity			
Promotional responsiveness			
Level of habit			
Customer number			
Market complexity			

Source: Dogramatzis, D., *Pharmaceutical Marketing: A Practical Guide*, CRC Press, Boca Raton, FL, 2001. With permission.

TABLE 8.11   How Do You Perform a Biopharmaceutical Product Attribute Analysis?

Product Attribute	Your Prescribers		Competitor A		Competitor B	
	Importance	Score	Importance	Score	Importance	Score
Efficacy						
Safety						
Tolerability						
Adv. events						
Onset						
Other						

	Your Patients		Competitor A		Competitor B	
	Importance	Score	Importance	Score	Importance	Score
Efficacy						
Safety						
Tolerability						
Adv. events						
Onset						
Other						

Source: Dogramatzis, D., *Pharmaceutical Marketing: A Practical Guide*, CRC Press, Boca Raton, FL, 2001. With permission.

TABLE 8.12   How Do You Create a Global Biopharmaceutical Market Data Template?

	2010A	2011E	2012E	2013E	2014E	2015E	Formula
A. Global market size							
Total # of indication patients							Global incidence
Total # of approved sub-indication patients							Global incidence
# of patients targeted for therapy							60%
# of patients on biotherapy							
Market penetration (actual)							
Market penetration (target)							
B. Patients on biotherapy							
Our product paying patients							
Our product free patients							
Total patients on our product							
Competitor A paying patients							
Competitor A free patients							
Total patients on Competitor A							
Competitor B paying patients							
Competitor B free patients							
Total patients on Competitor B							
Total patients on biotherapy							
C. Global sales (units)							
Our product							
Competitor A							
Competitor B							
Total biopharmaceutical units							

(continued)

TABLE 8.12 (continued)   How Do You Create a Global Biopharmaceutical Market Data Template?

	2010A	2011E	2012E	2013E	2014E	2015E	Formula
D. Global sales (thousand USD)							
Our product							
Competitor A							
Competitor B							
Total biopharmaceutical sales							
E. Market statistics							
Our product							
Patient number							
New patient number							
Growth rate in new patient number							
% of total new patients							
Market share (Units)							
Market share (values; USD)							
Market penetration							
Competitor A							
Competitor B							

Source: Dogramatzis, D., *Pharmaceutical Marketing: A Practical Guide*, CRC Press, Boca Raton, FL, 2001.

TABLE 8.13 How Do You Estimate a Biopharmaceutical Product's Global Market Potential?

	2010A	2011E	2012E	2013E	2014E	2015E	Formula
Total female population							
Female population 18–65 years							
% of female population with disease							
% of symptomatic female sufferers							
% of symptomatic female patients seeking Rx							
% of seeking female patients getting Rx							
Total male population							
Male population 30–65 years							
% of male population with disease							
% of symptomatic male sufferers							
% of symptomatic male patients seeking Rx							
% of seeking male patients getting Rx							
Total males + females on Rx (first-line)							
% total patients who fail on reference first-line							
% total potential patients for biotherapy							
Market breakdown data							
Total # potential patients for biotherapy							
% on therapy class A (Our product A)							
% on therapy class B (Our product B)							
% on therapy class C							

(continued)

TABLE 8.13 (continued)   How Do You Estimate a Biopharmaceutical Product's Global Market Potential?

	2010A	2011E	2012E	2013E	2014E	2015E	Formula
Our company sales potential by product line							
Potential patients on therapy class A							
Our Company market share %							
Potential patients on therapy class B							
Our Company market share %							
Potential patients on therapy class C							
Our Company market share %							
Potential patients on our product A							
Potential patients on our product B							
Total potential patients on our products							
Total market share (patients)							
Potential patients on our product A							
Average # of units per treatment cycle							
Average # of treatment cycles							
Potential product A units							
Potential patients on our product B							
Average # of units per treatment cycle							
Average # of treatment cycles							
Potential product B units							

Source: Dogramatzis, D., *Pharmaceutical Marketing: A Practical Guide*, CRC Press, Boca Raton, FL, 2001.

TABLE 8.14   How Do You Identify Biopharmaceutical Market Segment Attractiveness?

Criteria	Weight 1 = High, 5 = Low	Segment A GP	Segment B OB/GYN	Segment C Pediatric	Segment D Oncology
Disease incidence					
Disease prevalence					
Local patient population					
Patients treated					
Patients treated with product category					
Unit market size					
Annual market growth					
Reimbursement for indication					
Physician number					
Competition					
Differential advantage					
Attractiveness Score					

Source: Dogramatzis, D., *Pharmaceutical Marketing: A Practical Guide*, CRC Press, Boca Raton, FL, 2001. With permission.

Identifying a Market Segment's Attractiveness

When biopharmaceutical market segments, for example, several disease indications, are profiled in detail, comparisons can be made as far as their respective market attractiveness is concerned. Table 8.14 provides a useful market segment attractiveness template for comparing four separate therapeutic indications with each other while Table 8.15 provides insight into defining subsegments of a biopharmaceutical brand's potential market, a basic parameter in identifying a market segment's attractiveness.

The marketing literature abounds with several market attractiveness models in the form of matrices. Two of these, originally proposed by business consultants The Boston Consulting Group (BCG; http://www.bcg.com) and McKinsey&Company (http://www.mckinsey.com/) are especially well known in the biopharmaceutical industry and are shown in Figures 8.3 and 8.4, respectively. In the first, products are rated as "stars,

TABLE 8.15   How Do You Define Subsegments of a Biopharmaceutical Brand's Potential Market?

Total population		100%
Potential market	Disease sufferers	20%
	Asymptomatic	5%
Available market	Symptomatic	15%
	Not seeking treatment	5%
Qualified available market	Seeking treatment	10%
	Put under observation	1%
	Put on diet	3%
	Put on treatment	6%
	Treatment non-compliant	1%
Target market	Treatment compliant	5%
	Receiving traditional reference treatment	2%
Penetrated market	Receiving biopharmaceutical	3%
	Competitive biopharmaceutical	2%
Our market share	Our biopharmaceutical	1%

Source: Dogramatzis, D., *Pharmaceutical Marketing: A Practical Guide*, CRC Press, Boca Raton, FL, 2001. With permission.

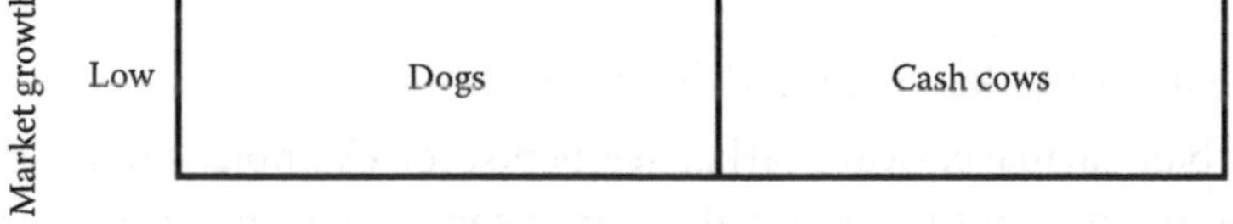

Relative market share (cash generation)

	Low	High
High	Question marks	Stars
Low	Dogs	Cash cows

Market growth rate (cash usage)

FIGURE 8.3   The BCG matrix.

cash-cows, question marks, or dogs" for their respective market attractiveness, while in the second the products' market attractiveness (high, medium, low) is plotted versus their respective marketing position (high, medium, low) to give a nine-square product comparison matrix.

Physician Profiling

The American Medical Association (AMA; http://www.ama-assn.org/ama/home/index.shtml) reports 815,000 U.S.-licensed physicians in

Market attractiveness

Criteria: Disease prevalence and incidence, healthcare dollars, pharmaceutical
treatment dollars, patent protection, disease awareness, disease diagnosis,
in-patient beds, access to care, market growing, reimbursement available,
fair pricing, distribution channels, advertising possible, opinion leader access,
local clinical trials, patient testimonials, celebrity spokespersons,
patient advocacy, marketing organization

		High	Medium	Low
Competitive position Criteria: First-in-class, efficacy, safety, tolerability, onset of action, duration of action, formulation, frequency of administration, contraindications, company brand, product brand, patient base, prescriber base, formulary inclusion, distribution agreements	High	Invest	Selective growth	Grow or abandon
	Medium	Selective growth	Grow or abandon	Harvest
	Low	Grow or abandon	Harvest	Divest

FIGURE 8.4   The GE/McKinsey matrix.

2009, belonging to dozens of medical specialties. This group is a definitive market segment for the biopharmaceutical industry; however, detailed market segmentation is essential before any biopharma embarks on marketing its products and services to the entire group. A simple calculation will verify the importance of physician market segmentation and profiling.

Let us hypothesize that American physicians are to be detailed by biopharma sales representatives, at a rate of five physician contacts per representative working day over 220 working days in a year (the rest is lost to holidays, leaves of absence, training, sales meetings, etc.). If every physician was to be visited at least twice monthly, the required total biopharma sales force would have to be

815,000 physicians	times
2 visits per month per physician	times
12 months	equals
19,560,000 total visits required in a year	divided over
1100 yearly visits per rep (5 × 220)	equal
17,782 biopharma reps required	

Nevertheless, biopharmaceutical products often target small patient populations (small market segments are called specialty or niche), biopharmas are typically small organizations, and the available sales and marketing budgets and organizations are limited. It becomes apparent that physicians need to be carefully identified, profiled, segmented, and the ideal segments to be preferentially focused on, so that the biopharmas involved manage to achieve the optimal promotional presence ("share of voice") with every physician involved.

Prescribing physicians can be segmented according to multiple variables, for example:

- Attitudes versus biopharma, e.g., apathetic, hostile, friendly, enthusiastic, collaborative.

- Attitudes versus patients, e.g., remote, strict, communicative, friendly.

- Benefits sought, e.g., efficacy, safety, tolerability, savings, adherence, and formulary.

- Brand loyalty, e.g., only others, only ours, mixed, balanced.

- Brand usage, e.g., light, medium, heavy, and dedicated.

- Disease characteristics, e.g., chronic, severe, debilitating, relapsing, progressive, final stage.

- Occasions used, e.g., in clinical trial, own usage, family usage, prescribing, advocating.

- Patient characteristics, e.g., age, years diagnosed, prior therapy, relapsing, non-adherent.

- Practice characteristics, e.g., patient base, indication base, biopharmas seen, reps seen, journals read, conferences attended.

- Prescriber characteristics, e.g., geographic, demographic, psychographic.

- Prescriber readiness to prescribe, e.g., unaware, aware, interested, prescribing.

- Product specific, e.g., chemical, traditional, reference, biochemical, revolutionary, experimental, most effective, safest.

- Requirements from biopharma, e.g., executive contact, rep visits, access to trials, samples, promotional material, grants.

- Scientific rationale, e.g., based on training, residency, opinion leader recommendations, treatment guidelines, latest literature, and conference announcements.

Table 8.16 summarizes some of the variables used to segment the prescribing physicians of a global biopharmaceutical brand, while Table 8.17 explains how prescribing physicians can be segmented according to their prescribing strength.

Creating a Biopharmaceutical Product Strategy
Having segmented their target physicians with some of the variables mentioned above, biopharmaceutical marketers may then set out to create targeted promotional strategies geared at satisfying the individual needs and wants of each prescriber group identified and profiled. For example, science-based prescribers may be offered access to clinical trials, inclusion into advisory boards or as trainers and speakers, or scientific journal subscriptions. Therapy-minded prescribers may be offered scientific bibliographies, medical reference textbooks, diagnostic tools and charts, and patient diaries and information to distribute. Finally, economy-minded prescribers may be targeted with patient adherence guidelines, pharmacoeconomic analyses, generic alternatives, etc.

Patient Profiling

According to the U.K.'s Multiple Sclerosis Society (MS; http://www.mssociety. org.uk/), the disease is the most common disabling neurological condition affecting young adults. Around 100,000 people in the United Kingdom have MS, of which approximately 20% have benign MS, 15% have primary progressive, and 65% eventually developed secondary progressive disease.

One of the most widely used methodologies for patient profiling includes the epidemiology tree analysis (commonly referred to as "patient flow" analysis). This is a method following every single patient along their disease progression, starting from undiagnosed patients, and moving into those seeking medical advice, those referred to a specialist, those not assigned to therapy, the patients receiving therapy, dropping out of therapy, switching medications, relapsing, worsening, etc. If every single disease probability is plotted on an epidemiology

TABLE 8.16 How Can You Segment the Prescribing Physicians of a Global Biopharmaceutical Brand?

Prescriber Characteristics					Prescriber Response				
Geographic	Demographic	Psychographic	Prescriber Readiness	Patient Base	Brand Usage	Brand Loyalty	Attitude	Benefits	Occasions
Global opinion leader	Sex	Knowledge-oriented	Unaware	Largest patient base	Light	Only our brand	Industry is evil	Tries all brands	Own participation in clinical trial
Continental	Religion	Clinical trials-oriented	Aware	Top prescriber "Class A+"	Medium	Only competitive brand	Remote	Personally selects more beneficial to patient	Own prescribing while training
Subcontinental	Age	Patient-oriented	Interested	Heavy prescriber or group with 80% of all prescriptions (20/80 rule) "Class A"	Heavy	Prescribes others	Apathetic	Selects more economical to hospital	Own usage when sick
Trade area (EU)	Family status	Team-oriented	Evaluation	Average prescriber "Class B"		Prescribes all brands equally	Communicative	Selects more economical to patient	Own experience from family
National	Seniority	Industry-oriented	Trial	Infrequent prescriber "Class C"		Periodically prescribes different	Friendly	Sticks to formulary	Own experience from saving patient life

Subnational	Career title	Remuneration-oriented	User	Under specialization—with potential "Class D"	Shifting away from us	Enthusiastic	Sticks to international guidelines	Own experience from mentor's influence
Capital	University	Only medicine in their life	Repeat user		Switched to competition	Objective	Selects only branded	Own acquaintance with industry executive
Metropolitan	Hospital specialist	Other interests	Dedicated user		Switched to us for first time	Subjective	Selects only generic	Nobel-prize winning science
Rural	Private specialist	Reserved			Switched back to us	Avoids reps but seeks industry executives	Selects only locally-produced	
Municipal	Family practitioner	Communicative				Listens to patient requests		
	Under specialization	Friendly				Listens to patient advocates		
		Advocate				Industry wining and dinning		

TABLE 8.17   How Do You Perform Physician Segmentation according to Their Prescribing Strength?

Key Account Category	Number of Prescribers	% of Total Prescribers	% of Total Prescriptions
Opinion leaders	5	0.048	5
Class A	50	0.48	35
Class B	3,000	29	45
Class C	7,000	70.47	20
Total	10,355	100	100

Source: Dogramatzis, D., *Pharmaceutical Marketing: A Practical Guide*, CRC Press, Boca Raton, FL, 2001. With permission.

tree, complete with detailed statistics and validated from various sources (medical societies, patient associations, medicines prescribed and consumed, patient hospitalizations, etc.), then a detailed patient profiling emerges.

Armed with epidemiology tree information, biopharmaceutical marketers may create targeted promotional actions tailored at individual segments. For example, for undiagnosed patients a campaign urging them to visit a physician, for patients on medication an adherence-improving campaigns, for patient families an educational campaign, etc. Let us not forget that biopharmaceutical marketing may depend on occasional market assumptions, but is far from being an abstract and subjective procedure. Instead, it is science-based, depends on continuous prescriber and patient surveys, is validated with multiple inputs, and tries to eliminate subjectivity and bias everywhere these may occur. Besides, the rise and fall of young biopharmas relies on the careful strategic analysis, including market segmentation, targeting, and positioning we are studying.

TARGETING AND POSITIONING

Targeting

Having identified and profiled all relevant target segments (including prescribers, patients, institutional buyers, influencers, and others), biopharmaceutical marketers embark upon the targeting process. Here, the main defining variable is market attractiveness; however, there are multiple other variables that play a role in targeting a given segment. Let us review some of them:

- *Market attractiveness*: current volume (biopharmaceutical dosages) and value (U.S. dollars) size, potential volume/value size, growth rate, profitability.

- *Competitor presence*: number, size, sales volume, sales growth, market shares, products, competitive advantages, competitive strategies.

- *Barriers to entry*: product approval, pricing and reimbursement, capital expenses, local market conditions, raw materials, laws and regulations, economies of scale.

- *Government restrictions*: clinical trials, marketing approval, pricing, reimbursement, formulary, pharmacovigilance, taxation, discounts required, local investment required.

- *Prescriber characteristics*: unmet needs, see above.

- *Patient characteristics*: unmet needs, see above.

- *Suppliers and buyers*: bargaining power, existence of alternatives, preferential relationships, local versus multinational.

- *Organizational capabilities*: intellectual property, period remaining under patent protection, product portfolio, competitive advantages, therapeutic area experience and expertise, opinion leader relationships, regulatory relationships, competitive strategy, available investments, know-how, priority, vision-mission-values, and more.

Based on all the above parameters, individual market segments are identified, profiled, and rated, while all relevant biopharma resources and capabilities are rated versus those of existing or expected competitors. The final outcome is the priority target segments (prescribers, indications, patients, institutional buyers, and local versus international) that need to be pursued by the biopharma according to detailed corporate strategy, business, and marketing plans that will be further discussed below. Figure 8.5 describes the biopharmaceutical targeting process we have just discussed.

Positioning

Advanced Therapies' core team was well into the second day of its strategic cascade deliberations. Having completed their market segmentation, profiling, and targeting, they were now confronted with positioning their experimental leading drug candidate, tentatively

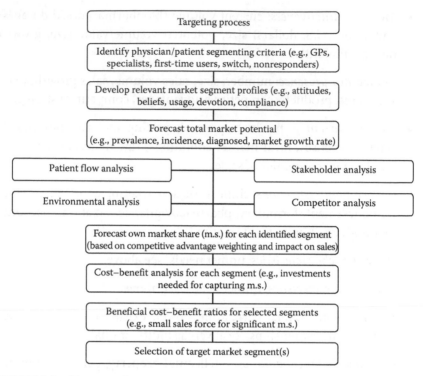

FIGURE 8.5   The targeting process.

named ADTHER57 (for Advanced Therapies' 57th drug lead and first to enter clinical trials). Once again, the CMO asked them to go through a useful marketing exercise. She specifically asked them to think of their own personally favorite nonsteroidal, anti-inflammatory drug (NSAID) and try to describe it in their own words. The descriptions gathered were almost identical: efficacious, kind to the stomach, quick onset of action, inexpensive. There it was, she proclaimed! The NSAID's positioning was born: safe, efficacious, quick-acting, and inexpensive. They now only had to repeat and expand this exercise for their ADTHER57. Let us follow up.

A biopharmaceutical product's positioning is "the place it occupies in its customers' minds." This position is primarily dictated by the product's own characteristics, for example, its intrinsic efficacy, safety, tolerability, onset of action, mechanism of action, and more. However, it is not only its basic pharmacodynamic and pharmacokinetic properties that find their way into the customer mind. It is also the word of mouth, from fellow disease sufferers and their families. It is the opinion and recommendation of medical experts, for example, the president of a medical association. It is the recommendation of a celebrity, who is either acting on its own, or has been employed by the biopharma as its spokesperson. It is also the product's pricing and reimbursement. It is the product's external thermo-insulated carrying case, its external packaging (white carton), the internal packaging (prefilled multi-injector device, its ease of use, its practicality for special patient groups, for example, kids' growth hormone or elderly patients' anti-Alzheimer's patch), and so on. Furthermore, it is the occasional unexpected moments (taken by a mother during pregnancy) taken by someone during its adolescent years, taken during a trip to the mountains, or purchased abroad. All in all, it is all those moments! Their collective influence (conscious and unconscious), own or that of others', stated or experienced, internal or external.

A biopharmaceutical's positioning encompasses all our life experiences with the given medicine. It is also relevant to the product's competitors' positioning. For example, we may consider our favorite NSAID the most effective, but unrealistically expensive (problematic positioning). Or, our own favorite brand may be the quickest to act, but with a syrup's taste to forget! "One more thing," the CMO pointed out. "Our product's positioning is for us to create in the mind of our prescribers and patients. This is the essence of our strategic focus for the next few hours!"

Positioning Process
The biopharmaceutical product positioning process is based on several distinct steps, for example: (1) detailed market segment profiling, for example, describing in depth the disease, the patients, the prescribers, and other stakeholders; (2) identifying the unmet and satisfied needs and wants of each stakeholder; (3) rating the importance of the identified product attributes; (4) rating the possession of these attributes by our own product and those of the competitors; (5) choosing our biggest competitive advantages that would most closely satisfy the needs and wants of our customers; (6) presenting these advantages in an easy to understand, easy to remember, patient-friendly, and compassionate manner; and (7) occupying the desired customer mind space, and repeating our messages, using various communication channels, in such a way that we eventually OWN that space.

A distinction needs to be made between biopharmaceuticals still in development and those already commercially available. In the first-case scenario (that of ADTHER57), our own positioning is based on clinical trial evidence (clinical endpoints, as well as on patient, prescriber, and nurse testimonials), which will suggest an initial positioning to be further refined during the marketing retreat. In the second-case scenario, commercial products already occupy a positioning that was conquered by the product characteristics themselves, as well as the biopharma's actions to "place it" at a certain positioning.

Positioning Strategy

As mentioned above, a positioning strategy is essentially based on the biopharmaceutical product's attributes, and how these better satisfy the unmet needs and wants of the product's target segments. Having chosen the best-suited competitive advantages, a positioning strategy then selects the proper communication messages, vehicles, and frequencies with which to be presented to the target segments. Table 8.18 details the major steps of coming up with a biopharmaceutical brand's positioning.

As far as the major product attributes to be used as potential competitive advantages versus the competition are concerned, the following list shows

TABLE 8.18   How Do You Come Up with a Biopharmaceutical Brand's Positioning?

1 Identify competitive products	Product category and brand
2 Identify determinant attributes	Features, benefits, applications, surrogates, salient
3 Measure existing perceptions	Unaided recall, aided recall, spontancity of brand recall, mental associations (brand and product class, brand and specific attributes)
4 Analyze relative position of alternatives	Identify prescription, non-prescription, and non-pharmacological alternatives
	Use product-positioning maps. Look for gaps
5 Determine preferred set of attributes	Rank all attributes according to their customer preference. Survey prescribers, patients, families, nurses, pharmacists, administrators
6 Define positioning	Competitive strengths of different brands and intensity of rivalry
7 Devise repositioning	Purchase intent share, growth of segments, evolution of ideal points, competitor positioning intensity and strategy, change in brand positions, emerging attributes, new brands, new segments

Source: Dogramatzis, D., *Pharmaceutical Marketing: A Practical Guide*, CRC Press, Boca Raton, FL, 2001. With permission.

a wide variety of potential biopharmaceutical positioning approaches that can be used across therapeutic categories or national markets:

Antidote	in case of overdose there is a specific antidote available.
Application	our product is the only one indicated for this symptom.
Attribute	our product has the fastest onset of action.
Benefit	it is the most efficacious medication for the disease.
Company	ethics we focus on improving the quality of life of our patients.
Competition	we are the uncontested market share leaders.
Competitor	it is just like another product you respect (generic positioning).
Compliance	the treatment allows the highest possible patient compliance.
Dependence	it induces sleep while causing the least possible dependence.
Disease mngmt	we are the only ones involved in disease management (DM), treatment guidelines for the disease.
Dosage	our product is indicated for a wide dosage range.
Endorsement	clinicians or medical societies endorse it.
Experience	of our long company history.
Expiry	our lyophilized product can last up to 3 years.
Formulation	our product comes in a patient-friendly, easy-to-use formulation.
Indication	our product is the only approved in this indication.
Innovation	we are introducing a new biological entity every 3 years.
Interactions	we have shown the lowest drug interaction rate in the therapeutic class.
Manufacturer	of who makes it.
No match	the product is the best, it has no equal.
Pharmacodynamics	the product has shown the best pharmacodynamics profile.
Pharmacokinetics	the product offers the optimal pharmacokinetics.
Price	our product is the most competitively priced.
Product Class	our new generation product sets a new standard of treatment.
Quality	our auto-injector device is the best in the world.

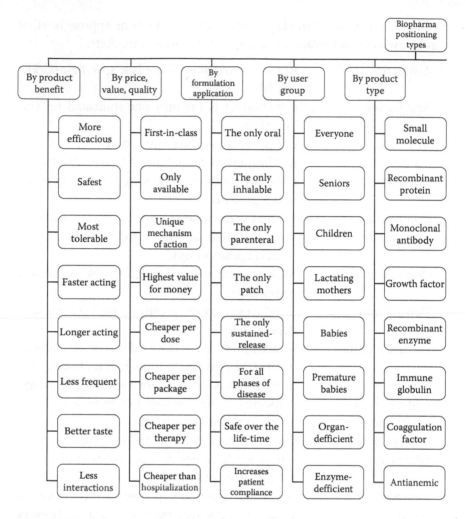

FIGURE 8.6   Types of positioning.

Rank	it is the best selling product.
Reimbursement	our product is the only reimbursed therapeutic option.
Safety	this therapy offers unsurpassed safety.
Service	we offer the best educational service to physicians.
Specialization	we are the only exclusive therapeutic category specialists.
Storage	our product does not require refrigeration, and is stored at room temperature.
Target	the product was created especially for patients like you.

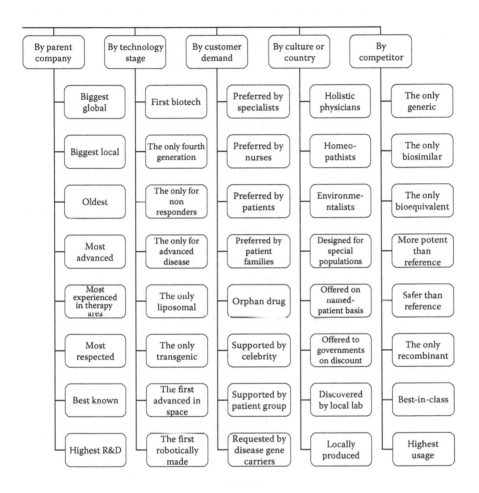

By parent company	By technology stage	By customer demand	By culture or country	By competitor
Biggest global	First biotech	Preferred by specialists	Holistic physicians	The only generic
Biggest local	The only fourth generation	Preferred by nurses	Homeo-pathists	The only biosimilar
Oldest	The only for non responders	Preferred by patients	Environme-ntalists	The only bioequivalent
Most advanced	The only for advanced disease	Preferred by patient families	Designed for special populations	More potent than reference
Most experienced in therapy area	The only liposomal	Orphan drug	Offered on named-patient basis	Safer than reference
Most respected	The only transgenic	Supported by celebrity	Offered to governments on discount	The only recombinant
Best known	The first advanced in space	Supported by patient group	Discovered by local lab	Best-in-class
Highest R&D	The first robotically made	Requested by disease gene carriers	Locally produced	Highest usage

Technology	of how the product was made (biotech, genomics, etc.).
Tolerability	the nasal spray is the best tolerated treatment.
User	we only specialize in your specialty area.
Value	we offer the best value for your hospital costs.
Variety	we offer the widest variety of dosage strengths and formulations.

Source: Dogramatzis, D., *Pharmaceutical Marketing: A Practical Guide*, CRC Press, Boca Raton, FL, 2001. With permission.

The Positioning Statement

Having completed the positioning process, Advanced Therapies' core team needs to come up with a single, brief, memorable, and powerful positioning statement, such as the following: "To (The Target Segment), Brand (X) is the (Frame of Reference) which provides a (Point of Difference)." A biopharmaceutical product's positioning may take several types, for example, based on product benefits, by user group, or compared to the competition. Figure 8.6 summarizes a plethora of biopharmaceutical positioning types.

For a biopharmaceutical positioning example see: ARANESP (AMGEN), http://www.aranesp.com/professional/crf/summary/summary.jsp

Based on the issues discussed above, Table 8.19 provides a concise example of coming up with a biopharmaceutical brand's targeting, profiling, and positioning statements.

Positioning a New Product versus an Existing Competitor

In our analysis above, positioning a biopharmaceutical was seen in the context of launching a new product in a market with one or more incumbents. Now let us take this process a step further. For example, do we always seek to replace the incumbent from its positioning throne and place ours there

TABLE 8.19 How Do You Come Up with Biopharmaceutical Brand Targeting, Profiling, and Positioning Statements?

Parameter	Targeting	Profiling	Positioning
Efficacy	Oncology specialists	Most efficacious in prolonging survival	First choice therapy for metastatic breast cancer
Safety	Gerontologists	Safest choice for patients under multiple Rx	For elderly insomnia sufferers
Tolerability	Pediatricians	No irritation and pain for your young patients	Children under injectable antibiotic treatment
Formulation	Gastroenterologists	Problem-free fever reduction	Antipyretic for patients with stomach side effects
Onset of action	Anesthesiologists	Highest versatility in all your OR procedures	For sleep induction, in anesthetic drug cocktails
Price	General pathologists	A nutritional supplement for all your out-hospital patients	Basic nutritional content, for ambulatory patients only

Source: Dogramatzis, D., *Pharmaceutical Marketing: A Practical Guide*, CRC Press, Boca Raton, FL, 2001. With permission.

instead? The answer is NO. Instead, we need to understand where our product demand will come from: (1) if the demand comes from capturing customers using the competitor product, then our positioning needs to dethrone the competitor; (2) if the demand comes from capturing users who tried and discontinued the competitor, then our positioning needs to outline our superior advantages and less disadvantages; (3) if the demand comes from growing the therapeutic area usage, then our positioning needs to create an entirely new positioning space, which is attempting to cover the previously unmet needs and wants of prescribers and patients.

Positioning a Biopharmaceutical Product Portfolio

Over the short life span of the biopharmaceutical industry to date, a select few biopharmas have managed to commercialize their first products, usually in collaboration with an out-licensing pharmaceutical partner. As the resulting sales royalties started to pour in, a biopharma eventually succeeded in launching its new products on its own, while lately the strongest biopharmas are well into the process of launching their second- and third-generation replacement products. When such an occasion occurs, the biopharmaceutical marketers are faced with the challenge of positioning a biopharmaceutical product portfolio from the base up. The name of the positioning game here is to undergo a detailed market identification, profiling, and positioning process for each product and then try to position them in a distinct and memorable positioning space that may be adjacent and collaborative to each other. For example, the third-generation, longer-acting, and more efficacious product may be positioned as such, while the original product may be placed as an economical solution for initial disease stages, or younger, or even patients with good adherence only. In the opposite case scenario, the different product generations may end up occupying superimposing and competing positioning spaces, resulting in product cannibalization, lost market shares, and lost incomes.

Positioning Our Marketplace Therapeutic Competition

In a different biopharmaceutical market scenario, two competing biopharmas are planning to enter a therapeutic area, each with a new product of its own. It goes without saying that their respective marketing departments will be hard at work devising their ideal product positioning. What happens, however, if the competitor's positioning is an identical or a superior product to our own? Obviously, the two positionings will duel each other and the minds of prescribers and patients will be partially or confusingly captured by the two competitors. In cases like this one, a biopharma may attempt to preemptively position the competitive product at either a different positioning space (e.g., less efficacious, second-line-only, cheaper alternative, generic) or even a negative positioning (e.g., less safe and highly intolerable), or even one that can easily be superimposed and eliminated by ours (e.g., only 5% more efficacious than the reference product, while our product is 30% more efficacious). At the end of the day, the positioning winner will command the therapeutic area and conquer higher market shares, even if the competitor is an improvement over the existing treatments to date.

Positioning a Disease Condition

When developing a new biopharmaceutical, a biopharma may realize that its candidate product may not fully satisfy the unmet patient needs and wants, or that it may be better suited for a niche market segment, or as a second line, or only in combination with another product, or ideal for a lifestyle problem that was not seen as a bona fide disease before. There are multiple examples, and some criticism, of biopharmaceutical companies vying for a positioning space that is not only occupied by the biopharmaceutical, but instead is defined by a new or different condition.

Let us think of some therapeutic condition examples. Makers of infertility, obesity, attention deficit hyperactivity disorder (ADHD), post-menopausal syndrome, erectile dysfunction (ED), overactive bladder (OAB), or AIDS-wasting medicines had to convince medical sceptics, patients and families feeling a taboo, previously uneducated media, or negative formulary committees who, for different reasons, thought that either the condition could not clearly be defined, or that a patient may continue her/his life without serious pathology, albeit with a limited quality of life. When such a scenario arises, biopharmaceutical experts are faced with the difficult task of positioning the condition in the customer's mind-set, for example, detailing its inconvenience, its reduced quality of life, its psychological impact on patients and families, etc. Here the main efforts of the marketers will have to rely on innovator clinical trial researchers, patient and family testimonials, celebrity spokespersons, and patient advocates who are willing to place the new condition under the research microscope or the public eye.

For a condition positioning example see: Erectile Dysfunction (ED), CIALIS U.S. Web site, http://www.cialis.com

For an illustrative summary of the S-T-P process, you may refer to Figure 8.7.

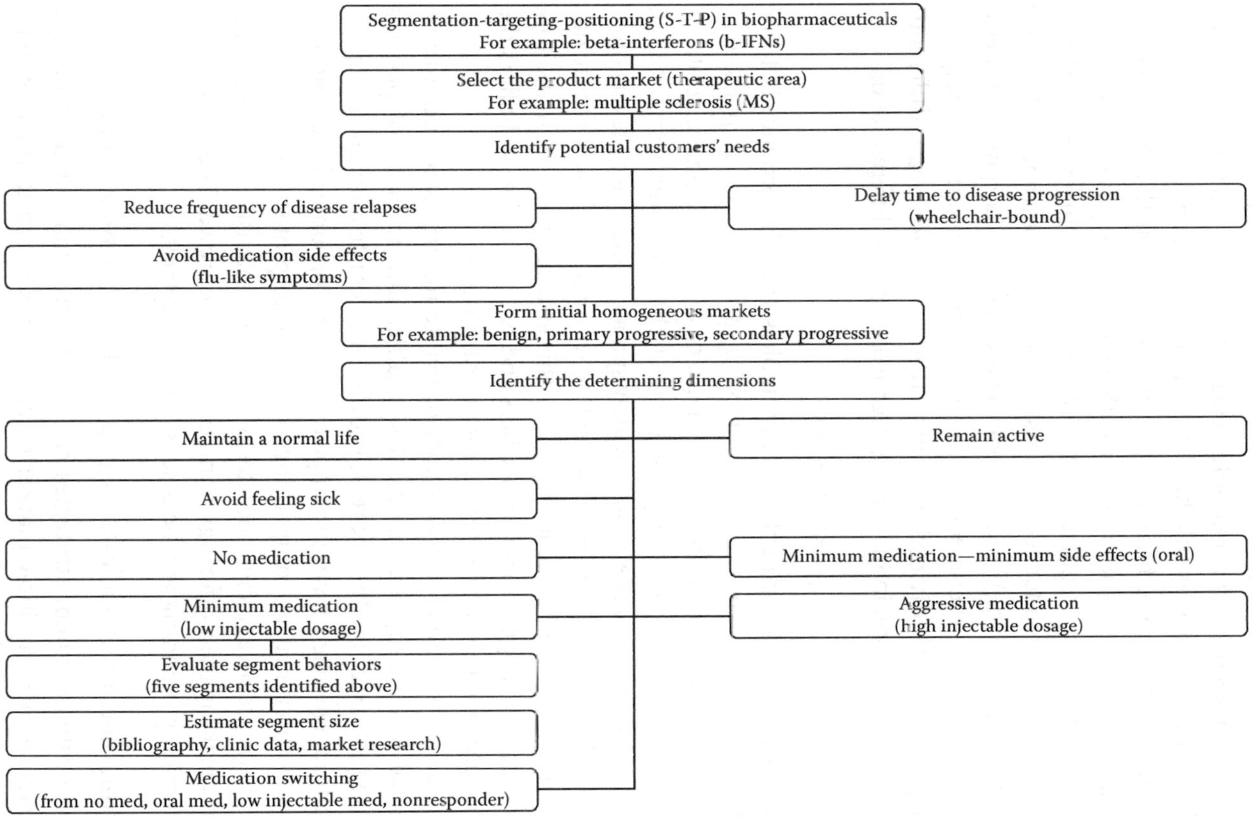

Segmentation-targeting-positioning (S-T-P) in biopharmaceuticals
For example: beta-interferons (b-IFNs)

Select the product market (therapeutic area)
For example: multiple sclerosis (MS)

Identify potential customers' needs

Delay time to disease progression
(wheelchair-bound)

Reduce frequency of disease relapses

Avoid medication side effects
(flu-like symptoms)

Form initial homogeneous markets
For example: benign, primary progressive, secondary progressive

Identify the determining dimensions

Remain active

Maintain a normal life

Avoid feeling sick

No medication

Minimum medication
(low injectable dosage)

Minimum medication—minimum side effects (oral)

Aggressive medication
(high injectable dosage)

Evaluate segment behaviors
(five segments identified above)

Estimate segment size
(bibliography, clinic data, market research)

Medication switching
(from no med, oral med, low injectable med, nonresponder)

FIGURE 8.7   The S-T-P process.

DIFFERENT SEGMENT STRATEGIES

Following the identification of unique market segments and the analysis of their economic attractiveness, competitive intensity, and differential product advantages in each, biopharmaceutical marketing departments must decide on the segment strategies suitable for each of their products. According to Dogramatzis (2001), the final selection may depend on the following factors: market characteristics (size, growth, competition, physician number, consumer attitudes), regulatory environment (reimbursement, pricing, cost containment), product characteristics (differential advantage, life cycle stage, branding, pricing), and company characteristics (corporate strategy, portfolio priorities, therapeutic category expertise, resources). Segment strategies are broadly divided into four categories, namely, mass, differentiated, niche, or custom, in increasing degree of segment differentiation.

Undifferentiated (or Mass Marketing)

An undifferentiated segment strategy implies that the product is to be marketed widely to the masses, employing a homogeneous marketing approach across all prescribing physicians, or dispensing pharmacists, or consuming patients. Obviously, the product characteristics support such a strategy by offering relief from a widely spread ailment (e.g., fever) often seen by all medical specialties, and acting through a safe and efficacious mechanism across all patient segments. This strategy requires marketing tactics that will appeal to all prescribers and patients alike, and offers the advantages of a universally homogeneous campaign.

On the other hand, vast amounts of marketing resources need to be budgeted toward multiple medical specialties and millions of patients around the world. Furthermore, it is difficult to create a unique competitive advantage when trying to appeal to a vast consumer base, and this increases the threat of competition. In trying to protect from competition, pharmaceutical conglomerates often rely on intensive branding campaigns, making their offerings stand out from the crowd. The significance and tactics of branding will be discussed in Chapter 9.

Differentiated (or Multiple-Market or Product-Variety Marketing)

Differentiated segment strategies call for the creation, implementation, and evaluation of multiple marketing campaigns aimed at different market segments. To illustrate the value of a differentiated strategy, let us envision a CNS-oriented biopharmaceutical company with a wide antidepressant portfolio. The company has identified the unique market segments of the adult depressed population, the elderly population, as well as the sufferers from obsessive-compulsive disorder (OCD) that may be helped by antidepressant therapy. In selecting its marketing strategies, the company may position a different antidepressant for each of the above segments (selective market strategy), or all products, at different prices or dosages, to a single segment (single market, product variety), or even one product (at different dosages) for all segments (single-product, multiple market).

Before such decisions can be made, however, the company has to consider the following: Can our product serve the needs of multiple segments? Can we successfully invest in and defend several segments simultaneously? And do we have the resources required? A differentiated segment strategy offers better chances of satisfying different customer needs, but may require increased marketing investments, compared to the undifferentiated strategy.

Single Segment/Niche (or Concentrated or Target Marketing)

Focusing on a single segment (niche market), by building a prohibitive competitive advantage within that segment, and defending against any potential entrant is a common strategy among many small or medium-sized biopharmaceutical companies which do not have the resources to compete with other giants on more and wider market segments. For instance, a biopharma may try to become a world's specialist company in Parkinson's disease, avoiding competing in other CNS therapeutic areas, and diversifying previously existing business units in oncology or rheumatology. Such a strategy offers unique advantages, such as focusing all resources in one therapeutic area, building a formidable portfolio, constructing barriers to entry for new competitors, and implementing a sharply focused marketing campaign.

A niche strategy, however, does not come without disadvantages. Strictly confined R&D programs have inherent risks of producing promising lead compounds failing to progress into marketable products, and thus delaying new product introductions for a long time. In addition, the niche market conditions may abruptly change, by either revolutionary new biological entities launched by a giant new entrant, or even a change in the regulatory environment leading to reduced prices or reimbursement coverage, sharply decreasing the biopharma's profitability. Furthermore, a niche market offers finite growth opportunities and limits the company's long-term financial stability and survival.

Custom (or Single Customer Marketing)

The dilemma of how small of a segment to focus on has also confronted other industry sectors, leading in some cases into the strategy called mass customization, meaning the micro-targeting down to the level of each individual consumer, such as in the case of custom-made blue jeans to fit the individual buyer size. One of the available techniques in targeting individual customers is database marketing, allowing the collection and management of large amounts of customer information. Furthermore, the new phenomenon of web marketing is heavily dependent on this approach, and will be discussed in Chapter 9.

Making multiple product types for multiple markets is not just a matter of transforming the biopharmaceutical discovery and development process. The industry will need to use completely different sales and marketing strategies. It will also need to forge much closer ties between its R&D and marketing operations, if it is to ensure that it creates products and services that are sufficiently good to surmount the rising threshold of innovation (Dogramatzis, D., *Pharmaceutical Marketing: A Practical Guide*, CRC Press, Boca Raton, FL, 2001. With Permission). The personalized medicine business model will be further presented in Chapter 13.

BIOMARKETING PLANNING

Strategic marketing and its incorporation throughout the drug development process is a key to the success of new product development at biopharmaceutical companies. There are several key marketing considerations that should be examined well in advance of a product launch. In order to optimize the marketing efforts in the development of new biopharmaceutical products, it is important for biopharmas to examine these factors while the product is in development.

Biomarketing Planning Phases

In the R&D phase, it is important to identify the intellectual property positions on the compounds and review the discovery efforts to ensure they are in line with the overall strategic priorities of the biopharma. Because Advanced Therapies is smaller and has limited funds for the very expensive development process, it must carefully select the potential products to pursue and then choose which ones to partner for and which ones to develop alone. To do this, the marketing team makes assumptions and builds estimates of the potential U.S. markets for the products and indications that might be coming out of its R&D department. It can then make more informed go/no-go decisions and be more knowledgeable for potential partnering and alliance negotiations.

During the preclinical phase, it is important for biopharmas to begin developing a vision for the potential product as well as to identify the key attributes and value drivers that will make the product succeed. Once they enter phase I clinical trials, the company should be able to identify the minimum attributes that the compound must demonstrate in order to achieve success. During phase I/IIa trials, the company should also start to examine the patient flow within the market they are hoping to enter, identify what clinical endpoints they will eventually have to achieve in order to effectively compete with products currently on the market, and begin to think about the potential economics and pricing of the product they are developing.

During phase IIa trials, the company may also want to begin targeting key physicians, patient groups, and thought leaders in order to solicit important market research information and to increase awareness and acceptance of what the company is developing. After collecting this information, the company should be able to make some informed management decisions regarding the clinical trial strategy going forward and garner more clarity into likely investment levels. The company should also have a solid understanding of the competitive landscape and what the positioning strategy of their product will be.

During the phase IIb/III stages of development, the company should be developing a publications plan, identifying and communicating with key opinion leaders, and finalizing pricing and reimbursement strategies. During filing, the company should work to ensure that they have a competitive label and an appropriate channel strategy. After launch, the company needs to begin the process of life cycle management and start to examine new claims, indications, and formulations for the product. In general, biopharmaceutical marketing tactics follow strategy, as can be seen in Table 8.20. As far as the biopharmaceutical planning process is concerned, Table 8.21 describes the main biopharmaceutical planning stages, while Table 8.22 describes the process of the annual global biopharmaceutical planning cycle.

Furthermore, Table 8.23 outlines the biopharma communication plan process, while Table 8.24 explains how you come up with a biopharmaceutical brand action plan. Finally, Table 8.25 provides a useful template for forecasting the marketing contribution for a biopharma launch.

TABLE 8.20 How Do Biopharmaceutical Marketing Tactics Follow Strategy?

Strategy	Tactics
Become market share leader	Hire and train 15 new sales representatives
Grow sales by 20% every year	Visit key accounts once weekly
Penetrate 10% of market in launch year	Prepare 3 new detail aids per year
Achieve 75% product awareness level	Organize launch symposium on Malta
Have sales force ranked among top 5	Conduct 4 prescriber focus groups
Capture 40% unit market share next year	Conduct DTC campaign during hay fever season
Gain product reimbursement fast	Distribute 1000 new product gimmicks

Source: Dogramatzis, D., *Pharmaceutical Marketing: A Practical Guide*, CRC Press, Boca Raton, FL, 2001. With permission.

TABLE 8.21 Which Are the Main Biopharmaceutical Planning Stages?

Identify and evaluate opportunities	Analyze market segments and select target markets	Plan a market position and develop a marketing mix strategy	Prepare a marketing plan— Execute the plan	Control efforts and evaluate the results
Identify unmet therapeutic needs	Situation analysis	Position product offering	Describe situation	Evaluate sales and shares
Assess total market size	Environmental scanning	Profile product offering	Present therapeutic arcas	Evaluate positioning
Construct patient journeys	Environmental monitoring	Develop product strategy	Describe positioning	Evaluate pricing
Identify target physicians	SWOT analysis	Develop distribution strategy	Define sales objectives	Evaluate distribution
Evaluate physicians' needs	Competitor analysis	Develop pricing strategy	Describe marketing tactics	Evaluate promotion
Identify pipeline candidate	Identify key success factor	Develop promotional mix	Allocate resources	Make adjustments
Assess candidate's profile	Identify leadership niche	Set marketing goals	Perform profit and loss	Measure changes

Source: Dogramatzis, D., *Pharmaceutical Marketing: A Practical Guide*, CRC Press, Boca Raton, FL, 2001. With permission.

TABLE 8.22 What Is the Process of the Annual Global Biopharmaceutical Planning Cycle?

Stage 1	Stage 2	Stage 3	Stage 4	Stage 5	Stage 6	Stage 7	Stage 8	Stage 9	Stage 10
March		April	May	June		July–August		September–October	
Board	Corporate Marketing	Corporate Ther Area	Region	Subsidiary	Subsidiary Marketing	Subsidiary Ther Area	Local Regions	Local Sales Areas	Consolidation and Submission
Vision	Ther areas	Product mix	Growth targets	Growth targets	Product mix	Product mix	Growth targets	Physician targeting	Bottom-up consolidation
Mission	Product mix	Product launches	ROI targets	ROI targets	Timings	Product launches	ROI targets	Physician segmentation	National ther area consolidation
Objectives	Product launches	Product withdrawals	Headcount targets	Headcount targets	Responsibilities	Product withdrawals	Headcount targets	Physician profiling	Subsidiary consolidation
Growth targets	Sales targets	Global internal analysis	Product mix	Product mix	Workshop schedule	Local internal analysis	Physician targeting	Physician prescribing targets	Subsidiary presentation to regional
ROI targets	ROI targets	Global stakeholder analysis	Marketing research update	Timings	Plan writing schedule	Local stakeholder analysis	Physician segmentation	Hospital prescribing targets	Subsidiary plans approved
	Timing	Global competitive analysis	Clinical trial update	Responsibilities	Consolidation schedule	Local competitive analysis	Physician profiling	District prescribing targets	Regional presentation to corporate
	Resource allocation	Marketing research update	Publication schedule	Planning deadlines	Local presentation schedule	Marketing research update	Activities for physicians	Local target consolidation	Regional plans approved

(continued)

TABLE 8.22 (continued) What Is the Process of the Annual Global Biopharmaceutical Planning Cycle?

Stage 1	Stage 2	Stage 3	Stage 4	Stage 5	Stage 6	Stage 7	Stage 8	Stage 9	Stage 10
	March	April	May	June		July–August		September–October	
Board	Corporate Marketing	Corporate Ther Area	Region	Subsidiary	Subsidiary Marketing	Subsidiary Ther Area	Local Regions	Local Sales Areas	Consolidation and Submission
		Clinical trial update	Congress schedule		Regional presentation schedule	Congress schedule	Activities for regulators	Local activities planned	Corporate marketing presentation to board
		Publication schedule	Marketing materials			Marketing materials	Activities for patients	Physician budgets planned	Other functional presentations to board
		Congress schedule	Opinion leader update			Opinion leader update	Activities for media	Sales targets proposed	Board approval of functional and regional plans
		Marketing materials	Organization chart			Marketing support	Sales call planning	Sales budgets proposed	Top-down global communication of targets
		Opinion leader update	Regional and corporate reporting			Marketing templates	Key account planning	Headcount proposals	External announcement of targets
		Marketing support	Timings			Financial templates	Budgets requested		
		Marketing templates	Responsibilities						
		Financial templates							

TABLE 8.23   What Is a Biopharmaceutical Company Communication Plan Process?

1	Communication plan	Who—what—how—when
1.1	Whom to communicate with	Opinion leaders, prescribers, physician associations, hospital and retail pharmacists, nurses, nursing associations, patients, consumers, patient associations, health authorities, wholesalers, journalists, financial community, other external stakeholders, internal audiences
1.2	What to communicate	Content and messages to deliver
1.3	How to communicate	Congresses, advisory boards, external speakers, internal spokespersons, press campaigns, internet, call centers, mailings, sales force, TV, newsletter, intranet
1.4	When to communicate	Phase II plan—pre-launch plan—launch communication plan
2	Communication matrix	Target populations and respective communication vectors
3	Draft phase II comm plan	Define the messages for each target. Messages are focused on company, disease, and compound
4	Final phase II comm plan	Define key messages per target, key communication activities and budget
5	Draft phase III comm plan	Evaluate previous communication actions and further define key messages per target. Messages are focused on product
6	Final phase III comm plan	Define key messages per target, key communication activities and budget
7	Draft launch comm plan	Define the messages for each target. Messages are focused on branding, positioning, messages, visuals, tagline, and promotional material
8	Final launch comm plan	Define key messages per target, key communication activities, and budget

TABLE 8.24   How Do You Come Up with a Biopharmaceutical Brand Action Plan?

Biopharmaceutical Brand:

Action Plan: 2011

Key Success Factor: **Objective:**

Key	Code	Budget Actual	Start	End	Response	JAN	FEB	MAR	APR	MAY	JUN	JUL	AUG	SEP	OCT	NOV	DEC	Impact

Marketing activity

TABLE 8.25 How Do You Forecast the Marketing Contribution for a Biopharmaceutical Launch?

Reporting Currency: USD	Year −3 2008	Year −2 2009	Year −1 2010	Launch 2011	Year +1 2012	Year +2 2013	Year +3 2014	Year +4 2015	Year +5 2016
Volume (units)									
Average unit price (ASP)									
Net sales									
Cost of goods (COGS)									
Gross profit									
Advertising									
Sales promotion									
Samples									
Market research									
Congresses									
Other									
Total marketing expenses									
Medical affairs									
Local clinical trials									
Outcomes research									
Other									
Total commercial expenses									
Marketing headcount									
Medical affairs headcount									
Selling headcount									
Total commercial headcount									
Brand contribution									
Sales force cost									
Consolidated contribution									
Contribution as % of sales									

QUESTIONS

1. Describe the marketing mix for a commercially available biopharmaceutical today.
2. Describe the major societal forces studied under the macroenvironmental analysis for a biopharmaceutical company.
3. Choose a prominent biopharmaceutical company, which is not based in your native country. Analyze the company to the best of your knowledge, and explain Porter's five forces that are shaping its course. A good way to start is to study their latest annual report in detail.
4. Which are the pharmaceutical environment's major stakeholder characteristics?
5. How do you perform a biopharma competitor analysis?
6. Which are some of the most common factors used in a biopharmaceutical SWOT analysis?
7. Describe the major biopharmaceutical segmentation variables, as well as the major steps involved in segmenting prescribers and patients.
8. Describe the BCG and GE/McKinsey matrices used in biopharmaceutical marketing.
9. Describe the biopharmaceutical product positioning process in detail.
10. Which are the main biopharmaceutical planning stages?

EXERCISES

1. Create a table that compares the respective vision, mission, and core values for 10 of the most prominent international biopharmaceutical companies today.
2. Our fantasy biopharma, namely, Advanced Therapies, will be active in the field of autoimmune diseases. As its first chief marketing manager, you need to create its vision, mission, and core values and present them to your board of directors for approval.
3. Choose a U.S.- and a U.K.-based biopharmaceutical company. Then, by studying the characteristics of their respective environments (e.g., Medicare/PBMs versus the NHS/NICE) describe their most important stakeholders and their characteristics.
4. You are a biopharmaceutical executive active in the therapeutic area of diabetes. Present a trend analysis of the most important issues (positive or negative) that are facing your therapeutic area over the next 3 years.

5. Take two global biopharmaceutical competitors in the oncology field. Then, by using their annual report and latest quarterly financials, construct a head-to-head competitive analysis of them.

6. You made it to the post of managing director of the U.K. subsidiary of a global biopharmaceutical, currently under review by the U.K.'s NICE organization. After studying the review progress of an actual program under review, present a SWOT analysis for your organization.

7. Choose a well-known biopharmaceutical and collect its sales evolution data over the last 5 years. Then, by collecting global epidemiology and patient treatment data, attempt to match the actual sales with your retrospective bottom-up sales projections over the same period.

8. You are about to launch your new biopharmaceutical into the vast U.S. market. By using the GE/McKinsey matrix, describe the market attractiveness for your endeavor.

9. You are launching a new recombinant erythropoetin and an orphan drug into the same pharmaceutical market. Which of the different segment strategies do you choose for either?

10. You are the European head of a major biopharma. What is the annual planning cycle that you would like to implement across all European subsidiaries? Who will be responsible for what and when?

REFERENCES

AMGEN Annual Report 2008, Thousand Oaks, CA, http://www.amgen.com

Biogen Idec Annual Report 2008, Cambridge, MA, http://www.biogenidec.com

Borden, N.H. 1965, The concept of the marketing mix, in G. Schwartz (ed.), Erectile Dysfunction (ED), *Science in Marketing*. New York: John Wiley & Sons, pp. 386–397.

Erectile Dysfunction (ED), CIALIS U.S. Web site, http://www.cialis.com

Dogramatzis, D. 2001, *Pharmaceutical Marketing: A Practical Guide*. Boca Raton, FL: CRC Press.

Freeman, E. 1983, Strategic management: A stakeholder approach, in R. Lamb (ed.), *Latest Advances in Strategic Management*, vol. 1. Greenwich, CT: JAI Press.

Porter, M.E. 1979, How competitive forces shape strategy. *Harvard Business Review* 57: 86–93, March/April.

Research and Manufacturers of America, 2008, *The Facts about Pharmaceutical Marketing and Promotion*. Washington, DC: PhRMA, July.

Tufts Center for the Study of Drug Development, 2009, Outlook 2009, Tufts CSDD, Boston, MA.

## CHAPTER 9

Biopromotion

U.S. advertising spend for prescription drugs declined 7.8% to $2.3 billion for the first six months of 2009 over the same period in 2008. Spending on TV ads by pharmas was down 6% to $1.5 billion for the period, while magazine ad spend dropped 20% to $610 million and newspaper ad spend plunged 33% to $49 million. On the other hand, formerly moribund Internet ad spend soared 205% to $119 million for the pharma sector, while radio ad spend rose 83% to $17 million.

Source: Arnold, M., Rx ad spend down 7.8% for first half of 2009, says TNS Medical Marketing & Media, September 16, 2009, Posted at: http://www.mmm-online.com/rx-ad-spend-down-78-for-first-half-of-2009-says-tns/article/149065/, 2009b.

IN CHAPTER 8, WE STUDIED the importance of market segmentation, profiling, targeting, and positioning. The latter attempts to place a biopharmaceutical product in a certain position in the customer's mind. The cumulative place that every biopharmaceutical occupies in the minds of a market's customers is also called a brand. Since this place is of paramount importance for the product's commercial success and profitability, brand management is specifically targeted at applying all pertinent marketing techniques in order to increase the biopharmaceutical product's perceived value to the customer.

By carefully and gradually building a valuable brand, biopharmaceutical marketers aim to increase the product's profitability and sustainability since a brand (1) increases the perceived value of the product in the customer's mind, (2) implies a higher product quality, which can dependably be purchased again in the future, (3) makes a product unforgettable, recognizable, and sought after, (4) increases customer loyalty, and (5) allows a product to be priced with a premium. Based on these factors, a brand can significantly increase a product's sales and profitability, both of which can be used as indicators of a brand's success.

According to Interbrand, one of the world's leading brand consultancies (http://www.interbrand.com/en/Default.aspx), "brands have the power to change the world and to change lives, especially in the health industry." Their brand valuation methodology is based on brand revenue (operating costs, taxes, capital costs), brand earnings, and a brand strength score (market leadership, trend diversification, support, stability, and protection), leading to a brand net present value (NPV). Furthermore, MedAdNews (http://www.pharmalive.com/magazines/medad/) has previously published a list of the global best-selling Rx brands, where biopharmaceutical brands feature prominently at numbers 4 (Enbrel), 5 (Remicade), 7 (Rituxan/MabThera), 15 (Herceptin), 18 (Aranesp), and more in Table 9.10.

BIOPHARMACEUTICAL BRANDING

We have just described a biopharmaceutical brand as the cumulative place it holds in all its customers' minds. These places are occupied by either (1) rational values (my medicine takes away my arthritis pain), (2) emotional values (my medicine allows me to be a full-time mom close to my kids, instead of being bedridden), (3) qualities (my medicine comes with a practical autoinjector device, and is fast acting, and well tolerable), or associated services (my medicine comes with free homecare support and a 24 h hotline). Furthermore, a biopharmaceutical brand may belong to a single product (a rheumatoid arthritis medicine), multiple products (a class of erythropoietic medicines), or a biopharmaceutical corporation (a corporate brand belonging to a California-based biotechnology pioneer).

As mentioned above, a brand is carefully and gradually constructed by biopharmaceutical marketers. This is achieved by providing memorable and enjoyable marketing communications, showcasing and strengthening the product's value and quality, while at the same time the actual customer experience is delivering upon these promises, which consistently satisfy the needs of its customers and increase its cumulative satisfaction and customer loyalty. Let us now review how a biopharmaceutical brand is comprised of multiple layers.

The Layers of a Brand

Biopharmaceutical brands are made up of four layers: the core product or service, the basic (actual) brand, the augmented brand, and the potential brand (see Figure 9.1). Let us see what these mean.

Biopharmaceutical brands are prescribed by physicians and taken by patients for the provision of a core effect(s). For example, a rheumatoid arthritis biopharmaceutical reduces the signs and symptoms of the disease, prevents further damage to one's bones, and helps one's ability to perform daily activities. The same product's actual brand is comprised of actual characteristics, for example, its external packaging, its patient information leaflet (PIL) insert, its autoinjector device, its accompanying instructions for usage, and obviously its pharmacy purchasing or home delivery at a refrigerated temperature, with a guaranteed quality (for example, free of contaminations, in a tamper-resistant packaging), etc. These are all basic product characteristics that the customer expects from this product, wherever it was purchased from. In addition to the previous two layers, the brand may also come with an augmented layer. For example, instead of making the painful trip to the pharmacy, an RA sufferer may expect free home delivery, several initial homecare nurse visits at the initiation of home therapy, easy-to-understand multilingual instructions (in paper or video/DVD), and also significant product reimbursement (or reduced/no patient co-payment).

Finally, the same biopharmaceutical brand may have a potential (or enhanced) layer. For example, the RA biopharmaceutical may have a patient advocacy network built around it, patient networking, patient adherence-improving tools and services, a very famous celebrity acting as its spokesperson, etc. These additional products and services, most of

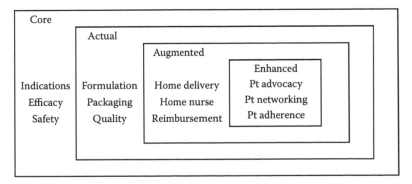

FIGURE 9.1   Layers of a biopharmaceutical product.

which are offered by the biopharmaceutical manufacturer at no additional cost to the patient or his or her insurance provider, make the collective value of the given brand so powerful and desirable that the customer feels a strong, lifelong relationship with the brand, leading to increased therapy adherence and customer loyalty.

BRAND ASSET MANAGEMENT

As mentioned above, by carefully and gradually building a valuable brand, biopharmaceutical marketers aim to increase the product's profitability and sustainability. The creation of such a brand is one of the responsibilities of brand asset management or brand management. Let us see what tasks are included within this critical marketing function. Brand building is the selection of a brand identity, including its name, associated trademark, images, colors, sounds, and other elements used to create a memorable and enjoyable brand experience. Table 9.1 provides a summary of assets used in building a biopharmaceutical brand identity.

Creating a global branding strategy (see Global Biobranding below) is the selection of common strategies, names, messages, images, and communication tactics that are to be used across the world, so that a powerful, global brand identity emerges and creates value for the brand in a proactive, strategic, consistent, multiethnic, and multilingual manner. Building brand architecture indicates the existence of multiple product brands, or product family brands, or corporate brands that need to be carefully constructed so that they complement and support each other, in a clear, strategic, and consistent manner (see product width, length,

TABLE 9.1   How Do You Create a Biopharmaceutical Brand Identity?

1 Description of the brand
2 Audience
3 Tone of voice
4 Background
5 Brand objectives
6 Our customer emotional values
7 Barriers
8 Bonds
9 Communication objectives
10 Positioning promise
11 What will make the customer believe the promise?

TABLE 9.2   How Do You Brand a Biopharmaceutical Product toward Its Various Stakeholders?

Stakeholders	Product	Category	Corporate	Industry
Consumers	+++	+	++	+++
Managed care customers	+++	++	+	+
Payers	+++	++	+	+
Physicians	+++	+++	++	+
Academia	++	++	++	+
Alliance partners	++	+	+++	+
Employees	++	+	+++	+
Advocacy groups	++	+	++	++
Media	+++	+	+++	+++
Stockholders/investors	+	+	+++	+++
Regulators/governments	+++	++	+	+++

and depth below). For example, Table 9.2 provides a concise guide on how to brand a biopharmaceutical product toward its various stakeholders.

Brand rationalization refers to the occasional reduction of the promoted brands, either due to a product discontinuation at the end of its life cycle (see Chapter 12) or an abrupt product withdrawal due to serious side effects, or the introduction of an improved version (new dosage, administration route, formulation, etc.). In this case, the biopharma's brand portfolio needs to be carefully realigned, so that the new products overtake the old one in the mind of the customer, without causing confusion, or allowing a competitor to capture that valuable space.

Brand repositioning (or rebranding) indicates the attempt of a biopharma to reinforce a product's image, by either improving its positioning and moving its position in the mind of the consumer, or attempting to prevent the damage from a competitive brand launching, or moving its positioning due to changing customer demands (for example, patients demanding an increased quality of life, and not only high efficacy with severe side effects). Let us think of an established biopharmaceutical powerhouse, for a minute. The company has been in operation for over 30 years, it currently boasts 20 different commercialized biopharmaceuticals, belonging to six therapeutic areas. It is obvious, that multiple products exist within the same therapeutic area; some of them launched 20 years ago and recently having lost their patent protection, while the respective replacements are competing for the same indication customers. When such a situation occurs, a thorough brand repositioning needs to be carefully designed, validated, and executed, with one goal in mind: multiple brands, possessing clearly defined and adjacent brand positionings, vying for different placements within the customers' minds, and adding to the company's profitability, in a strategically sound, non-confusing, and consistent manner.

The brand repositioning, or portfolio alignment effort, involves three distinct steps: (1) what is the brands' positioning today—how are they perceived: disease-modifying, symptom-reducing only, safe, quick onset, cheap, quality; (2) where should the brands be positioned in the future for maximum cross-coverage—brand A as disease-modifying, first-line, powerful treatment, brand B as second-line, combination-only, and brand C as cheapest generic alternative for uninsured, out-hospital, or low-reimbursement patients and (3) what brand moves are necessary for the portfolio realignment, for example, what clinical trials, opinion leader articles, or patient testimonials can gradually establish these moves?

Brand orientation refers to the importance given to brand management by a biopharmaceutical corporation and its brand management dedication and expertise. For example, a young biopharma launching its first commercial product with limited branding support may lose valuable market share opportunities, even if it has a beneficial product profile (second-generation product), over the older, but more established and better supported existing biopharmaceutical (first-generation) brand.

Biopharmaceutical Brand Width, Length, and Depth

In building biopharmaceutical brand architecture, we have previously mentioned about the existence of multiple branding strategies. Let us see what these may be. Table 9.3 summarizes six different branding approaches, for example, a centralized versus a noncentralized approach, as well as

TABLE 9.3   Biopharmaceutical Brand Strategies (Fictitious Brand Names)

Line extension	Brand extension
Existing brand—Existing product, e.g., new formulation, new dosage	Existing brand—New product, e.g., new longer acting molecule administered once monthly
Multibrand	New brand
Existing product—New brand, e.g., growth hormone for a new indication	New product—New brand, e.g., new coagulation factor acting at different step
Centralized	Decentralized
Artitropin A, Artitropin B, both made by company ARTION	Fertitropin, Artitropin, Erythrotropin made by MICROPROT

TABLE 9.4   Product Mix

Biopharmaceutical Product Mix		
Product Width	**Product Length**	**Product Depth**
Number of different product lines	Number of products within the lines	Number of versions of same product
Long-acting molecule	100 International Units (IU) per vial	100 IU single vial package
Median-acting molecule	50 IU per vial	100 IU 3-vial package
Short-acting molecule		100 IU 5-vial package
		100 IU 10-vial package
		100 IU 3-vial package with autoinjector
		100 IU 5-vial package with autoinjector

launching a new brand versus a brand extension strategy. Furthermore, Table 9.4 introduces the meanings of product width (number of different product lines), product length (number of products within the lines), and product depth (number of versions of the same product).

Biopharmaceutical Brand Portfolio Example: Johnson & Johnson
Fourth largest global biotech company with 2008 sales over USD 6 billion.

> Major brands include: Remicade (Infliximab), Eprex (Epoetin Alfa), Procrit (Epoetin Alfa), ReoPro (Abciximab), Simponi (Golimumab), and Stelara (Ustekinumab). Courtesy of J&J, New Brunswick, NJ, http://www.jnj.com

GLOBAL BIOBRANDING

International government healthcare regulation is imposing, widely diverse, and constantly changing. For example, every single aspect of biopharmaceutical markets is regulated in some way, including clinical trials, brand naming, marketing approval, pharmacovigilance, pricing, reimbursement, formulary inclusion, prescribing, advertising, and more. In addition, global populations are diverse, with different values, attitudes, needs, wants, standard of living, purchasing power, and more. Why then do more and more biopharmaceutical companies adapt global biobranding strategies, under the light of such diverse customer segments, living under different conditions or regulations?

Why Global Biobranding

Despite the diverse conditions mentioned before, the reasons for global biobranding are multiple: (1) Disease manifestations are identical in their nature, excluding minor ethnic differences among populations; (2) global political and economic country unions are constantly expanding (e.g., European Union, British Commonwealth, NAFTA, ASEAN), bringing the standards of living and applicable regulations closer together; (3) increased patient mobility leads to common needs and wants; (4) increased patient access to Internet searching, e-mail, social networking, web telephony, and web conferencing bring patient networking to new levels, never before possible; (5) the patient advocacy movement is becoming stronger, more proactive, highly educated, and media-adept, leading to new demands for increased quality of life across national borders; (6) Opinion leader and prescriber mobility and web access lead to the creation of widely accepted treatment guidelines; (7) international regulatory agencies are moving closer to global harmonization; (8) biopharmaceutical products take longer to develop, leaving reduced time under patent protection, thus necessitating the globally simultaneous commercial launches in every market; (9) as more patient populations enter the global healthcare markets (due to higher standard of living and increased education and transparency), biopharmas are faced with enormous promotional campaign expenses, if they were to be nationally implemented, instead of in a global cascade manner; and (10) increased industry competition, more biopharmaceutical players in every therapeutic area, and rising commercialization risks make the global biobranding strategies a must.

Creating a Global Branding Strategy

Faced with the changing geopolitical and healthcare conditions mentioned above, biopharmaceutical marketers are driven toward the strategic, proactive, global, and coherent biobranding model across all reachable commercial markets. The process of creating a global campaign, however, is not an easy task by itself, and is far from a corporate team devising and cascading its proposal across remote biopharma subsidiary operations. Instead, global biobranding is primarily focused on six contributing elements: (1) the corporate R&D scientists, (2) external opinion leader input, (3) global patient input, (4) dedicated and specialized external marketing consultants (marketing research, pricing, naming, reimbursement, formulary, positioning, and others), (5) corporate therapeutic area executives, and (6) core subsidiary therapeutic area experts (United States, EU, Japan, Asia–Pacific, LATAM). If all these elements are proactively and strategically invited to participate and contribute, through a series of

TABLE 9.5 Global Branding Characteristics

Most Important Components in Defining a Global Brand	Existing Barriers to the Development of Global Brands
Same name	Market differences
Same positioning	Affiliate resistance
Same logo	Legal/regulatory
Same message	Customer preferences/needs
Same brand personality	Different approval times by country
Same target	Varying competitive set by locale
Same look/style to advertising	Central/local budget conflicts
Similar price	Management structure
Same advertising executions	Appropriate marketing talent
Same distribution approach	Lack of a worldwide/networked communications partner

successive biobranding strategy formulation meetings, the final outcome is a globally acceptable, prescriber-validated, patient-driven, and corporate/subsidiary-adapted branding for maximum global impact. Table 9.5 provides a practical summary of some of the required biopharmaceutical global branding characteristics.

BIOBRAND NAMING

One of the most important aspects of biopharmaceutical branding is its naming. Drug names need to be submitted and approved by the relevant regulatory agencies. In addition, they must be distinctive, suggestive of product benefits and qualities, as well as easy and global in their characteristics. Table 9.6 gives several examples of the drug naming prerequisites.

Biopharmaceutical Naming Process

Industry marketers, together with specialized external branding and naming specialists, start working on biopharmaceutical names during Phase II clinical trials. Armed with the initial clinical trial results, they start constructing the product's pharmacodynamic and pharmacokinetic profile that gives rise to distinct competitive advantages. Following a process of physician and patient weighting, the product's unique characteristics are rated versus the competition, and its unique selling points (USPs) start to emerge.

Initial naming candidates focus on the product's USPs, which are either core, actual, or augmented (see layers of a product, above). These USPs may remind the patient of the product's core benefits (e.g., efficacy, safety,

TABLE 9.6   Powerful Biopharmaceutical Brand Names

Distinctive	Suggestive of Product Benefits	Suggestive of Product Qualities	Easy	Global
Bold	Epo...	Effective	To remember: Remindful of disease, human, age, stage, problem, organ, mechanism, zenith	Multilingual
Decisive	Gene...	Safe	To recognize: Synthetic, biotech, natural, pure, nothing like it, life, neo..., advanced, medical	Multiethnic
Inspiring	Huma...	Fast acting	To pronounce: Short, phonetic, rhyming, playful, joyful, artistic	Accent free
High tech	Rec...	Tolerable		Not judgmental Not nationalistic Respectful

Note: Epo... = erythropoietin; Gene... = biosynthetic (through gene alteration); Huma... = human growth hormone; Rec... = recombinant insulin.

onset of action, mechanism of action), its actual characteristics (e.g., a unique dosage and formulation), or its expected—augmented—benefits (e.g., increased mobility, leading to more family-time, and a better quality of life). The naming candidates then follow the following arduous process: (1) individual interviews and focus groups with prescribers, pharmacists, nurses, patients, and their families, (2) preliminary trademark (patent office) and regulatory (FDA) screening, (3) short-listing by biopharma executives, (4) full legal and regulatory search, (5) global linguistic analyses (for being multiethnic, accent-free, not judgmental, and respectful), and (6) final name selection by the biopharma.

Eventually, the chosen biopharmaceutical name is submitted to the authorities for approval (FDA's Guidance for Industry, February 2010). Quite often the submitted names are rejected, leading to significant delays in the product's marketing authorization approval, usually for being similar to other approved products, which tends to lead to prescribing and dispensing errors, with serious consequences.

Naming Techniques

There are various biopharmaceutical naming techniques used by branding experts. Before delving into some of them, we briefly mention the use of sophisticated naming software, which are basically constructed around three pillars: (1) multilingual dictionaries, including ancient languages and even slang, (2) the ability to construct new variants, often combining multiple words or devising a new one, and (3) the ability to prescreen these word constructs for spelling, linguistic, and phonetic user-friendliness.

Armed with this technology, naming experts rely on certain naming techniques that may follow naming trends and fashions. Some of the most commonly used naming techniques are: (1) using an ancient language such as Latin, to borrow a word that means dreaming as indicative for a sleeping aid, (2) a word indicative of the product's attributes, e.g., its mechanism of action, its quick onset, its efficacy, its amino-acid sequence, its enzyme interaction, (3) a word indicative of the product's chemical/biochemical composition, e.g., acid, basic, phenol, monoclonal antibody, (4) an inspirational word, e.g., life-, neo-, mobile-, vivacious-, energy-, joy-, (5) a male-sounding word, e.g., referring to strength, stamina, musculature, competitiveness, (6) a female-sounding name, referring to youth, beauty, motherhood, kindness, caring, (7) a kids-sounding name, referring to truthfulness, exuberance, playing, joy, a smile, (8) a molecular-sounding word, e.g., protein-, gene-, antibody-, inhibitor-, blocker-, and more.

Now let us focus on some actual biopharmaceutical names, for inspiration:

- Avastin, a cancer vasculature inhibitor

- Elegard, an anticancer agent sounding cool and elegant

- Enbrel, enabling relief

- Fuzeon, a fusion inhibitor

- Herceptin, a monoclonal antibody blocking the HER-2/neu enzyme

- Iressa, an anticancer agent with a lovely and calming sound

- Namenda, an NMDA (N-methyl-D-aspartate) receptor inhibitor

- Selzentry, an anti-AIDS medicine blocking cell sentry

- Sutent, an anticancer agent generically named sunitinib

- Zometa, an anticancer agent generically named zoledronate

HOW ARE BIOPHARMACEUTICALS PROMOTED?

Advanced Therapies' team is now well into their third day of marketing strategy deliberations. It appears that their leading biopharmaceutical drug candidate, ADTHER57, has shown promising results in preclinical and Phase I clinical trials to date, and they are now faced with the new task of implementing a new critical function in-house, that of marketing their product portfolio and their company to multiple stakeholders.

In general, a biopharmaceutical firm has four major promotional tools in its possession: (1) personal selling, (2) public relations and publicity, (3) sales promotion, and (4) advertising. Some of these tools may be implemented only after a product's marketing authorization approval, while others may be implemented even during the research and development phase. Furthermore, promotional activities may be directed toward the product portfolio, or the biopharmaceutical company itself. Let us look at these activities briefly.

1. *Personal selling* involves the use of company sales personnel who directly interact with the company's stakeholders, mostly medical professionals, other healthcare professionals, and regulators, in the stakeholder's working setting, and inform them about the company's and product's characteristics and benefits. The sales personnel are usually life-sciences graduates who receive additional company training on the disease, product, company, and competition attributes so that they interact better with the stakeholders. The essence of personal selling is building a personal relationship and eliciting an interaction that is aimed at satisfying the stakeholder's needs and wants, either for information, education, company interaction, inclusion into clinical trials, etc.

2. *Public relations* and publicity involves all the company's activities aimed at interacting with the wider public, for example, the disease prescribers, patients and their families, patient advocates, the general public, the media, financial analysts, investors, and others. The aim is that the company's values, intellectual property, innovation, therapeutic areas, products, and services are widely known, and they in turn elicit a greater awareness, interest, willingness to try, usage, and eventually loyalty to the company's offerings. The essence of public relations is reaching wider audiences, in a more lay, easy-to-understand, and friendly manner.

3. *Sales promotion* usually refers to the consumer goods, where a manufacturer may offer price discounts, or purchase refunds, or free offers,

expecting wider awareness, trial, and hopefully usage of its products. In the biopharmaceutical industry per se, the product pricing is often state-regulated and price discounts and offers are often limited or prohibited all together. However, biopharma manufacturers may offer free services associated with their product's purchase, such as free homecare support, telephone hotlines, reimbursement assistance, and more.

4. *Advertising*, either product- or company-related, can be used where allowed, since product promotion to the general public (direct-to-consumer-advertising or DTCA) is not allowed in most biopharmaceutical markets. Instead, biopharmas may only advertise to medical and healthcare professionals, through their industry publications, conferences, etc.

All the above elements of biopharmaceutical promotion are further discussed below. Table 9.7 summarizes the main characteristics of the four elements of the biopharmaceutical promotion.

We have previously mentioned that while personal selling is aimed at creating personal relationships and eliciting customer interactions, public relations is aimed at reaching wider audiences and eliciting customer awareness and interest. It is easy to understand that all biopharmaceutical promotional activities can thus be rated according to customer interaction and intimacy, forming an advertising and promotion pyramid, such as the one shown in Figure 9.2.

PHARMACEUTICAL PROMOTION IN NUMBERS

IMS Health (http://www.imshealth.com) is the world's leading provider of market intelligence to the pharmaceutical and healthcare industries. According to the company, IMS receives data from more than 139,000 data suppliers covering 730,000 individual dispensing sites worldwide. Data sources include drug manufacturers, wholesalers, retail pharmacies, hospitals, long-term care facilities, and healthcare professionals. IMS Health is also involved in monitoring healthcare-related promotional spending, producing spending data as total U.S. promotional spending between 2004 and 2008 (see Table 9.8) and the U.S. DTC versus R&D costs between 2001 and 2007 (see Table 9.9).

Based on global sales data from 2008, pharmaceutical brands have been ranked by the MedAdNews publication, giving the world's 100 best-selling prescription brands, as shown in Table 9.10, among which several biopharmaceutical brands have been mentioned in this chapter's introduction.

TABLE 9.7   What Are the Characteristics of the Four Elements of Biopharmaceutical Promotion?

	Personal Selling	Advertising	Public Relations	Sales Promotion
Advantages	High credibility and impact sale can be closed	Massive reach Proactive planning	Diverse audiences Large impact	Direct influence on usage Effect on final customer
Communication objective	Indirect sales through prescribers by specialized representatives	Boost image (brand/ corporate) Inform, persuade, remind, sell	Gain public understanding and acceptance	Provide short-term incentive to prescribe/ purchase (trial/rebuy)
Cost per contact	High	Low	Low	Low
Direct feedback	Yes	No	No	Yes
Disadvantages	High cost Inconsistency in message delivery	High overall cost Inflexible message	No immediate effect Diverse audience needs	Significant logistical needs May cause discount war
Market environment	Customer needs more info Product is complex After-sales service is important	Dispersed customers Information and service not critical	Different stakeholder needs Negative industry/ company image	Competitive Price sensitive High switching
Marketer control over message	High	High	High	Low
Message flexibility	High	Low	High	Low
Mode of communication	Direct contact	Indirect	Direct and indirect	Indirect
Regular and recurrent activity	Yes	Yes	Yes	No
Sponsor identified	Yes	Not always	Not always	Yes

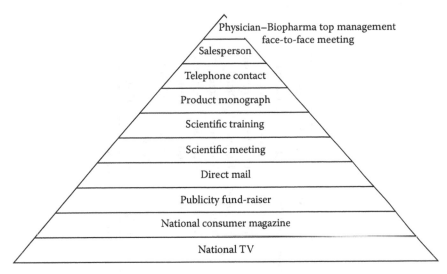

FIGURE 9.2 The advertising and promotion pyramid.

TABLE 9.8   Total U.S. Promotional Spend by Type between 2004 and 2008 (in $ Million)

	2004	2005	2006	2007	2008
Professional promotion	8,064	7,438	7,457	6,905	6,838
Direct to consumer advertising	4,026	4,251	4,897	4,900	4,429
Total promotion	12,090	11,689	12,354	11,805	11,267
Professional journal advertising	544	476	527	470	387
Sales rep details	7,520	6,962	6,930	6,435	6,451
Professional promotion	8,064	7,438	7,457	6,905	6,838
Direct to consumer advertising	4,026	4,251	4,897	4,900	4,429

Source: Courtesy of IMS Health, Norwalk, CT, http://www.imshealth.com/deployedfiles/imshealth/Global/Content/StaticFile/Top_Line_Data/U.S._Promo_Spend_Data_2008.pdf

TABLE 9.9   U.S. DTC versus R&D Costs during 2001–2007 (in $ Billion)

	2001	2002	2003	2004	2005	2006	2007
R&D	30	31	34	39	40	43	45
DTC	2.7	2.7	3.3	4.0	4.2	4.9	4.9

Source: Courtesy of IMS Health, Integrated Promotional Services, Norwalk, CT.

TABLE 9.10 World's 100 Best-Selling Prescription Brands in 2008

1–10	11–20	21–30	31–40	41–50	51–60	61–70	71–80	81–90	91–100
Lipitor	Actos	Avastin	Neulasta	Spiriva	Eloxatin	NeoRecormon	Symbicort	Pegasys	Lucentis
Plavix	Singulair	Cozaar	Crestor	Topamax	Prograf	Tamiflu	Gardasil	Erbitux	Botox
Advair	Protonix	Copaxone	Procrit	Prevnar	Lupron	Arimidex	Humalog	Casodex	Pravachol
Enbrel	Seroquel	Aricept	Levaquin	Zetia	Avonex	Ambien	Pulmicort	Kaletra	Detrol
Remicade	Herceptin	Pariet	Lantus	Zyrtec	Valtrex	CellCept	Toprol	Zometa	Coreg
Nexium	Prevacid	Humira	Vytorin	Celebrex	Lyrica	Rebif	Yasmin	Neupogen	Duragesic
Rituxan	Effexor	Gleevec	Avapro	Lamictal	Tricor	Xalatan	Betaseron	Evista	Cialis
Diovan	Aranesp	Fosamax	Taxotere	Micardis	Viagra	Gemzar	Keppra	Flovent	Prilosec
Zyprexa	Lovenox	Lexapro	Abilify	Benicar	Anandia	Truvada	Flomax	Atripla	Zpsyn
Risperdal	Atacand	Norvasc	Epogen	Cymbalta	Actonel	Depakote	Imigran	Harnal	Cerezyme

Source: Courtesy of Med Ad News, Med Ad News 200: World's best selling medicines, Med Ad News, 15(7), July 2009.

As far as DTC advertising is concerned, it has been argued that it has increased consumers' awareness of drugs and companies. DTC communication was allowed in the United States in 1985 (Palumbo and Mullins, 2002), and has grown substantially to the present day, increasing from an initial spend of $152 million in 1993 to an estimated $2 billion in 2002. Table 9.11 lists the top 20 pharmaceutical products in terms of spending on DTCA in 2005, while Table 9.12 describes the DTCA spending by media between 2006 and 2008.

TABLE 9.11   Top 10 Brands by DTC Spending

Company	Brand	Moving Annual Total (MAT) to November 2008 ($ Million)
Eli Lilly & Co.	Cymbalta	194
GlaxoSmithKline	Advair Diskus	189
BMS/Sanofi-Aventis	Plavix	179
Sanofi-Aventis	Ambien CR	164
Eli Lilly & Co.	Cialis	159
Pfizer	Lyrica	157
BMS/Otsuka	Abilify	136
Pfizer	Lipitor	123
Pfizer	Viagra	122
Sepracor	Lunesta	117

Source: Reproduced from Arnold, M., *Medical Marketing & Media*, 2009. Copyright 2009. Reproduced with permission of Haymarket Media Inc. in the format Other book via Copyright Clearance Center.

TABLE 9.12   DTC Spending by Media ($ Million)

Media	2006	2007	2008 (MAT to November 2008	Share (%)
TV	2,951	2,942	2,993	62.5
Magazines	1,875	1,881	1,530	31.9
Newspapers	199	97	125	2.6
Internet	166	157	125	2.6
Radio	45	24	15	0.3
Outdoor	8	3	2	0.1

Source: Courtesy of Arnold, M., DTC report: Between screens. *Medical Marketing & Media*, 44(4), March 15, 2009, Posted at: http://www.mmm-online.com/dtc-report-between-screens/article/129756/, 2009a.

Since the introduction of DTCA in the United States, there has been debate about DTCA in Europe, which has been prevented by EU legislation. However, in July 2001, the European Commission ruled that DTCA communications would be allowed within Europe for a trial period of 5 years (effective from 2002) for three disease areas: asthma, diabetes, and HIV/AIDS. Dolan et al. (2008) have reported that in 2008 the European Commission has proposed the establishment of a harmonized legal framework on how pharmaceutical manufacturers make information available for the benefit of patients. [Directive and a Regulation of the European Parliament and of the Council as regards information to the general public on medicinal products subject to medical prescription, COM(2008)662 and COM(2008)663.]

PUSH AND PULL STRATEGIES

When applying biopharmaceutical promotion, there are two different approaches that a manufacturer can apply, commonly known as push and pull strategies (see Figure 9.3).

When using a push strategy, a manufacturer transmits direct information to the consumer, in an effort to raise awareness, interest, trial, usage, or loyalty. For example, "our molecule is the most efficacious, safe, and fast-acting, try it for yourselves." Because the information is transmitted from the manufacturer to the customer, it is "pushed," thus the strategy name describing it.

In a different approach, a biomanufacturer is not directly promoting its medicine to the customer. Instead, a product ad may ask: "have you been suffering from this ailment recently? A new biopharmaceutical made by

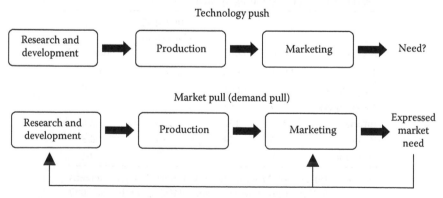

FIGURE 9.3 Technology push versus market pull.

our company may be able to help you. Why do not you visit your physician and ask him about it?" In this situation, the information is not "pushed," but instead it is "pulled" by the patient asking the prescriber. Let us take a closer look at these two approaches below.

Push Strategy

In using a push strategy, a biomanufacturer seeks to send custom-tailored product information, promoting the product's competitive advantages through the promotion of its USPs. This approach is based upon the premise of common diseases, affecting a large number of patients, where alternative treatments have been used for some time, but the patients still have several unmet needs and wants. For example, if patients are suffering from an autoimmune disease (e.g., rheumatoid arthritis, ulcerative colitis, psoriasis, or multiple sclerosis), they may have been using traditional immunosuppressive medicines that left them wanting for the following—then missing—product characteristics: increased mobility, a delay in disease progression, less side effects, and an enhanced quality of life.

Since the introduction of an innovative disease-modifying biopharmaceutical, the previously missing product attributes have been greatly achieved, and so the product's unique attributes make it an ideal treatment candidate. A push strategy then undertakes to communicate these improved attributes to the patients (where DTCA is allowed) or their prescribers, increasing the customer awareness, interest, and willingness to try. As previously mentioned, a push strategy may be utilizing a mass medium (radio or television) and exclude the possibility for customer interaction. Alternatively, if patient interaction and input is critical, then a more interactive promotional medium may be utilized, such as personal selling to prescribers by company sales professionals, or phone and web marketing that give the opportunity for interaction through phone, e-mail, social networking, or web conferencing technologies.

Prescription Medicine Buying Groups

Having selected a push strategy, biomanufacturers are then faced with the selection of customer audiences to be targeted, communication media to be implemented, as well as the frequency and detail of the promotional information. As far as the customer audiences are concerned, depending on the applicable legislation, a biomanufacturer may target four different audiences. First, medical opinion leaders, prescribers, and referring *physicians* who are directly or indirectly involved in suggesting and selecting the final treatments. Medical audiences are usually targeted through trade press and conferences, or with personal selling. Second, *patients*, their families, patient advocates, and the general public need to be informed about the disease characteristics, self-diagnosis instructions, the availability of effective treatments, and their respective competitive advantages leading to more awareness, interest, and trial. The usual methods of reaching this audience is with DTCA (where allowed), through medical experts or celebrity spokespersons who call on the patients to be diagnosed and treated, or with educational campaigns (TV, radio, printed media, and web) where "advertorials" inform about the disease and its treatments.

A third audience for biopharmaceutical promotion is *healthcare professionals* who are associated with first interacting with, diagnosing, referring, or treating a disease sufferer who may or may not know about his or her disease yet, for example, pharmacists, nurses, physical therapists, psychologists, and others. The promotional approaches used are either personal selling (to pharmacists, nurses, etc.) or trade journals and conferences. A fourth audience is increasingly becoming more important to biopharmaceutical promotion: The *administrators* and regulators who are responsible for reimbursing a biopharmaceutical medicine, including it into treatment guidelines, or prescribing guidelines (formularies), or healthcare coverage regulations. This audience is very diverse, comprising of political, financial, medical, and other health professionals who are responsible for healthcare policy, drug consumption, and cost containment. The usual methods of biopharmaceutical promotion to them are through personal selling or other targeted communications, focus groups, and conferences.

In addition to push versus pull, and target-oriented marketing, there is one more distinction of biopharmaceutical marketing approaches, as Table 9.13 indicates. Specifically, a product's marketing may be traditional (e.g., fever, mass market), or high density (e.g., Alzheimer's, treated only by specialists), and even targeted (e.g., a rare metabolic syndrome, treated by only super specialists in a few medical centers). The respective biopharmaceutical marketing approaches are called either multisource, limited source, or sole source, indicating the nature of the marketing efforts toward the respective prescribing/medical expert base.

TABLE 9.13   How Is the Present-Day Biopharmaceutical Marketing?

Traditional	High Density	Targeted Treatment
First line	Second line	First and second line
Usually oral	Specialist administered	Range of delivery systems
Mass populations	Clinically defined populations	Targeted populations
Mainly NCEs	Mainly biologics	Diagnostics and biologics
Chronic conditions	Mainly chronic conditions	Chronic and acute conditions
Mostly symptom relief	Mainly disease modifying	Disease modifying and preventative
Multisource	Limited source	Sole source
Primary care and specialists	Focus secondary care	Primary and secondary care
Grow share/existing market	Grow new markets	Outcomes-based pricing
Features and benefits	Outcomes oriented	Higher targeted marketing
Mass marketing/high DTC	Education and targeted marketing	Smaller and smarter sales force
Low price per dose	Smaller and smarter sales force	Cooperation with MCOs
Large sales force	Higher quality sales calls	
High volume sales calls	Premium per treatment	
Price erosion	Reimbursement is key	

Source: Courtesy of IBM Business Consulting Services, Pharma 2010, Armonk, NY, http://www-935.ibm.com/services/jp/bcs/pdf/lspharma/pharma2010.pdf

The majority of biopharma's marketing budget is targeted at doctors and others with prescribing power, who are effectively the gatekeepers to drug sales. In the European Union, only OTC drugs are promoted directly to consumers. Examples include analgesic preparations and some ailment-specific drugs such as hay fever remedies. In the United States, all drugs may be promoted to consumers, but in practice, DTCA focuses on OTC and common-ailment-targeted prescription drugs.

Physician-Targeted Promotion

However enormous the implications of DTCA of drugs and the budgets devoted to this, the issue of physician targeted promotion is significantly greater on all fronts, both financially and in terms of eventual outcomes. According to Buckley (2004), promotion and marketing to doctors makes up a quarter to a third of their annual budgets totaling more than $11 billion each year in the United States alone. It is estimated that, of this, about $3 billion is spent on advertising and $5 billion on sales representatives, while expenditure per physician is believed to be over $8000. This activity includes advertising, gift giving, and support for medically related activities such as travel to meetings and support for conferences.

There is good evidence that clinicians choose drugs in a similar way to "ordinary consumers" choosing "ordinary" consumer goods, however, if choices were rational, only the most effective or cheapest products would be used. Clearly, this is not the case for many medical conditions. In addition to addressing the customers' rational needs in choosing a medicine, we must therefore identify and recognize the other needs underlying the customer's choice of medicine.

Physician Needs upon Prescribing

Having focused on medical prescribers as the primary focus of biopharmaceutical promotion, Advanced Therapies' team had to further elucidate their primary needs when prescribing. As Table 9.14 indicates, there are primarily three classes of factors physicians consider when prescribing: First, patient or treatment needs, for example, disease chronicity, morbidity, and severity, the patient's own requests, financial status, and medication co-payment, as well as the biopharmaceutical's efficacy, safety, tolerability, and remaining characteristics. Second, the applicable healthcare

TABLE 9.14 Factors Physicians Consider When Prescribing

Shelf	Patient	Third-Parties
Medical knowledge	Disease condition	Patient insurance coverage
Clinical experience	Prior therapy	Applicable formularies
Peer influence	Concurrent therapy	Prior authorization restrictions
Biopharmaceutical advertising	Patient requests	Insurance company information
Medical congresses and continuing education	Financial status	Pharmaceutical benefit managers (PBM) information
Biopharma sales reps	Medication co-pays	Public opinion
Clinical practice guidelines	Patient family requests	Medical employer of physician
Peer-reviewed medical literature	Patient compliance to therapy	
Life beliefs and attitudes	Patient age and family status	
Western medicine versus holistic approach		

legislation, medical treatment guidelines, insurance, reimbursement, and formulary restrictions, patient employer, and prescriber employer limitations. Third, the prescriber's own characteristics, needs, and wants, for example, medical and clinical knowledge, peer influence, life attitudes and beliefs, compassion, willingness to experiment and innovate, information provided by the industry, and more.

It becomes immediately apparent that identifying and satisfying the most prescriber needs and wants in an ideal manner enhances the possibilities for a biopharmaceutical manufacturer to have its products prescribed by the physicians. In order to do so, a personal relationship with the prescriber needs to be gradually and carefully built, the descriptive prescriber's input needs to be invited, collected, and analyzed, and finally tailored biopharma solutions need to be delivered to each prescriber. These tailored solutions may be more information, education, access to the company's clinical trial program, interaction with the company's R&D specialists, inclusion as advisory board member, a trainer, or a spokesperson, networking, research grant assistance, and more.

As far as the biopharmaceutical product's offerings are concerned, the product may be combined with additional information, education, and services toward the prescribers, healthcare professionals, patients, and their families, aiming for better treatment guidelines, better patient education, diagnosis, and treatment, better caring, enhanced adherence to therapy, and more. The process of combining a product's basic offering (efficacy, safety, tolerability, formulation, ease of use, and pricing) with additional products and services is often called disease management, and has been credited with not only increased patient satisfaction, adherence, and quality of life, but also with healthcare cost containment and with biopharmaceutical industry's increased product sales and customer loyalty.

Pull Strategy

When following a pull strategy, a biopharmaceutical market segment has often the following characteristics: (1) low disease diagnosis, (2) significant disease-related stigma (e.g., for psychosis, multiple sclerosis, psoriasis, AIDS), (3) decades without any real therapeutic innovations, (4) lack of patient awareness for the availability of effective treatments, (5) unfavorable disease depiction in the media, or (6) lack of public education and other factors. In such cases, a pull strategy is better designed around the market segment's characteristics, by inviting the patients and their families to "come out of the closet," visit their physician, undergo new diagnostic tests, try new and effective medicines, and also be further trained for increased adherence to prescribed treatment, increased self-diagnosis of disease relapses, treatment discontinuation upon side-effect manifestation and more. Here the message is primarily "visit your physician, ask about the disease, overcome the stigma, and stay on the medication."

ADVERTISING

Prescription-Only versus Over-the-Counter Pharmaceuticals

When it comes to pharmaceutical advertising, there are two main classes of products that are regulated differently when it comes to their promotion. On one side, prescription-only medicines (POM) are those whose pharmacy purchasing requires the patient showing a valid physician prescription. The promotion of these medicines (biopharmaceuticals are usually POMs) is regulated in the United States by FDA, the same agency responsible for their clinical trial and marketing authorization approval (see Chapter 6).

On the other side, over-the-counter (OTC) pharmaceuticals are those whose purchasing is neither dependent upon a medical prescription, nor the interaction and scrutiny from a pharmacy personnel, and in some countries may be even available outside a pharmacy setting, for example, a supermarket. Thus, POMs are usually kept "behind the pharmacy counter," while OTCs are kept "over the counter" or in front of it, and can be purchased more easily and without a prescription. The promotion of these products in the United States is overseen by a different agency, the Federal Trade Commission (FTC; for more information visit http://www.ftc.gov/whocares). While DTC advertising of POMs is allowed in only a few countries around the world, OTC DTC advertising is allowed in many more countries, but even this is prohibited in other states.

As far as other pharmaceutical markets are concerned, the United Kingdom recognizes three pharmaceutical categories: (1) prescription only medications, (2) pharmacy-only medications, e.g., various chemicals and OTC strengths that require special information and general sales list (GSL) which are available off the shelf. In most countries, there even exists legislation that allows a medicine to switch from POM to OTC status, after several years of safe and effective use.

As far as pharmaceutical advertising is concerned, the FDA recognizes several different types of advertising components, such as the product claim advertisements, reminder advertisements, help-seeking advertisements, other product claim promotional materials, and risk disclosure requirements for different types of advertisements, which we study below.

Product Claim Advertisements

According to the FDA (http://www.fda.gov/Drugs/ResourcesForYou/Consumers/ PrescriptionDrugAdvertising/ucm072077.htm), product claim ads are the only type of ads that name a drug and discuss its benefits and risks. These ads must not be false or misleading, they have to use understandable language, and must include certain key components within the main part of the ad: (1) the name of the drug (brand and generic), (2) at least one FDA-approved use, (3) the most significant risks. Furthermore, they must present the benefits and risks of a prescription drug in a balanced fashion; print product claim ads must include a brief summary about the drug and the following statement: "You are encouraged to report negative side effects of prescription drugs to the FDA," and broadcast product claim ads must include the following: the drug's most important risks presented in the audio, and either all the risks listed in the drug's prescribing information or a variety of sources for viewers to find the prescribing information for the drug.

Reminder Advertisements

Reminder ads give the name of a drug, but not the drug's uses. These ads assume that the audience already knows the drug's use. A reminder ad does not have to contain risk information about the drug because the ad does not say what the drug does or how well it works. Unlike product claim ads, reminder ads cannot suggest, in either words or pictures, anything about the drug's benefits or risks. For example, a reminder ad for a drug that helps treat asthma should not include a drawing of a pair of lungs, because this implies what the drug does. Reminder ads are not allowed for certain prescription drugs with serious risks. Drugs with serious risks have a special warning, often called a "boxed warning," in the drug's FDA-approved prescribing information.

Help-Seeking Advertisements

Help-seeking ads describe a disease or condition but do not recommend or suggest a specific drug treatment. Some examples of diseases or conditions discussed in help-seeking ads include allergies, asthma, erectile dysfunction, high cholesterol, and osteoporosis. The ads encourage people with these symptoms to talk to their doctor. Help-seeking ads may include a drug company's name and may also provide a telephone number to call for more information. When done properly, help-seeking ads are not considered to be drug ads and FTC regulates them. If an ad recommends or suggests the use of a specific drug, however, it is considered a product claim ad that must comply with FDA rules.

Other Product Claim Promotional Materials

Apart from advertisements, other promotional materials are used to promote the use of a drug. These are called "promotional labeling" and include brochures, materials mailed to consumers, and other types of materials given out by drug companies. If these materials mention the drug's benefit(s), they must also include the drug's prescribing information.

Biopharmaceutical Advertising Objectives

We have previously mentioned about POM versus OTC advertising, as well as the different requirements from different types of pharmaceutical advertisements. Table 9.15 summarizes some of the most common biopharmaceutical advertising message objectives.

As far as the biopharmaceutical advertising messages, commonly referred to as "hooks," are concerned, Table 9.16 lists some of the most important ones, either product related, physician related, clinical use, or

TABLE 9.15   What Are the Most Common Biopharmaceutical Advertising Message Objectives?

Informative	Persuasive	Reminder
New therapeutic products	Pharmaceutical brand preference	Mature products
New therapeutic indications	Growth products	Product availability
New strengths, formulations, packagings	Attitudes on product benefits	First choice
Low adverse events	Talk to sales representative	Most-widely prescribed medication
Educational services	Long-term cost-effectiveness	Low price
Disease management	Prescribe/try now	Purchase more for home/office use
Company image: Therapeutic category expertise, global leadership, vision, and ethics	Brand switching from competitive products	
Administration instructions		
Compliance promotion		
Eliminating fears of adverse events		
Switch to OTC status		

TABLE 9.16 What Are the Main Biopharmaceutical Advertising "Hooks"?

1 Product related	Efficacy, safety, innovation, mechanism of action, route of administration, cost-effectiveness, formulation, packaging
2 Physician related	Specialists involved in clinical trials, publications, advisory committee recommendations
3 Clinical use	Safety, tolerability, dependability, clinical illustration, before and after
4 Patient related	Compliance, quality-of-life, preference, patient group endorsement
5 Manufacturer related	Leadership, innovation, image, history, patient orientation, services
6 Nonrational	Empathy, humor, curiosity, unusual image, self-gratifying, patriotism

Source: Dogramatzis, D., *Pharmaceutical Marketing: A Practical Guide*, CRC Press, Boca Raton, FL, 2001. With permission.

TABLE 9.17 What Are the Advertising Objectives over the Biopharmaceutical PLC?

	Pre-Introduction	Introduction	Growth	Maturity	Decline
Promotional objective	Set objectives Design tactics Set budgets	Establish awareness Enhance demand	Support product liking and preference	Maintain loyalty Encourage switching	Promote new uses, new strengths
Advertising strategy	Concept testing Media selection	Develop intend to prescribe/buy Inform trade	Increase spending Increase intensity Fight competition	Promote repeat purchases Remind and differentiate	Decrease spending if withdrawal Advertise replacement
Message objective	Tease Prepare market	Inform	Persuade	Remind	

other characteristics that are involved. Furthermore, we should not forget that as a biopharmaceutical product progresses through its lifecycle (see Chapter 12), advertising objectives change with time and lifecycle period, as explained in Table 9.17.

DIRECT-TO-CONSUMER ADVERTISING

Creating Direct Pull

To help offset revenue losses due to fewer new drug launches and generic entries, manufacturers try to maximize performance of existing brands (Provost Peters, 2004). Product promotion is a critical element of this effort.

In 2008, drug manufacturers spent more than $11 billion on total product promotion, including drug detailing and DTCA. Manufacturers are allocating a large portion of marketing resources to physician detailing; however, the traditional detail-based marketing model for professional promotion is being challenged since physicians increasingly use the Internet for medical information and point-of-care decision tools like electronic prescribing.

Although the overwhelming majority of promotional spending is geared toward providers, DTC spending is a subject of ongoing debate. According to IMS Health (see Table 9.8), between 2004 and 2008, while total U.S. professional promotion decreased from $8.1 billion to $6.8 billion, DTC advertising increased from $4 billion to $4.4 billion. According to Provost Peters (2004), manufacturers tend to spend the most on consumer ads for drugs used to treat chronic conditions that require treatment over extended periods of time such as asthma, depression, allergies, arthritis, and diabetes. Drugs with low occurrence of mild side effects are also better candidates because there is less information on risk that needs to be conveyed to the consumer.

DTCA Proponents and Critics

DTCA has had numerous proponents and critics ever since its introduction in the United States in 1985. Proponents claim that (1) it increases patient and patient family awareness, (2) it decreases disease-associated stigma, (3) it increases the number of patients seeking physician advice and eventually disease diagnosis, (4) it increases patient adherence to treatment, (5) it increases patient participation and empowerment, and also (6) it increases freedom of choice and self-management of disease.

Fierce criticism has been expressed by various sources based on the following potential disadvantages: (1) DTC may increase utilization and unnecessary medicine-related spending, (2) it may increase self-medication and side effects, (3) it may drive consumers to pharmacological-only treatments and away from other potential approaches, (4) it may drive consumers to higher priced medicines, (5) it may tend to higher medicine prices due to their expensive marketing costs, (6) it may drive to new lifestyle problems being treated with unnecessary medicines, and (7) it may take away public resources from life-saving treatments or critical life-sciences R&D initiatives. Table 9.18 summarizes the main advantages and disadvantages often associated with DTCA.

For a pull strategy example see: Why Rebif, http://www.mslifelines.com/rebif/why-rebif/indexjsp

TABLE 9.18   Disadvantages and Benefits of DTCA

Disadvantages	Benefits
Leads to unsustainable pharmaceutical expenditure without improving health outcomes	Improves patient and public awareness about health conditions and treatment options
Many advertisements are misleading and of poor educational value	Prompts consumers to talk to their doctors for the first time about particular medical conditions or illnesses
Exploits the weakest and most vulnerable members of society	Helps patients to be more involved in decisions about their health care
Undermines the provision of drug information from other sources	May reduce costs associated with under-treatment of certain conditions
Leads patients to pressure their doctors to prescribe unnecessary or inappropriate drugs	Provides patients with essential information about a drug that no-one else has any incentive to provide
Damages the doctor–patient relationship	Encourages health professionals to keep up with current prescribing information
Increases frequency of unnecessary visits to the doctor	Improves patient compliance with a prescribed drug regimen
Promotes pharmaceutical solutions for problems that could be solved by a change in lifestyle	Heightens consumer awareness of the inherently risky nature of virtually all prescription drugs
Encourages a belief that there is a drug for every condition	Provides the pharmaceutical industry with an important means of correcting erroneous information provided by other sources
Reduces patient's confidence in their ability to get better and stay well	

PERSONAL BIOPHARMACEUTICAL SELLING

As previously mentioned, the biopharmaceutical personal selling process involves the use of industry sales personnel in directly interacting with medical prescribers or other industry stakeholders, and mobilizing them across the prescription decision model, a model created to describe the potential position of a prescriber toward a given medicine. According to this model, a prescriber may be at one of the following distinct process steps: (1) lack of awareness, (2) product awareness, (3) considering to prescribe, (4) willing to prescribe, (5) trial, (6) usage, (7) repeat usage, (8) product loyalty, and (9) product championship. The relative position of each prescriber along this model is driven by the patient needs and wants, the prescriber's own needs and wants, as well as the applicable healthcare legislation, rules, and regulations.

TABLE 9.19   Top 10 U.S. Pharmaceutical
Sales Details (MAT July 2008)

GlaxoSmithKline	9,349,081
Pfizer	8,722,967
Merck	6,417,848
AstraZeneca	5,236,353
Novartis	4,686,745
ScheringPlough	4,653,845
SanofiAventis	4,497,137
Eli Lilly	4,138,208
Johnson & Johnson	3,517,216
Forest Pharmaceuticals	3,212,233

Source: Vecchione, A., Loop of faith,
Medical Marketing & Media, 38–45,
November 2008.

Pharmaceutical and biopharmaceutical sales forces have grown steadily over the recent years. For example, Table 9.19 numbers the U.S. pharmaceutical sales details during 2008.

Despite their similarities, however, biopharmaceutical sales forces are significantly different than those seen in big pharma. Figure 9.4 summarizes some of the most prominent differences among the two industries' sales forces.

The Decision Matrix

As mentioned above, the idea is to get your customers to the next stages of the decision process, using the messages below in the right order, from the right sources. So, if you are going after early adopters, read across the early adopter row and get people's word of mouth in the order prescribed (see Table 9.20).

BUILDING A BIOPHARMA SALES FORCE

In the pharmaceutical industry, the most effective and expensive promotional element of a successful brand strategy is an experienced, well trained sales force. The process of sizing, staffing, training, and deploying a sales team requires thoughtfulness, significant market research, as well as competitive and market analysis. When built thoroughly and thoughtfully, a sales force will provide the level of market share and ROI that justifies its expense. Currently, there are approximately 80,000–90,000

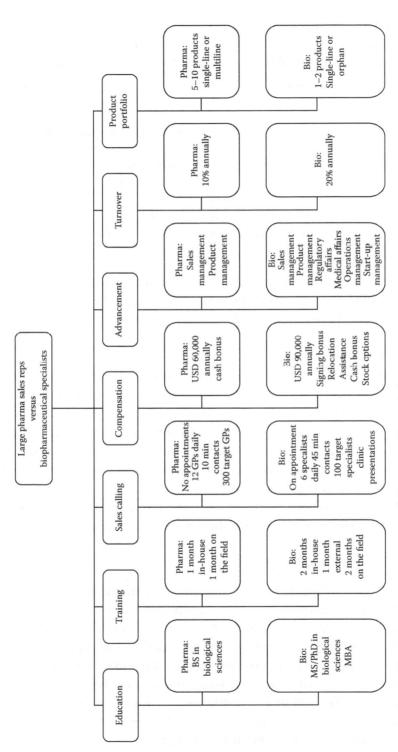

FIGURE 9.4 Sales force differences between pharma and biotech firms.

TABLE 9.20   The Buying Decision Matrix

Infrequent Prescribers	Refill Prescribers	Specialists	Therapy Champions
N/A	N/A		Clinical trial and research collaboration
N/A	N/A	Therapeutic category/clinical specialists	
N/A	N/A	Group practice and patient management	
N/A	N/A	Speakers in peer-to-peer programs	
N/A		Sales force details	
		E-detailing	
		Mailing of product samples, script pads, etc.	
		Web-based product and therapeutic-category information	

pharmaceutical sales representatives calling on the medical community in the United States (Evangelista et al., 2008). Figure 9.5 depicts the biopharmaceutical sales planning and execution process.

Sales Force Sizing

In building a sales force for any specialty, the key is understanding which segments or subsegments of the medical community are most valuable for your brand business and understanding, where they are located, how responsive they are to promotion and the frequency of message delivery required to change prescribing behavior. Market research is key to understanding the segments. Table 9.21 provides a complete example of a biopharmaceutical sales force sizing.

Table 9.22 describes a simple template for ranking your national/regional/global key account prescribers of a biopharmaceutical product.

BIOPHARMA MEDIA RELATIONS

The U.S.-based Biotechnology Industry Organization (BIO; http://www.bio.org) reported in its (http://bio.org/speeches/pubs/milestone08/2007-2008_BIO_Milestones_WEB.pdf) Milestones 2008 publication that in 2008 their membership increased by 100 organizations, to 1200 members, of which almost 70% includes R&D-focused member companies. It is easy to envisage these companies competing with each other for state incentives, private and institutional investors, corporate partners, products to in-license, clinical trial patients, commercial patients, prescribers, public awareness, and media attention.

The multiple audiences mentioned above (publics) thus become focus of each and every biotechnology organization in its quest to compete more effectively and efficiently. Public relations (PR) is the management of communications between each organization and its publics. According to the audiences targeted, a biopharma may have to conduct investor relations, government relations, media relations, and more. The most important aspects of the rigorous public relations program that needs to be implemented by each biopharma are shown in Table 9.23.

The company stage at which a public relations program needs to start being implemented is often a matter of debate. On one hand, there is an early need for the organization to promote its competitive advantage and its growth opportunities, as early as possible, so that potential investors, employees, and partners are attracted. On the other hand, a start-up biopharma is often strapped on cash and devotes almost its entire budget in R&D progress. As a rule of thumb, a biopharma's PR program needs to be in place, in a gradual fashion, as early as an important external or internal audience needs to be influenced, and a complete and vigorous, multitasking PR program needs to be in place as soon as the organization is approaching the completion of critical milestones in its company evolution.

Public Relations

In general, public relations attempts to attract public exposure of an organization to its audiences (publics) by using mutual interest topics and news. Furthermore, public relations attract each public's interest and endorsement, without direct payment for the endorsement gained (as opposed to paid direct advertising, personal selling, etc.). Eventually, PR seeks to establish direct relationships with the organization's multiple publics, on a long-term mutually rewarding basis. That is, the biopharma gains awareness, interest, usage, preference, and loyalty, while the targeted audiences gain information, education, additional services, and they also gain the privilege of closely interacting with the organization and even influencing its future direction (new products), or improve its social responsibility, etc.

At Advanced Therapies, the PR process began with their external and internal analysis, which led to the identification of their diverse audiences and their respective interests, needs, and wants. Furthermore, it led to the definition of individual company objectives from each and every external and internal audience, as well as the future stage of each one of these relationships. Having defined their future objectives, the company team then

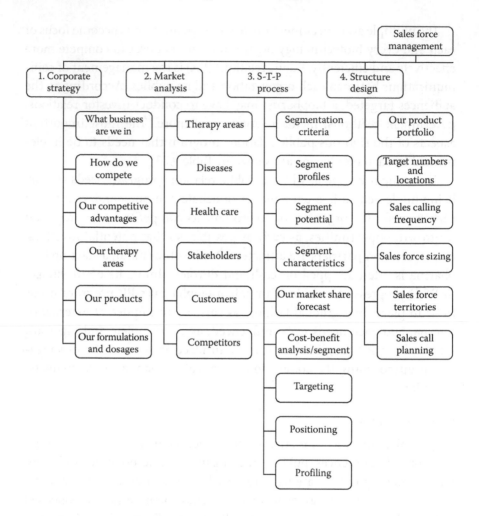

FIGURE 9.5   Sales planning and execution process.

preceded in identifying potential PR angles, stories, and news that may interest their respective audiences.

For example, potential investors might be interested in the company's unique research platform and future valuation; its potential employees might be interested in the company's academic "easy going" atmosphere and lovely premises location, while its future prescribers and patients might be interested in its primary drug candidate's initial efficacy and safety results. Armed with these stories, additional angles could be created, for example, why the research platform might lead to exceptional financial

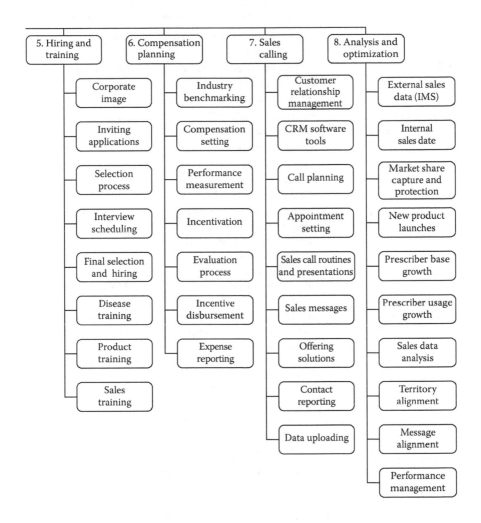

returns in the future, or why the product characteristics might eventually improve the patients' quality of life. By carefully crafting the company image to complement their audiences' needs and wants, Advanced Therapies was then well in its way of crafting its first PR program, and assigning tasks, responsibilities, and budgets to each employee interacting with an external audience. The PR program had to be multi-audience focused, to involve most of the company's human resources, to use multiple stories and angles, and to proactively manage the public image to be created by every planned PR activity.

TABLE 9.21 How Do You Estimate a Biopharmaceutical Sales Force Size?

Task	Parameter to Be Determined	Number
Allocation of sales effort, i.e., how many calls to cover the target	Number of prescribers (accounts and prospects)	2,000
	Average sales call frequency	10 times/year
	Total sales effort required $(2,000 \times 10 = 30,000)$	20,000 calls
Sales force size, i.e., how many Reps	Average daily sales call frequency by a representative	10 calls/day
	Average number of Rep working days	200 days/year
	Number of Reps required $(20,000/200 \times 10 = 10)$	10 Reps
Territory creation, i.e., how many territories	Ten territories are needed to ensure proper coverage. In most countries of the world, pharma companies define territories in IMS territory.	10 territories
	If 30 IMS territories in country	3 IMS territories/Rep
Actual territory design, i.e., which territories per Rep	The sales force must be given balanced territorial groups, according to number of territories, number of customers, value size of district, growth potential of district Determining factors are salesperson's home, number of large accounts, and number of metropolitan areas	Rep A in North Rep B in Central Rep C in South sectors, three territories each

Source: Dogramatzis, D., *Pharmaceutical Marketing: A Practical Guide*, CRC Press, Boca Raton, FL, 2001. With permission.

TABLE 9.22 How Do You Rank Your National/Regional/ Global Key Account Prescribers of a Biopharmaceutical Product?

Region	Class	Prescriber	Center/Clinic	Total Prescriptions	Our Market Share (m.s.)	Our m.s. Potential	Competitor A m.s.	Competitor B m.s.	Competitor C m.s.	Our Local Rep	Remarks
	A										
	B										
	C										

TABLE 9.23 How Does a Biopharmaceutical Company Manage Its External Relations?

Investor Relations	Other Relations	Public Relations	Legal and Ethical Issues
Bank relationships	Government contact and information exchange	Define PR strategy	Health and safety requirements
Analysts/credit rating	Regulatory relations	Global PR programs	Environmental requirements
Shareholders relationships	Industry relations	Corporate PR program	Other legal requirements
	Patient organization relations	Corporate PR material	
	Medical community relations	PR events	

Why a PR Firm?

One of the critical issues that had to be discussed was Advanced Therapies' need for choosing and liaising with an experienced external PR agency that was both well connected in the biotechnology arena, but also held similar views and understood the company's changing PR needs, at this early stage of company development. The advantages from using an external PR partner were multiple. First, there was a need for an experienced partner to guide their PR priorities and provide new and independent viewpoints on Advanced Therapies' unique characteristics. Second, the PR firm would bring important awareness, multiple PR opportunities, new contacts and media, and significant networking. Third, the external partner would be able to create new strategies, and provide in-house skills (e.g., creative writing) that were missing from the biopharma. Fourth, a PR firm would be able to capitalize on new techniques and tools, for example, the emerging Web 2.0 communications, which we discuss below.

The initial timing for hiring an external PR partner also had to be discussed. Advanced Therapies was now entering Phase I clinical trials, a fact that created an immediate need for clinical investigators, human volunteers, media attention, and also additional investors. Thus, the timing was deemed appropriate for an initial contact, and the CMO was tasked with inviting the proposals of five candidate PR firms, from which the final partner would be chosen. The exact timeline included the following steps: (1) defining Advanced Therapies PR objectives, (2) building an initial company PR brochure, backgrounding all the company's achievements and major characteristics, (3) identifying PR agency candidates (based on their defined clientele, size, history, achievements, etc.), (4) inviting the short-listed companies to present, (5) meeting the short list, (6) brainstorming on the merits of each collaboration, (7) making the final selection, and (8) signing a detailed PR contract.

PR Responsibilities

The PR responsibilities, either on the biopharma's or the external partner's side, are multiple and require thorough planning. For example: (1) analyst relations (trade analysts, financial analysts); (2) corporate/media auditing; (3) counsel regarding distribution and timing of press releases; (4) crisis management; (5) FDA advisory committee meeting support; (6) industry/competitor auditing/monitoring; (7) internal/employee communications; (8) investor relations/financial community expertise; (9) media backgrounding; (10) media outreach in support of news announcements; (11) media relations (proactive efforts, daily communications, editorial calendars); (12) message development/corporate positioning; and (13) ongoing media relations in addition to (14) planning and counseling; (15) press and collateral materials development; (16) press release development/distribution; (17) press tour planning and support; (18) pursuit of opportunistic media; (19) satellite media tours; (20) satellite symposia coordination/execution; (21) scientific/medical conference support; (22) speaker placement/industry expert profiles; (23) speaker presentation/media training; (24) speakers board assembly; (25) tailored messages; (26) tradeshow/special event support (on-site support, press room staffing); (27) Web site development; and (28) writing (press releases, press kit development, and collateral).

Very often, Advanced Therapies will be faced with important upcoming company, product, or service announcements. The planned timetable for each of these important PR opportunities has been commonly created, and will follow the program below.

Six months before product launch (announce the company): Identify and brief key analysts. Announce the company, funding, investors, executives, company direction.

Three months before product launch: Develop market segment positioning and messaging. Gain endorsement of analysts, customers, and partners as references. Conduct embargoed briefings with large pool of analysts and longer lead press.

One week: Conduct embargoed briefings with short leads and biotechnology bloggers.

Product announcement: Include market demand, value proposition, differentiation, pricing, reimbursement, availability.

Constant, long-term biopharma company and product visibility: Create opportunities for thought leadership, company visibility, personnel achievements, scientific distinctions, and product reviews.

As far as potential media stories are concerned, here is a representative list of some of the future PR opportunities to be exploited with Advanced 'Iherapies' diverse audiences:

Sample media "stories": Straight news (news announcements, earnings), industry trends, primer/overview (Q&A), profiles, or product stories (product overviews, product reviews, hits, and misses).

Measuring the Effectiveness of PR

Following their PR strategy brainstorming, the company is wondering how to measure the effectiveness of their newly decided PR strategy, as well as their collaboration with the external PR partner. On the detailed measurement proposal of the partner, and the modifications and additions proposed by the CMO, Table 9.24 is reviewed and approved by all the marketing retreat's participants.

TABLE 9.24   Measuring the Effectiveness of Biopharmaceutical PR

Budget	Awareness	Attitude	Media Coverage
Versus budget	Pre- and post-PR	Pre- and post-PR	Broadcast frequency
Versus last year	awareness, liking,	stakeholder	Broadcast time
Versus total	preference,	attitudes versus	No. of newspapers
promotion	conviction of	company,	Media clippings
Versus competitors	customers	products,	
		management	

Positioning	Response Generation	Share Price	Sales
Perceptual mapping	No. of phone calls,	Level	Units and values
of own company/	faxes, or e-mails	Liquidity	New accounts
products versus	New prospect leads	Range	Orders per account
competitors	New patients treated		Order size per
			account

BIOPHARMA WEB AND SOCIAL MARKETING

According to current Internet world statistics (http://www.internetworld stats.com/stats.htm), an estimated 25.6% of the total world's population (6.8 billion) are Internet users, representing a 380% growth between 2000 and 2009, with the highest penetrations observed in North America (74%), Oceania/Australia (60%), and Europe (52%). Furthermore, according to DomainTools (http://www.domaintools.com/internet-statistics/) on March 28, 2010, there were almost 117 million domains, belonging to the .com, .net, .org, .info, .biz, and .us extensions. A large proportion of these sites are health related, and so the creation of a distinctive web strategy and its implementation with focus and dedication is a must for every healthcare biotechnology organization today.

Biopharma Web Strategy

A biopharma web strategy involves several prerequisites, which are listed below. According to Nalen (2007), building a brand is like putting together a jigsaw puzzle, where each piece fits into the overall larger picture. Some integral and essential points include the following: (1) align the brand's online message with offline programs, (2) get site visitors to identify, (3) make sure the user experience is an enjoyable one, (4) have a ubiquitous web presence, and (5) take care of the bottom line.

What Are Your Target Audiences Searching For?

Almost two-thirds of people seeking health information online use a search engine rather than directly inputting a URL, according to a 2002 survey conducted by the Boston Consulting Group (von Knoop, 2003). Because a search engine plays a huge role in directing customers to sites, marketers are paying increased attention to how information seekers carry out searches, and to how search engines process queries and rank results. These techniques are known as search marketing.

Table 9.25 describes what a biopharmaceutical product Web site contains, while Table 9.26 lists what a corporate biopharmaceutical company Web site contains.

The Power of Social Media

Social media has enhanced the power of the assertive and informed consumer who has access to extensive health information. Currently, there

TABLE 9.25 What Does a Biopharmaceutical Product Web Site Contain?

1. Disease Education	2. The Product	3. Medication Guide	4. Treatment Support	5. Patient Networking	6. Patient Access
Overview	Development history	Formulation and dosages	*Medication Journal*	Disease portals	What to ask your insurance provider
Living with the disease	Mechanism of action	Treatment regimen	*Adverse Event Journal*	Patient associations	Find out whether this medication is on your provider's list
Disease progression	Clinical data	How to store and transfer	*Self Evaluation Journal*	How to enroll in your regional patient association chapter	Reimbursement denials and appeals
Common problems	Benefits of therapy	How to prepare	Contacting your health care provider	Patient association events calendar	Find out your co-payment
Available treatment	Common side effects	How to administer	Contacting and informing your physician	Patient association resources	Getting your prescription
Choosing a treatment	Contraindications	Treatment monitoring	What to ask your physician	Finding a patient mentor	Getting prior authorization
Frequently asked questions	Special warnings	How to treat adverse events	Finding a prescriber	Becoming a patient mentor	Recertification
Disease glossary	Patient information leaflet (PIL)		Finding an infusion center		Registering for medication home delivery

(continued)

TABLE 9.25 (continued)   What Does a Biopharmaceutical Product Web Site Contain?

1. Disease Education	2. The Product	3. Medication Guide	4. Treatment Support	5. Patient Networking	6. Patient Access
	Frequently asked questions		Concomitant medications and supplements		Receiving your first medication supply
			Treatment team member contacts		Ordering your refill supplies
			Travel checklist		Product spoilage and return
			Homecare nursing support		Billing and coding
			Online support		Assistance for the uninsured
			Hotline support		Co-payment assistance
			Educational resources		Reimbursement glossary
			Informational resources		

7. Caregivers	8. Physicians	9. Pharmacists, Nurses	10. Sitemap	11. Search	12. Privacy Terms
Disease overview	Registration and verification	Registration and verification	Our web pages	Search our site	Disclaimer
Living with a sufferer	Product development history	Formulation and dosages		Search for publications	Terms of use

(continued)

			Search the web
Administering medication	Detailed clinical data	Treatment regimen	
Identifying and treating symptoms	Contacting a treatment expert	Contraindications	
Feeding the patient	Mechanism of action	Special warnings	
Cleaning the patient	Treatment guidelines	How to administer	
Psychological support	Diagnostic tools	Treatment monitoring	
Contacting the physician	Formulation and dosages	How to treat adverse events	
Contacting the health care provider	Treatment regimen	What to inform patients and caregivers	
Contacting the nurse	Contraindications	Managing treatment expectations	
Educational support	Special warnings	Identifying treatment failures or disease relapses	
Finding a caregiver mentor	How to administer	Keeping a patient registry	

TABLE 9.25 (continued)   What Does a Biopharmaceutical Product Web Site Contain?

7. Caregivers	8. Physicians	9. Pharmacists, Nurses	10. Sitemap	11. Search	12. Privacy Terms
Staying positive	Treatment monitoring	Full prescribing information (SPC)			
	How to treat adverse events	Frequently asked questions			
	What to inform patients and caregivers				
	Managing treatment expectations				
	Identifying treatment failures or disease relapses				
	Keeping a patient registry				
	Full prescribing information (SPC)				
	Frequently asked questions				

TABLE 9.26   What Does a Corporate Biopharmaceutical Company Web Site Contain?

1. Our Company	2. Foundation and Philanthropy	3. Our Pipeline	4. Marketed Products	5. Partnering	6. Investors
Overview	Our foundation	Research ethics	Products by therapy area	In-licensing	Investors' calendar
Our history	Therapy foundation	Research vision	Products by name	Out-licensing	Stock information
Mission and values	Our vision	Biotechnology principles	Physician testimonials	Our alliances	Financial reports
Board of directors	Our initiatives	Medicine development	Patient testimonials	Academic researchers	SEC filings
Organization graph	Advisory board	Our technologies	Our products in the news	Venture funding	Investor's kit
Leadership team	Science education	Our patents		Suppliers	Analyst coverage
Ethics	Continuing med education	Preclinical research		Exports	Financial webcasts
Sustainability	How to support us	Therapy areas		Wholesalers	Annual meeting
In the community	How to get a grant	Our scientists			Investor contacts
Governance principles		Clinical trial program			Share transfer agent
Our views on public policy		Patient enrollment			Informational resources
Our awards					Request for materials
Informational resources		Advisory board			Frequently asked questions
		Informational resources			
Locations		Postdoctoral program			E-mail alerts
Our Web sites					

(continued)

TABLE 9.26 (continued) What Does a Corporate Biopharmaceutical Company Web Site Contain?

7. Media	8. Careers	9. Sitemap	10. Search	11. Privacy Terms	12. Contact Us
Press releases	Working with us	Our web pages	Search our site	Disclaimer	By function
Media kit	Working benefits		Search for publications	Terms of use	By therapy area
Media agency	Available positions		Search the web		By product
Media contacts	How to apply				By subsidiary
In the news	Locations				Maps and directions
Your news feedback	Diversity policy				
Informational resources	Trainee program				
Twitter contact	University recruiting				
Facebook contact	Agency recruiting				
	Conference presence				
	Workplace awards				
	Our employees				
	Our alumni				
	Our newsletter				

arefour types of social media content creators who are having the most impact on public perceptions of pharmaceutical companies and their products. Unfortunately, for the industry, much of this content has not been very flattering. Social media has provided an outlet for a range of whistle blowers, industry insiders, and drug industry critics to express their dissatisfaction with industry practices. However, it has also created a new support network where patients share perspectives on their condition and treatment options.

Table 9.27 outlines the significance of Web 2.0 communications for the biopharmaceutical industry, while Table 9.28 describes some of the new media platforms being used by the biopharmaceutical industry today.

TABLE 9.27   What Is the Significance of Web 2.0 Communications for the Biopharmaceutical Industry?

#	Description	Significance for Biopharma
1	Platforms that connect people together (social networks). Examples: Facebook, MySpace, LinkedIn, Second Life	Physicians, nurses, pharmacists, patients, and caregivers can enlist in social networks, and share experiences, give mentoring, provide support, furnish referrals, and be a sounding board for each other
2	Ability to produce and share content with others (social media). Examples: YouTube, Twitter, Flickr	Individuals and companies can share testimonials, e-mails, pictures, sounds, and videos, to inform, educate, and entice each other
3	Platforms that facilitate participation, not only individual uploading. Examples: Healthcare-related blogs	Individuals can share their experiences online and in real time, reaching the far corners of the world within seconds from an event happening
4	Platforms that facilitate information sharing (collective intelligence). Example: Wikipedia	Humans having progressively mastered the papyrus, typography, faxing, bulletin boards, the Web 1.0, and e-mailing, can now upload, comment, correct, and constantly update information, producing a collective knowledge that is taking humanity to new heights

TABLE 9.28 What Are Some of the New Media Platforms Being Used
by the Biopharmaceutical Industry?

#	Title	Description
1	Blogs	An electronic diary posted on the web and open for comments, updated daily with new content and responses to comments
2	Corporate Web site	Company Web sites as described above
3	E-mail alerts	Frequent e-mail alerts to anyone interested in specific subjects (disease, product, company) and submitting their own e-mail to be included in mailing list
4	Mobile messaging	Content delivered wirelessly to connected mobile devices (web PCs, portable PCs, PDAs, smart phones)
5	Online advertisements	Company/product advertisements posted on popular Web sites (health and news portals) where direct-to-consumer ads are allowed, paid for by the time period
6	Pay per click	Company/product Web site links posted on popular Web sites and paid for by the number of unique user clicks toward the company site
7	Podcasts	Sound or video content delivered through the web or wirelessly to mobile iPod devices
8	Product Web site	Product Web sites as described above
9	Search engine marketing	Companies paying search engines to display an advertisement with a link to all users interested on relevant search topics (e.g., disease)
10	Search engine optimization	Incorporation of key words into corporate Web site coding that attracts search engine attention and makes the Web site be displayed at the top of search results
11	Second life	A virtual reality Web site, where individuals and corporations can create alter egos that behave according to instructions, interact with other alter egos (e.g., prescribers and patients), and promote the company's agenda
12	Social networks	Web sites that facilitate the social networking between individual users and companies, by recording personal details, receiving comments, allowing the creation of friends' lists, or eventually actual personal interaction if the two parties agree
13	Video on demand	Video content posted on company or external servers and downloaded on demand (usually free of charge) by interested web users
14	Viral video	Video content posted on special sites that facilitate the storing and exchange of user content, bypassing the downloading from corporate or personal sites
15	Webinars	Instructional video, usually by a health professional or a fellow patient, that is preannounced to occur at certain time intervals and is attended by connected users
16	Wikis	Web sites encouraging the posting of information by anyone, changes to this information by others, thus leading to a collective intelligence source

QUESTIONS

1. What are the layers of a biopharmaceutical product?
2. What are the various possible biopharmaceutical brand strategies? Provide an actual example for each.
3. What are the most important components in defining a global brand?
4. What are the main advantages and disadvantages of the main biopharmaceutical promotional strategies?
5. Which are the major factors physicians consider when prescribing?
6. What are the advertising objectives over the biopharmaceutical PLC?
7. Which are the main advantages and disadvantages of DTCA?
8. What are the steps involved in sales force sizing? Use your own example.
9. Which are some of the parameters used in measuring the effectiveness of biopharmaceutical PR?
10. What are some of the new media platforms being used by the biopharmaceutical industry? Use one actual product example as it is presented on each platform.

EXERCISES

1. Biopharmaceutical products are often associated with U.S. web pages, as local regulations allow DTCA. By visiting one of them, describe the layers of a biopharmaceutical brand based on its web presence.
2. How do your brand, a biopharmaceutical product used to treat infertility toward its various stakeholders? Use a commercially available product example.
3. Can you describe the product width, length, and depth of the following biopharmaceutical brands: Enbrel, Humira, and Eprex? Define which national market you are using as example.
4. You are launching a new oncology biopharmaceutical globally, aimed at the breast and lung cancer therapeutic areas. Now suggest three potential brand names, search for international conflicts, and describe the naming application process with FDA, EMEA, and the JMHLW.
5. An immune system–stimulating biopharmaceutical is being launched by your organization in the U.S. market. Describe your suggested push- and pull-promotional messages to be approved by your board of directors.
6. You are in charge of a biological antiretroviral in the U.S. market. What main advertising "hooks" would you use for your product versus its multiple audiences?

7. Look at your home country. Find statistical data on a given medical specialty. Now attempt to size and organize the regional bases of your sales force to launch a new biopharmaceutical aimed at the given specialty. Explain your rationale.

8. Advanced Therapies is a start-up biopharma active in the field of autoimmune diseases. Design an organization graph outlining its corporate Web site under creation.

9. Are you Web 2.0 savvy? Then embark on a mission to make a new biopharmaceutical more well known. What tactics will you use?

10. You are involved in the web marketing of a new antiretroviral. Which Web 1.0 or 2.0 fora are the most important? Name 10 examples each.

REFERENCES

Arnold, M., 2009a. *Medical Marketing & Media*, Haymarket Media Inc. in the format Other book via Copyright Clearance Center.

Arnold, M., 2009b. Rx ad spend down 7.8% for first half of 2009, says TNS. *Medical Marketing & Media*, September 16, 2009. Posted at: http://www.mmm-online.com/rx-ad-spend-down-78-for-first-half-of-2009-says-tns/article/149065/

Biotechnology Industry Organization, 2008. *2007–2008 Milestones*. BIO: Washington, DC. Posted at: http://bio.org/speeches/pubs/milestone08/2007–2008_BIO_Milestones_WEB.pdf

Buckley, J., 2004. Pharmaceutical marketing—Time for change. *EJBO Electronic Journal of Business Ethics and Organization Studies* 9(2): 4–11.

Dogramatzis, D., 2001. *Pharmaceutical Marketing: A Practical Guide*. CRC Press: Boca Raton, FL.

Dolan, A., Neal, A., Liptrot, N., and Graham, S., 2008. *Assessing Corporate Brands and Product Brands in Pharmaceuticals—A Quick Look to Bridge to True Insight*. Adelphi International Research: Macclesfield, Cheshire, U.K.

Evangelista, W.S., Poulin, M., Geissler, C.T., and Andrew, J., 2008. Pharma's new U.S. commercial model: Promoting the science not the swag. Deloitte. Posted at: http://www.deloitte.com/assets/Dcom-UnitedStates/Local%20Assets/Documents/us_Consulting_ScienceorSwagDebate_121409.pdf

Food and Drug Administration (FDA), 2010. Guidance for industry—Contents of a complete submission for the evaluation of proprietary names, February 2010. Posted at: http://www.fda.gov/downloads/Drugs/GuidanceComplianceRegulatoryInformation/Guidances/UCM075068.pdf

IBM Business Consulting Services, Pharma 2010, Armonk, NY, http://www-935.ibm.com/services/jp/bcs/pdf/lspharma/pharma2010.pdf

IMS Health, Integrated Promotional Services, Norwalk, CT.

J&J, New Brunswick, NJ, http://www.jnj.com

Med Ad News, 2009. Med Ad News 200: World's best selling medicines. *Med Ad News*, 15(7): July 2009.

Nalen, P.H., 2007. Online brands. PharmExec guide to branding, October 15, 2007. Posted at: http://pharmexec.findpharma.com/pharmexec/article/articleDetail.jsp?id=465566&sk=&date=&%0A%09%09%09&pageID=2

Palumbo, F.B. and Mullins, C.D., 2002. The development of direct-to-consumer prescription drug advertising regulation. *Food and Drug Law Journal*, 57 (3): 423–443. Posted at: http://www.kff.org/rxdrugs/loader.cfm?url=/commonspot/security/getfile.cfm&PageID=14372

Provost Peters, C., 2004. *Fundamentals of the Prescription Drug Market. National Health Policy Forum Background Paper*. NHPF: Washington, DC, August 24, 2004.

Vecchione, A., 2008. Loop of faith. *Medical Marketing & Media*, 38–45, November 2008.

von Knoop, C. et al., 2003. *Vital Signs: E-Health in the United States*. Boston Consulting Group: Boston, MA. Posted at: http://www.bcg.com/impact_expertise/publications/files/Vital_Signs_E_Health_United_States_Jan2003.pdf

## CHAPTER 10

Biopricing

Biologics in 2008 comprised a mean 13.7% of pharmacy benefit expenditures. A mean 11.7% of 2008 total biologic costs under the pharmacy benefit were paid for by the consumer.

Source: Bristol-Myers Squibb, *2009 Biotechnology Monitor & Survey*™: *Marketplace Policies, Practices, and Perspectives*, New York, 2009, Posted at: http://www.biotechmonitor.com/Publication.asp

W E HAVE PREVIOUSLY STUDIED the research and development efforts, the manufacturing techniques, as well as the promotional efforts required by a biopharmaceutical manufacturer to commercialize its product. Moving along the four Ps continuum, we now proceed into price and place dimensions. The focus of this chapter is biopharmaceutical pricing, one of the major determinants of healthcare costs, and most closely, drug expenditures.

The parameters we have just mentioned, namely, pricing and expenditures, are multidimensional, and often competing with each other. On the one side, biopharmaceutical enterprises are entirely leveraged, require in excess of $1 billion to commercialize a biopharmaceutical, and are thus looking for profit maximization and risk reduction, characteristics indicating higher biopharmaceutical prices. On the other hand, state governments or employer/private insurance funds are faced with increased life expectancies, the maturing of baby boomers, and sky-rocketing healthcare costs, an important contributor of which is drug expenditure. Faced with these dilemmas, regulators are seeking to maintain costs, by either controlling biopharmaceutical prices, or product usage, or company profitability. In this chapter, we will discuss global biopharmaceutical pricing regulation, as well as the methods involved in defining biopharmaceutical prices, and achieving reimbursement in an ever more regulated and restricted healthcare environment. Under this environment, increased efficacy and safety are confronted with higher costs or limitations in the use of newer, more innovative biopharmaceuticals.

FACTORS CONSIDERED IN DRUG PRICING

Before we embark on analyzing the biopharmaceutical pricing methods in place, we need to study a millennia-old pricing truth: "a product's pricing is ideal when it maximizes the producer's profitability at a pricing level that is deemed as appropriate and fair valued by the consumer." This axiom contains two important truths. First, a profit-oriented biopharma organization is driven to profit maximization by its multiple stakeholders (mainly investors). Second, the organization's customers will pay for a product as much of a price as possible, until the product's competitive advantages are matched by alternative products that possess an even higher price, that is where the consumer thinks the product is "fair valued."

Now let us turn our attention to the two opposing forces driving modern-day biopharmaceutical pricing. On the one side, factors driving higher product prices are R&D costs, manufacturing costs, administrative costs, as well as the product's patent protection, competitive advantages, degree of differentiation, disease characteristics, patient characteristics, prescriber characteristics, and biopharma strategy objectives.

On the other hand, factors driving lower product pricing are competitive alternatives, disease–patient–prescriber characteristics, economies of scale, the biopharma's cost differentiation, prescription regulation, loss of patent protection, and marketing monopoly. We will review most of these factors below. As far as drug expenditure is concerned, Figure 10.1 summarizes some of the most important factors influencing drug expenditures today.

U.S. HEALTHCARE COST NUMBERS

Unregulated versus Regulated Markets

Although not easily realized by consumers, various markets exist according to the price-setting limitations (or lack of) for the products sold in these markets. In a *seller's market*, a seller may define its pricing at will, for example, because there is no alternative, and the market is a monopoly.

In a *buyer's market*, the buyer sets the pricing; because there are multiple sellers with identical products that need to be sold, or they risk becoming obsolete (e.g., a farmer's market). In an oligopoly, there are a few competitors (in my native language *oligon* means a few, while *polo* is to sell). A biopharmaceutical market is usually an oligopoly, where high barriers to entry (e.g., high R&D costs; see Chapter 8) limit the number of existing competitors. Finally, in a *free market*, there is a multitude of competitors, where open competition drives the product prices lower (due to price transparency and alternatives' existence). An example of free markets is Internet sales, and the existence of price-comparison search engines.

In all of the examples mentioned above, we have assumed that each seller sets a certain price level at which he or she offers their products in a given market. However, a large market is rarely homogeneous, meaning there exist multiple distinct market segments within the given market (see Chapter 8). When this occurs, as in the case of biopharmaceutical markets, biomanufacturers usually adapt their product prices accordingly, matching the individual market segment characteristics to the pricing levels offered.

The existence of various market segments, even for a single therapeutic indication, for example, Parkinson's disease, is due to various factors: (1) the different standards of living among nations; (2) the existence of import/export barriers, having to do with the protection of public health; (3) the existence of varying numbers of locally active competitors; (4) the existence of various reimbursement and formulary regulations; (5) the existence of various biopharmaceutical industry regulation policies; (6) the existence of different prescriber and patient needs across markets; (7) the offering of various price or volume discounts by the industry; (8) the existence of various non-biopharmaceutical remedies (e.g., Chinese medicine); and more. For all these diverse reasons, biopharmaceutical pricing is complex, diverse, non-transparent, and highly regulated across the world's therapeutic markets.

An additional biopharmaceutical market designation is the labeling of regulated versus unregulated. Under *regulated*, there are a large number of international markets that major aspects of healthcare and medicinal policies (e.g., IP protection, clinical trials, marketing authorization, pricing, and reimbursement) are regulated by the state. In contrast, under *unregulated*, there are also a large number of nations that exert lesser or no regulation on major healthcare policies, for example, by not imposing strict patent-protection laws or allowing the free setting of medicinal prices upon their commercial introduction. We will mention examples of both regulated and unregulated biopharmaceutical markets in the following sections.

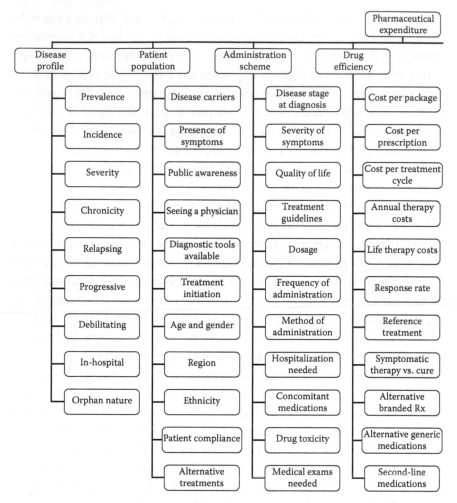

FIGURE 10.1 Factors influencing drug expenditures. (From PRIME Institute, in Pharmaceutical Research and Manufacturers of America, *Pharmaceutical Industry Profile 2009*, PhRMA, Washington, DC, 2009. With permission.)

The U.S. Healthcare Market

The discussion of the world's most significant biopharmaceutical markets would not be appropriate without first discussing the characteristics of the largest healthcare market in the world, namely, that of the United States of America. Let us take a brief look into some of its impressive characteristics, as provided by various, well-respected sources. According to the Organization for Economic Collaboration and Development (*Source: OECD, OECD Health Data 2008*, Paris, France, 2008, http://www.oecd.org. With permission.), during 2007 the United States had

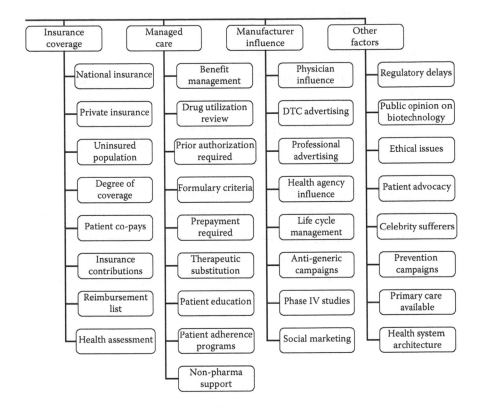

- 16% of GDP allocated to health expenditure ($7290 per capita)
- 12% of total healthcare expenditure allocated to pharmaceutical expenditure ($878 per capita)
- 2.43 practicing physicians and 10.57 practicing nurses per 1000 population
- 3.1 hospital beds per 1000 population
- Life expectancy at birth (2006 data) was 80.7 years (females) and 75.4 (males)

In addition, according to IMS Health (http://www.imshealth.com) during 2008 in the United States

- Total prescription market was $291.5 billion

- Top therapeutic class by value sales was Antipsychotics with $14.6 billion

- Top pharmaceutical corporation by value sales was Pfizer with $20.5 billion, and top biopharmaceutical corporation was Amgen with 13.4 billion

- Top pharmaceutical product by value sales was Lipitor with $7.8 billion, and top biopharmaceutical product was Enbrel with 3.4 billion

- Total prescription market by number of dispensed prescriptions was 3.84 billion prescriptions, of which 2.05 were dispensed by chain pharmacy stores, 0.77 were dispended by independents, 0.48 were dispensed by food stores, 0.31 were dispensed by long-term care, and 0.24 were dispensed by mail order.

Furthermore, the U.S. Centers for Medicare and Medicaid Services provide data on the U.S. Health Expenditures by Object 2003–2006 (USD billion) in Table 10.1 (2009), and the National Association of Chain Drug Stores provide data on the U.S. pharmaceutical prescription costs in 2007–2008 (USD) in Table 10.2 (2009). Finally, the Pharmaceutical Research and Manufacturers of America provide data on how each healthcare dollar is spent in 2008 in Figure 10.2.

We have previously mentioned the terms of unregulated versus regulated markets. So, which side of the spectrum does the U.S. biopharmaceutical market belong to? The answer is, surprisingly, both! On the side of IP protection, clinical trials, and marketing authorization, the U.S. market is arguably the highest regulated market in the world. Simultaneously, on the issue of biomanufacturers being able to set their products' selling prices, the U.S. market is unregulated, that is, it does not impose an initially state-mandated price, nor does it compare international prices, nor does it demand deflationary repricings in the future.

At the end of the day, however, the lack of initial pricing regulation has led to high biopharmaceutical prices in the U.S. market. Proponents and critics of the pricing regulation have their own opposing views. Let us try to neutrally review them for a moment. On the one side, free pricing

TABLE 10.1   U.S. Health Expenditures by Object 2003–2006 (U.S.$ Billion)

Object of Expenditure	2003	2004	2005	2006	2007
Total	1734.9	1854.8	1980.6	2112.7	2241.2
Spent by:					
Consumers	828.3	880.8	937.0	986.3	1043.5
Out-of-pocket	224.6	234.9	247.0	255.0	268.6
Private insurance	603.7	645.9	690.0	731.3	775.0
Public	779.0	839.9	899.0	973.0	1035.7
Other	127.6	134.2	144.6	153.4	162.0
Spent for:					
Health services and supplies	1623.1	1733.1	1850.4	1976.1	2098.1
Personal health care expenses	1447.5	1550.2	1655.1	1765.5	1878.3
Hospital care	527.4	566.8	607.5	649.3	696.5
Physician and clinical services	366.7	393.6	422.2	449.7	478.8
Dental services	76.9	81.5	86.4	90.5	95.2
Other professional services	49.0	52.9	56.0	58.7	62.0
Home health care	38.0	42.7	48.1	53.0	59.0
Prescription drugs	174.2	188.8	199.7	216.8	227.5
Other nondurable medical products	32.1	32.7	34.0	35.3	37.4
Durable medical equipment	22.4	22.8	23.8	24.2	24.5
Nursing home care	110.5	115.2	120.6	125.4	131.3
Other personal health care	50.4	53.3	56.9	62.5	66.2
Public administration and net cost of private health insurance	121.9	128.8	138.7	150.4	155.7
Public health activities	53.7	54.0	56.6	60.2	64.1
Medical research	35.5	38.8	40.2	41.3	42.4
Medical structures and equipment	76.3	83.0	90.0	95.2	100.7

Source: U.S. Centers for Medicare and Medicaid Services, Office of the Actuary, "National Health Statistics Group."

TABLE 10.2   U.S. Pharmaceutical Prescription Costs in 2007–2008 (USD)

	2008	2007	2008 vs. 2007
Average brand name prescription price	137.90	121.18	13.8
Average generic prescription price	35.22	32.60	9.4
Average prescription price	71.69	68.77	4.2
Of $71.69 manufacturer receives	55.68		
Of $71.69 wholesaler receives	2.51		
Of $71.69 retailer receives	13.50		

Source: Industry Facts at a Glance: material pulled from NACDS website http://www.nacds.org/wmspage.cfm?parm1=6536 (February 6, 2010). NACDS shall not be liable for any errors or omissions in content. © National Association of Chain Drug Stores, Inc. ("NACDS"). Used with permission. All rights reserved.

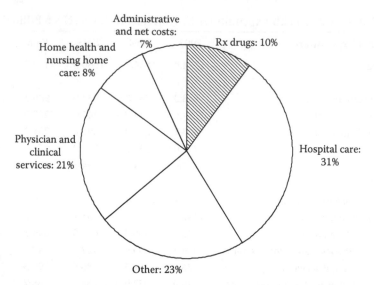

FIGURE 10.2   How each healthcare dollar is spent in 2008. (From Pharmaceutical Research and Manufacturers of America, *Pharmaceutical Industry Profile 2009*, PhRMA, Washington, DC, 2009; U.S. Centers for Medicare and Medicaid Services, 2009. Office of the Actuary, National Health Statistics Group, National health expenditure data, Posted at: http://www.cms.hhs.gov/NationalHealthExpendData/, accessed September 2009. With permission.)

(1) is an incentive for higher R&D costs, leading to national industry innovation; (2) allows U.S. biopharmaceutical enterprises to focus on the largest pharmaceutical market in the world with strong patent protection and recuperate a vast proportion of R&D costs, before reaching other markets; (3) gives U.S. patients an increased access to innovative health therapies and choices; (4) allows the U.S. federal and state governments to offer the highest possible quality of biopharmaceutical medicines to their respective constituents; and (5) allows the industry to maximize their profits as any other organization in other industries would do.

On the other side of the biopricing dilemma, critics charge that (1) biopharmaceutical R&D costs are not as high as those argued by the industry; (2) the highest prices are not due to high R&D costs, but instead to significant promotional costs, due to increased competition; (3) increased prices limit the government healthcare choices; (4) increased prices reduce the patients' actual choices (due to high co-payments); and (5) it is unethical for biomanufacturers to attempt to recuperate the majority of their costs from unregulated countries, while still selling their products with profit in heavily regulated markets.

As far as actual biopharmaceutical prices are concerned, there is a high variability in prices found at different distribution channels (see Chapter 11). A basic distinction can be made between the private and public-funded biopharmaceutical markets. At the highest end of the spectrum, we find prices for pharmaceuticals paid by patients themselves (private customers). At the next level, prices of biopharmaceuticals may vary for privately insured patients (either under a personal plan, or an employer-provided plan). Here, the biopharmaceutical prices are fully or partially reimbursed by the insurance plan, in what is called a "multitier" model. For example, a cheaper, generic alternative may demand a low patient co-pay (Tier 1), a recommended, or "preferred," branded patent-protected alternative may demand a higher co-pay (Tier 2), while an excluded, branded alternative may demand the highest co-pay (Tier 3—a disincentive).

When it comes to the government-reimbursed market segment, there are also a multitude of biopharmaceutical pricing levels. In general, big government programs, such as Medicare, Medicaid, and the Veterans' Health Administration cover large populations and, thus, have an increased bargaining power versus the biomanufacturers, leading to increased discounting, for example, a 15.1% discount on the average manufacturer price (AMP). As Table 10.2 indicates, a biomanufacturer usually receives 75% of the product's retail price, the wholesaler receives 5%, and the retail pharmacist receives 20% of that price.

MECHANISMS TO ENSURE COST-EFFECTIVE DRUG CONSUMPTION

Most healthcare systems use a combination of price and rationing to control healthcare costs. Mechanisms used to ensure cost-effective drug consumption include the use of co-payments, formularies, and controls on the prices paid for drugs, on prescribing physicians, and on pharmacists.

Factors Considered When Setting Prices in the European Union

According to the European Commission's Pharmaceutical Sector Inquiry Final Report (2009), in general, national pricing policies consider three key factors: (1) The price level ex-factory, which determines the main cost factor for the medicine. To arrive at the retail price level, the margins for the wholesalers and pharmacists as well as the VAT are added. (2) The reimbursement level, expressed as a percentage of the retail price. This will determine how much of the retail price is paid by public funds. The remaining part, also referred to as co-payment, is paid by the patient or his private supplementary insurance. The reimbursement level can often be decisive for the question whether a medicine is accessible to the patient (group) concerned. (3) Potential restrictions on stakeholders such as doctors or pharmacists, which will determine how often and under what conditions a medicine can be prescribed, dispensed and used.

These three issues are often considered jointly when a decision on the price level for a medicine is taken. They allow the authorities to control the overall budget per medicine, which is mathematically defined as (a) price per medicine at retail level × (b) reimbursement level in % × (c) volume of medicines used. In some cases, authorities and companies agree immediately on an overall budget instead of the three separate factors.

Supply- and Demand-Side Country Practices

The European commission has reported that EU member states adopt a long list of practices that affect pricing decisions. There are practices focusing on (1) prices and/or (2) reimbursement levels, which are generally referred to as "supply-side practices." And there are practices focusing on (c) use of the medicine called "demand-side practices." Some policies combine supply- and demand-side practices. The most important practices are summarized in Table 10.3. It is however important to note here that the pricing landscape is dynamic.

International Price Comparisons

When using international reference pricing, a government reviews price levels for each new biopharmaceutical in reference countries and sets the local price according to a local legislated formula, for example, lowest among EU countries, average among Commonwealth countries, using a standard-of-living adjustment formula, etc. For example, a large number of countries reference U.K. biopharmaceutical prices (often Commonwealth countries). There are several issues to be confronted here though, for example, the standard-of-living adjustments, the currency fluctuations, and the different strengths, dosages, and formulations used in the compared markets.

As a direct consequence of international price comparisons, the issue of "parallel importation" has arisen, that is, the movement of goods from a low-priced country to a higher-priced one, usually by large multinational wholesalers or Internet pharmacies. While the practice is fully legal among the EU countries, there are still important limitations in importing foreign medications into the large U.S. market, and even those originating from neighboring Canada. As far as the U.S. market prices are compared with international prices, it appears that (1) branded biopharmaceuticals

TABLE 10.3   What Kind of Price Regulation Policies Do Biopharmaceutical Companies Face from National Governments around the World?

#	Type	Description	Market Example
A	*Price barriers*		
1	Price setting by Government	Governmental pharmaceutical pricing committee sets the official local price (usually the local wholesale price) from which the manufacturer-to-wholesaler and retail prices are set using set formulas	
2	International reference pricing	Government reviews price levels for each new biopharmaceutical in reference countries and sets the local price according to a local legislated formula, e.g., lowest among EU countries, average among Commonwealth countries, using a standard-of-living adjustment formula.	Greece
3	Therapeutic class reference pricing	Government reviews price levels of all locally available medicines within the same therapeutic class and sets a maximum price reimbursement level for the new biopharmaceutical, e.g., the class average or a pre-agreed price reimbursement ceiling	Netherlands
4	Price-volume limitations	Local price reimbursement level is set for a maximum sales volume. If the sales volume is exceeded, the biopharmaceutical manufacturer is mandated to retroactively reduce reimbursement prices for that year, or return a given percentage of value sales to the State	Italy
5	Profit control	Government sets a maximum profit level for any product or manufacturer within a year. If these profit targets are exceeded, the manufacturer is mandated to return a given percentage of profit to the state	United Kingdom
6	Price floor	Government sets a price floor for every off-patent pharmaceutical (e.g., 80% of on-patent level), in order to incentivize the domestic generic industry. If the price level was to be left unaltered, then prescribers would feel reluctant to pay same price for a no-brand alternative. Also, if price level was completely liberalized, the branded manufacturer would reduce the price level to a significantly lower level, blocking the sales of generics due to their lack of volume efficiencies	

(continued)

TABLE 10.3 (continued)   What Kind of Price Regulation Policies Do Biopharmaceutical
Companies Face from National Governments around the World?

#	Type	Description	Market Example
7	Tendering	Government purchases annual quantities of each therapeutic area medicines, requiring the submission of sealed tenders, leading to price-only comparisons of all medications, and ignoring efficacy, safety, tolerability, long-term cost effectiveness and innovation criteria	Israel
B	*Approval barriers*		
8	Marketing approval delay	Government applies local clinical data requirements, time delays, high fee cost barriers, drug master file content regulations, and approval criteria that are designed to either delay entry of newer high-priced medicines, or unfairly incentivize less regulated domestic generic manufacturers	
9	Pricing approval delay	Government requires submission of detailed cost-of-goods data, or multi-country price lists, officially validated by its local embassies, which are then analyzed and compared by designated price committees, leading to significant delays. Here, manufacturers may delay price submission from low-priced countries, or Governments may dictate price submission from mostly low-price countries in a pricing regulation tug-of-war	
10	Reimbursement approval delay	Following marketing and pricing approval, reimbursement approval may require extended periods of time, effectively limiting the sales of newer highly priced biopharmaceuticals, as opposed by low-priced chemical reference treatments	
11	Cost-effectiveness approval delay	Following the marketing, pricing, and reimbursement approvals (three hurdles), the fourth hurdle mandates the cost-effectiveness comparison of all medications within the same therapeutic class, which obviously relies on Government-imposed cut-off points as far as life prolongation or QoL are concerned, often leading to Government–industry confrontations on patient access to new medicines (e.g., why some EU patients have access and not others)	United Kingdom

TABLE 10.3 (continued)   What Kind of Price Regulation Policies Do Biopharmaceutical
Companies Face from National Governments around the World?

#	Type	Description	Market Example
C	*Dispensing and prescribing barriers*		
12	Formulary requirements	Formularies may be imposed by state insurance plans, regional health authorities, municipal authorities, or individual hospitals limiting the prescribing of highly priced medicines. The formularies may be "positive," i.e., allowing the use of all included medicines, "negative," i.e., prohibiting the use of included medicines, "tiered," i.e., allowing different levels of patient co-payments, or "restrictive," i.e., allowing up to an annual maximum number of patients	United States
13	Prescribing guidelines	Prescribing guidelines may apply strict treatment guidelines, i.e., who receives what, how often, and how much, prescriber limitations, e.g., only prescribed by reference hospitals, or community specialists, diagnosis limitations, e.g., initial diagnosis only by medical committees, brand substitution, e.g., prescriber recommends only class of medicines, statins, and pharmacy can substitute for lower-priced generics, hospital-only distribution and not retail.	
14	Prescribing budget	Individual prescriber monitoring, leading to prescribed patient limitations, refill limitations, prescribed unit limitations, prescribed value limitations, prescribed classes limitations, or prescribed percentage of generics requirements. Regulations may include board disqualifications, insurance plan disqualifications, or tax penalties for overprescribing, and salary incentives for under-prescribing	United Kingdom
15	Promotional obstacles	Government-imposed limitations on promotional activities to physicians, medical conference attendance subsidies, direct industry-to-prescriber bank payments, perks, and gimmicks limitations, consultancy fee limitations, clinical trial fees, etc. The limitations may also cover direct-to-consumer advertising, advertising to other health professionals, etc.	

sold in private channels are higher priced, (2) the same products sold to government programs are equally priced with international government purchase prices, and (3) U.S. generic prices are usually lower than those in comparable international markets, probably due to economies of scale and increased competition.

Co-Payments and Reimbursement Policies

Individual patients suffering from chronic and severe diseases, often treated with biopharmaceutical medications, face different restrictions in their usage across nations. For example, a patient may be insured or noninsured, when insured, he or she may enjoy a limited reimbursement level, leading to a significant co-payment out of his or her pocket, or a biopharmaceutical may be reimbursed up to a certain limit (reference), or a biopharmaceutical may be excluded from a formulary, etc. In some countries, it is even common for a patient to change employers or the location of residency, in search of better disease reimbursement conditions, a phenomenon criticized by patient advocates as treatment inequality. In fact, the same phenomenon has given rise to the "medical tourism" movement, where patients suffering from a disease choose to travel to foreign countries, in search of better pharmaceuticals, surgery, services, and more.

Formularies

As previously discussed, state and private insurance schemes often utilize a biopharmaceutical drug formulary, where all commercially available formulations are either fully reimbursed, or partially reimbursed, or even non-reimbursed for their members. In other cases, the formularies take the form of either "positive" (medications are covered), or "negative reimbursement lists" (listed medications are excluded or not covered). In the majority of cases, there is a multitiered model in effect, according to which medications listed at different tiers are covered at different percentages (explained above).

Price Controls

There are various methods of governmental price setting of biopharmaceuticals in different markets. First, prices can be set at cost-of-goods plus allowed profit. Second, they can be set at international price level (referred to as a "basket of reference countries") adjusted by a formula. Third, they can be set equal to the price of a previously priced substitute. Fourth, they can be priced freely, but reimbursed up to a certain limit (price band).

Fifth, they can be priced at a certain premium over a standard treatment. Sixth, they can be priced at a price discount, over a branded original (often mandated for newer off-patent generics). Seventh, they can be priced higher than local alternatives (in support of the local industry). Eight, they can be re-priced higher by a set percentage, or lower by a set percentage by an across-the-board re-pricing decree. Ninth, they can be priced higher, provided a detailed pharmacoeconomic analysis has proven that over the long term they are more cost effective than existing alternatives.

Finally, as an emerging phenomenon, biopharmaceuticals can be priced at a conditional pricing, for example, higher priced if efficacy endpoints are observed in practice (see later into this chapter). Whatever the means of governmental price control is, there are various criticisms expressed. For example, price controls may stifle innovation, may reduce access to new medicines, or may create treatment inequality among populations.

Controls on Physicians and Pharmacists

There are various government-imposed schemes of prescriber practices. For example, (1) following treatment guidelines; (2) following restrictive formularies; (3) sophisticated biopharmaceuticals prescribed by only disease specialists, or even state hospital clinic directors; (4) prescription monitoring, limiting the number of vials prescribed, or the overall prescription value; (5) annual physician prescription ceilings; (6) prescriber incentives on generics usage; (7) fixed annual reimbursement of physician services, irrespective of patient visits; (8) competition among family physicians for lowest fees required to service a given patient population; (9) prior authorization of prescription by the patient's insurance fund; or (10) mandatory inclusion of patients into adherence-improving programs.

On the other side, profit and dispensing limitations have been imposed on pharmacists too. For example, (1) substitution rights with cheaper bioequivalent medicines, often recommended or even mandated by the government; (2) reduction of retail profit margins; (3) expensive biopharmaceuticals often dispensed only through state hospital pharmacies; or (4) patient adherence to treatment monitoring. One of the well-known international government-regulated pricing systems is the U.K. Pharmaceutical Price Regulation Scheme (PPRS) described below.

Pharmaceutical Price Regulation Scheme Example: U.K.'s PPRS

According to the U.K.'s Department of Health (DH), the health departments of the United Kingdom and the Association of the British

Pharmaceutical Industry have a common interest in ensuring that safe and effective medicines are available on reasonable terms to the NHS. It is important to both parties that the pharmaceutical industry is strong, efficient and profitable. Therefore the objectives of the scheme are to:

- Deliver value for money for the NHS by securing the provision of safe and effective medicines at reasonable prices, and encouraging the efficient development and competitive supply of medicines.

- Encourage innovation by promoting a strong and profitable pharmaceutical industry that is capable and willing to invest in sustained research and development to encourage the future availability of new and improved medicines for the benefit of patients and industry in this and other countries.

- Promote access and uptake for new medicines.

- Provide stability, sustainability and predictability to help the NHS and industry develop sustainable financial and investment strategies.

Overall, under the PPRS scheme, pharmaceutical prices are renegotiated every five years with biopharma industry, there is free pricing for new biological entities, there are restrictions on profits, it is difficult to obtain price increases, and renewals of PPRS often involve agreement on across the board price reductions.

Source: United Kingdom Department of Health—Department for Business Innovations and Skills, Life sciences in the U.K.—Economic analysis and evidence for "Life sciences 2010: Delivering the blueprint." DH: January 2010, Posted at: http://www.berr.gov.uk/files/file54303.pdf. With permission.

VALUE-BASED PRICING

Biopharmaceutical pricing, even though apparently complex and sophisticated follows four basic contributing parameters. First, the estimated cost-of-goods (COGS) per unit of product sold. Second, the product's competitive advantages over the competitive products (present and anticipated), and their respective prices. Third, the price level that either reimbursement agencies or patients (co-payments) will be willing to pay for the product's competitive offerings, often called willingness-to-pay. Fourth, the desired return-on-investment (ROI), that the biopharma has set for the given product, taking into consideration the following components: (1) overall R&D

costs, including costs for the failed drug candidates within the same thera-peutic area; (2) expected total product sales on- and off-patent protection until its market withdrawal; and (3) total lifetime product sales, marketing, and administrative costs. In general, market pricing assessments lead to indicative upper biopharmaceutical price levels, while the company's strat-egy and product assessment leads to the lowest acceptable pricing levels. Both assessment approaches will be further discussed below.

Market Perspective and Value-Based Pricing

We will start from the market perspective of a biopharmaceutical, which is based on its competitive advantages and the value the customer is will-ing to pay for it. Let us see how this can be expressed with a formula: *Value = Reference Price ± Differentiation*.

Here the value of a biopharmaceutical to its customer equals the refer-ence price of a therapeutic alternative plus/minus the new product's dif-ferentiation, where some product characteristics would be advantageous over the reference offerings (positive differentiation), while others might be inferior (negative differentiation). It is imperative that, if there is a posi-tive differentiation, a higher price can be sought (a premium), while if the differentiation is negative, a lower price (a discount) may be requested. At the end of the day, if we constantly ask "is this product worth the premium price?," then so can a biomanufacturer ask its prescribers and patients "what premium would you be willing to pay for such a differentiation?"

Value-based pricing, therefore, involves four distinctive steps: (1) defining the product, (2) demonstrating the value, (3) quantifying the value, and (4) communicating the value. Let us see how these steps are done.

Defining the Biopharmaceutical

As previously described, a biopharmaceutical is defined mainly through a well-designed, controlled, long-term, thorough, and multinational, mul-ticenter, and multi-patient clinical trial program. As more trials are com-pleted and analyzed, more product attributes become apparent, and some of them hopefully offer differentiation to the product.

An additional dimension in biopharmaceutical differentiation is the multiple clinical trial settings used. For starters, a new biological entity (NBE) may be simultaneously tested in three therapeutic indications, three disease states (early, stable, progressive), three patient age popula-tions (paediatric, adult, elderly), alone or in combination, four dosage strengths, and two routes of administration! Where is the product value here? The answer is that the biopharmaceutical comes out from the clinical trial program with different product values in different patient segments.

How should our own Advanced Therapies price its leading NBE candidate then? Let us think of a scenario where their first autoimmune biopharmaceutical is active in rheumatoid arthritis, ulcerative colitis, and rheumatoid psoriasis. It appears that ADTHER57 has three distinct product values, one each per indication chosen. Which one is higher? The one where the product is targeted against the indication with the highest unmet patient needs.

"OK, fine, so our NBE may be launched with differential prices in different indications, right?" proclaims one of their board members. "Not that easy," answers the marketing executive. The reasons being that (1) government pricing agencies may object to highly differential pricing for the same product, (2) differential pricing would require differential branding and promotion, (3) it would seem unethical, and be accused as predatory pricing, to price the product X for RA, and 2X for colitis, and (4) unauthorized, off-the-indication brand switching may occur if the price differential is too high.

Not to despair, there are certain strategic moves that Advanced Therapies may follow when it eventually launches ADTHER57 into the marketplace: (1) launch in unregulated (free pricing) country markets; (2) launch in regulated markets all at the same time, so that sales under patent protection are maximized (requires simultaneous marketing authorizations, too); (3) launch the product in the indication with the highest unmet need first, where the product enjoys the highest differentiation; (4) launch the product in therapeutic areas with lesser product value later, but if clinical trial results allow, position the product in a higher severity subsegment, where a higher dosage is beneficial, so that cost per treatment per patient per year resembles that of the first-launched indication; (5) increase product differentiation between therapeutic areas (e.g., with different routes of administration and formulations) so that off-the-indication brand switching is limited; (6) increase product differentiation between national markets (e.g., with different external packaging and language used) so that parallel exports are discouraged; (7) use promotion that differentiates, differentiates, differentiates (!), so that different product positionings are successfully endorsed; and (8) discourage indication switching and cross-border imports by any means (usually lobbying in the United States, or legal action and limiting shipments to lower-priced countries in the European Union).

Demonstrating a Biopharmaceutical's Hidden Value

The major method of demonstrating the value of a new biopharmaceutical product in development is the careful design of its clinical trials' program. Let us think about this proposition for a while. An old marketing adage would proclaim, "In order to increase any product's sales, you need to (1) increase product differentiation, (2) increase the number of users, (3) increase usage per user, (4) increase frequency of usage, (5) increase user adherence, or (6) increase user loyalty."

Let us see how these principles apply to the clinical trial setting in a pharmacologically sound and ethical way (prerequisites): (1) differentiation needs to be shown in terms of statistically significant differences versus placebo or reference drug(s); (2) multiple indications need to be tested and proven effective for the biopharmaceutical in question; (3) higher efficacy with acceptable tolerability at higher dosages needs to be shown; (4) increased frequency of dosing needs to be proven beneficial, while still avoiding under- or over-dosages; (5) increased patient adherence needs to lead to higher treatment response rates, as indicated by lower efficacy observed in treatment dropouts; (6) increased loyalty needs to be shown as beneficial, by designing "cross-over" treatments, where patients switch therapy groups after a period of time and continue to be monitored; (7) the patients' vital signs, disease endpoints, but also their perceived quality of life (QoL) need to be shown to improve with the new biopharmaceutical; and (8) the product differentiation, apart from its "core attributes," namely, efficacy and safety, can be further improved by the use of new administration devices (e.g., painless multi-injector devices, or inhalation versus injection). Table 10.4 describes the launch pricing options for a new biopharmaceutical product.

TABLE 10.4   What Are the Launch Pricing Options for a Biopharmaceutical?

		Price		
		Premium	**Adjusted Premium or Parity**	**Penetration**
Innovation	High	First-in-class/high unmet need	Market-adjusted premium	N/A
	Medium	Low reimbursement, life-enhancing drug	Dominant competitor	Late entrant
	Low	Higher tolerability	Dominant competitor	Successor brands

Quantifying a Biopharmaceutical's Value to Various Stakeholders

We are now entering the third step in value-based pricing. Clinical trial results will have given Advanced Therapies' board initial indications of their product's value. What comes next is quantifying that value by going directly to the customer, either the prescribing physician or the patient. There are, however, some potential caveats to this approach: (1) the biopharmaceutical may be targeted at therapeutic categories that are usually fully reimbursed, so that prescribers and patients may not have the price as a limiting factor, as opposed to the country's price regulators who also need to be involved in the process; (2) the procedure lends itself susceptible to lack of objectivity, especially when the unmet disease needs are high; (3) unregulated markets may tend to higher prices accepted, while regulated markets may tend to indicate lower prices, even below what the regulators may accept based on long-term cost-to-benefit analyses; and (4) ethnic differences may lead to distortions in acceptable prices, for example, some markets only desiring the very best, while other markets being more "reserved" and mindful of the country's common economic situation versus the disease burden.

The problems mentioned above lead to the following strategies: (1) Approach all involved parties, be it the prescribers, patients, families, price regulators, formulary committees, health authorities, insurance funds, or hospital administrators, and assign weighting and ratings to each one of these influencers; (2) define early into the process the biggest unmet needs and their relative significance for prescribers and patients; (3) study the competition's attributes (present and anticipated) and value them with the help of prescribers and patients; (4) conduct multinational pricing surveys as early as possible; (5) take into account historic pricing precedents within each country, for example, how much premium was previously allowed and for what therapeutic advantage; and (6) incorporate more objective value-estimating methodologies and tools, such as detailed pharmacoeconomic analyses.

Pharmacoeconomic Analysis

According to the U.K.'s National Institute for Health and Clinical Excellence (NICE; http://www.nice.org.uk/), from a theoretical perspective, pharmaceutical prices should be set on the basis of cost-benefit analysis, also known as pharmacoeconomic analysis (OECD, 2001. With permission). The pharmacoeconomic value of a new pharmaceutical product is generally measured by a comparison of the change in total healthcare and other costs with the change in health outcomes that are associated with the use of the new product. Changes in costs include the acquisition and administration costs for the new product compared with those for the drugs that the new therapy might replace, as well as changes in the costs that are associated with the treatment of the disease and with side effects. Also included might be changes in productivity-related costs and other indirect costs.

For a drug-value analysis, changes in health outcomes are most commonly measured in changes of quality-adjusted life years (QALYs), which are computed on the basis of the level of well-being in alternative health states and the duration of time in each alternative health state, both with and without the new drug. The ratio of changes in costs divided by changes in QALYs is computed to calculate a cost per QALY for the new drug. Many countries now incorporate a review of pharmacoeconomic evidence as part of their assessment of whether to recommend reimbursement or usage of a new product at the price that is requested by the manufacturer. In the United Kingdom, NICE uses a threshold of £30,000 per QALY to set the upper limit on willingness to pay for therapeutic advances. NICE produces guidance in public health, health technologies (including biopharmaceuticals), and clinical practice in the United Kingdom.

By conducting the relevant analyses, manufacturers can use such metrics to estimate a price at which a new therapy falls within the accepted range. For additional information on the field of pharmacoeconomics, you may visit the International Society for Pharmacoeconomics and Outcomes Research (ISPOR; http://www.ispor.org), as well as the London School of Economics (LSE)—Department of Social Policy (http://www2.lse.ac.uk/socialPolicy/Home.aspx) Web sites.

Communicating a Biopharmaceutical's Value with a Core Value Dossier

The traditional pharmaceutical marketing communication channels, such as the sales force, journal advertising and scientific publications, all have a role in communicating the value of a new product to its customers. However, these traditional channels tend to focus on either top-line product messages, or specific aspects of the product or disease profile. Increasingly, the vehicle that is used for communicating the most complete picture of the differential value of a product is a *core value dossier* (CVD), which is aimed specifically at the payer, and focuses on the clinical and economic differentiation of the product in the context of the contemporary treatment environment. This is particularly important for products that are expected to have a large effect on the drug budget, and/ or if the current burden of the disease is not well understood and needs to be highlighted. Several healthcare consultancies and Contract Research Organizations (CROs) are able to help young biopharmaceutical organizations with the creation of a CVD.

Providers and scientists will communicate in advance of discovery. Providers know the needs of their patient population and can bring valuable insight to focused discovery. Companies should consider focus groups of potential end users early in the development process.

Positioning Importance on Reimbursement Example: Tacrolimus and Pimecrolimus in the United Kingdom

1.1. Topical tacrolimus and pimecrolimus are not recommended for the treatment of mild atopic eczema or as first-line treatments for atopic eczema of any severity.

1.2. Topical tacrolimus is recommended, within its licensed indications, as an option for the second-line treatment of moderate to severe atopic eczema in adults and children aged 2 years and older that has not been controlled by topical corticosteroids (see Section 1.4), where there is a serious risk of important adverse effects from further topical corticosteroid use, particularly irreversible skin atrophy.

1.3. Pimecrolimus is recommended, within its licensed indications, as an option for the second-line treatment of moderate atopic eczema on the face and neck in children aged 2 to 16 years that has not been controlled by topical corticosteroids (see Section 1.4), where there is a serious risk of important adverse effects from further topical corticosteroid use, particularly irreversible skin atrophy.

1.4. For the purposes of this guidance, atopic eczema that has not been controlled by topical corticosteroids refers to disease that has not shown a satisfactory clinical response to adequate use of the maximum strength and potency that is appropriate for the patient's age and the area being treated.

1.5. It is recommended that treatment with tacrolimus or pimecrolimus be initiated only by physicians (including general practitioners) with a special interest and experience in dermatology, and only after careful discussion with the patient about the potential risks and benefits of all appropriate second-line treatment options.

Source: United Kingdom NHS—National Institute for Health and Clinical Excellence (NICE), Final guidance on tacrolimus and pimecrolimus for atopic eczema (TA82), 2004, Posted at: http://guidance.nice.org.uk/TA82/Guidance. With permission.

DETERMINING THE GLOBAL LAUNCH STRATEGY

Let us not forget: a biopharmaceutical's pricing depends on (1) cost of manufacturing, (2) differential value, (3) willingness to pay, and (4) desired profitability. The cost of manufacturing a biopharmaceutical has been analyzed in Chapter 7, while differential value and willingness to pay were discussed above. Let us now focus on the desired profitability, directly mandating the biopharma's pricing objectives.

Biopharma Pricing Objectives

There are three distinctive pricing objectives that a biopharmaceutical manufacturer may have for a new product introduction. First, the product is deemed as far superior to any present or anticipated competitive alternative, thus targeting a significant price premium, over and above the alternatives, in a pricing objective called "market skimming." Second, the new product is considered as therapeutically equivalent to existing or anticipated alternatives, lacking any significant competitive advantages, thus targeting a similar price to the closest alternatives, a strategy called "price parity." Third, the product is internally deemed as inferior to existing competitive alternatives, thus having a negative differential value, and leading to a lower price (offered at a discount), in a strategy aimed for maximum market penetration or market share capture, a strategy called "penetration pricing."

Launch Price Strategy

The biopharmaceutical launch price strategy follows the following steps:

1. The cost-of-goods are estimated in detail, as in capital-fixed-variable expenses. Furthermore, future economies of scale (achieved at higher sales volumes) are entered into the pricing formula.

2. The product's competitive advantages (differential value) are weighted versus the competition's, valued, and entered into the estimation.

3. The pricing objective emerges (premium–parity–discount) and entered into the estimation.

4. The biopharma's expected ROI is entered into the estimation, for example:

   a. Total R&D Costs + Approval Costs + Manufacturing Costs + Selling and Marketing Costs + Administrative Costs = Total Product Costs + Desired Profits = Total Sales Revenues Targeted

   b. ÷ Total Units Sold over the Product's Lifetime =

   c. Target Unit Price (Minimum)

5. Alternative pricing scenarios are developed (it is imperative that all three scenarios are above 4c:

   a. Highest for Unregulated Markets

   b. Average for Slightly Regulated Markets

   c. *Lowest for Toughest-Regulated Markets* (usually tender markets—"cut-throat")

6. Biopharma representatives are involved in direct negotiations with local pricing authorities over the submitted CVDs (see above).

7. Based on price negotiations above, several *pricing segments* are identified.

8. External market research agencies are involved in assessing prescriber and patient price elasticities (see sub-chapter below).

9. Pricing options 5a, 5b, and 5c are evaluated by creating price-elasticity demand curves for regulators–prescribers–patients (see sub-chapter below).

10. Based on the price elasticity demand findings (# 9), *a global price band* (or "price corridor") is developed, for example, between $136 and $400/vial.

11. Based on preexisting parallel export patterns, additional *price corridors* are created (e.g., a European, Latin American, Middle Eastern), where the EU corridor may be $187–$277/vial.

12. Within each price corridor, the highest–average–lowest scenarios are also tested and the parallel exports predicted, together with overall European profitability estimates.

13. Final pricing levels to be submitted to each local pricing authority are created and internally reviewed and approved.

14. A country-by-country launch timing plan is created, where unregulated countries come first and toughest-regulated come last.

It becomes immediately apparent that international export insight, local market knowledge, therapeutic area expertise, pricing strategy, tactical know-how, external expertise, and sophisticated pricing software are all critical in defining a new biopharmaceutical product's ideal pricing. A summary of the launch price strategic steps is described in Table 10.5.

Country Prices

Assuming appropriate preparatory work has been conducted throughout the development process, in terms of estimating price potential and concurrently optimizing product development to maximize the pricing/commercial opportunity, development of the final launch price for a new product generally occurs between registration and technical approval. For countries without formal price controls (such as the United States, the United Kingdom, and Germany), a manufacturer is free to launch at its desired price immediately after attaining marketing approval. Before this, the company normally conducts price-sensitivity testing with physicians, patients, and/or payers (depending on the product) to validate the planning price estimates and set a profit-maximizing price. For price-controlled markets, such as France, Spain, and Italy, if reimbursement is sought then price negotiations with government authorities are required to set an agreed price at which the product can be launched. For both "free-price" and price-controlled markets, the probable actions or reactions of competitors can be an important consideration.

Global Optimization

Given the interdependency between prices across countries, the finalization of individual country prices without considering the global effect is unwise. To ensure that prices in certain countries do not inadvertently result in negative effects elsewhere in the world, many global manufacturers conduct global pricing optimization exercises, which take into account individual optimal country prices, price-referencing mechanisms, and probable parallel trade patterns, to determine a set of prices (and, usually, a price corridor or price floor) that are optimal for the company at the global level.

TABLE 10.5 How Does a Biopharmaceutical Company Prepare for Pricing
and Reimbursement in Advance of an Upcoming Product Launch?

1	Objectives	Achieve a high premium price and achieve reimbursement in highest number of markets launched, with minimum delay possible
2	Process start	During phase II
3	Process completion	When priced, launched, and reimbursed in all markets targeted
4	Set up task force	A pricing and reimbursement task force, to include corporate clinical, manufacturing, marketing, financial (pricing), regulatory, and legal expertise, as well as select subsidiary resources, e.g., U.K. NICE input, Middle East tendering input, U.S. Medicare/Medicaid input.
5	Early pricing assumptions	The existing target product profile (TPP) contains a very specific pricing assumption
6	Evaluate clinical results	Several identified clinical attributes (e.g., efficacy, safety, tolerability, onset of action, duration of action, frequency of administration, route of administration, storage) mandate the future product price when benchmarked versus the reference chemical treatment or other, previously launched biopharmaceuticals
7	Estimate cost of goods	Receive preliminary manufacturing input from the production of clinical batch supplies and adjust for lower full-scale manufacturing costs at time of launch
8	Define desired global price band	Based on existing data, define a preliminary global price band, in order to satisfy all stakeholders involved (prescribers, patients, payers, regulators, media)
9	Conduct PE studies	Collect all possible pharmacoeconomic data in support of the anticipated price negotiations with various pricing authorities around the world
10	Finalize price band	Based on previous assumptions and data collected, finalize the global price band
11	Define submission sequence	In order for a high premium price to be achieved, it is preferable to launch first in unregulated pricing markets (e.g., United States, United Kingdom, Germany), then follow with regulated markets (e.g., France, Italy, Spain, Greece), and finally launch in co-modified tender markets (Middle East, Africa, Former Soviet Union). Respectively, launch first in high standard-of-living markets, without strict reimbursement/formulary restrictions (e.g., Scandinavia, Switzerland), keeping clear of strict negative reimbursement markets (make-or-break so-called fourth hurdle, e.g., United Kingdom)
12	Set up corporate submission dossier	To include unmet patient needs, disease burden, price band, COGS, site of manufacturing data, distribution conditions and costs, prize-winning research, clinical superiority data, effect on patient survival, effect on patient QoL, hospital cost savings, cost-effectiveness superiority data, customer testimonials, media excerpts

TABLE 10.5 (continued)   How Does a Biopharmaceutical Company Prepare
for Pricing and Reimbursement in Advance of an Upcoming Product Launch?

13	Local lobbying	In anticipation of future submissions, contact and collect feedback from pertinent opinion leaders, regulators, politicians, or patients who may be predisposed for or against the new price levels set by the biopharmaceutical to be launched
14	Locally adapt dossier	Adapt dossier to give emphasis to local mandates and irregularities, also emphasize local drug impact on state cost savings, prescriber testimonials, patient testimonials, other drug impacts on savings, local employment, reduction of patient absenteeism, freeing of health personnel time and resources, value-added services (e.g., free home delivery and nurse training), availability of free samples or donation to local health authorities
15	Undertake local submissions	In collaboration between corporate and local biopharma personnel, local consultants, lobbyists, and legal experts undertake the pricing and reimbursement submissions
16	Participate in local negotiations	Follow-up with regulatory queries, attend negotiation meetings, get corporate approval for slight price reductions within the secret in-company price band, and achieve reimbursement and formulary inclusion by individual health authorities, insurance companies, or hospitals
17	Request corporate approval	Submit a pricing approval form back to corporate to inform of all the pricing levels, time adjustments, volume discounts, tendering specificities, or additional services mandated by the local regulators before the local price is to be locked
18	Get local approval	Be included in local, state, national, or regional price list; inform and thank all stakeholders involved in the negotiation process, announce price to all members of the distribution channels and prepare for launch
19	Enrich and return the corporate dossier	After inclusion of local authority information, negotiations' fine points, solutions offered, authority comments and requests (occasionally hard bargaining)
20	Prepare for future product extensions	Update the local submission to include upcoming product line extensions, new formulations, etc.

Pricing Timetable

We have just described the essential steps in devising the launch price strategy for a new biopharmaceutical. Furthermore, the exact pricing timetable by clinical phase of development is detailed in Table 10.6.

Biopharmaceutical Price Variability

Biopharmaceutical prices may vary widely, based on the following factors: (1) therapeutic area segment, (2) distribution channel, (3) private versus

TABLE 10.6 Pricing Timetable for Biopharmaceuticals, by Clinical Phase of Development

Preclinical	Phase I	Phase II	Phase III	Launch
Indication chosen	Target product profile (TPP)	Detailed physician pricing research	Patient price sensitivity	Market launching per country sequence (unregulated first)
Comparator products chosen	Corporate and subsidiary pricing teams	Physician price sensitivity	Detailed product forecasting	Finalize reimbursement
Initial product positioning	Opinion leader advocates	COGS analysis	Product advocacy activities	Finalize formulary discounting
Unmet medical needs identified	Patient association advocates	ROI assessment	Optimal price setting	Study competitive responses
Product attribute compared and weighted	Pricing and reimbursement advisory board	Pharmacoeconomic assessment	Global price band	Adjust pricing accordingly
	Payer assessment	Competitive analysis	Regional and national price corridors	Economies of scale
	Physician assessment		Prepare reimbursement CVD	ROI analysis
	Patient assessment			

institutional buyer, (4) and product life cycle stage. Let us review some of the available prices, as listed by the U.S. Department of Health and Human Services—Health Resources and Services Administration (http://www.hrsa.gov/opa/glossary.htm. With permission):

- Actual Acquisition Cost (AAC): The net cost of a drug paid by a pharmacy.

- Average Selling Price (ASP): The weighted average of all non-federal sales to wholesalers and is net of charge backs, discounts, rebates, and other benefits tied to the purchase of the drug product, whether it is paid to the wholesaler or the retailer.

- Average Manufacturer Price (AMP): The average price paid to a manufacturer by wholesalers for drugs distributed to retail pharmacies.

- Average Wholesale Price (AWP): A national average of list prices charged by wholesalers to pharmacies.

- Best Price (BP): The lowest price available to any wholesaler, retailer, provider, health maintenance organization (HMO), nonprofit entity, or the government.

- Ceiling price: The maximum price that manufacturers can charge covered entities participating in the U.S. Public Health Service's 340B Drug Pricing Program. Compared to a drug's Average Manufacturer Price (AMP), covered entities receive a minimum discount of 15.1% for brand name drugs and 11% for generic and over-the-counter drugs, and are entitled to an additional discount if the price of the drug has increased faster than the rate of inflation.

- Copayment: In some Medicare health plans, this is the amount a Medicare beneficiary must pay for each medical service he or she gets, like a doctor visit.

- Dispensing fee: The dispensing fee represents the charge for the professional services provided by the pharmacist when dispensing a prescription (including overhead expenses and profit).

In the U.S. market, the AWP is based on information provided by drug manufacturers, distributors, and other suppliers and sold by commercial publishers of drug pricing data, such as First DataBank (http://www.firstdatabank.com/) and Thomson Medical Economics (http://medicaleconomics.modernmedicine.com/about). Figure 10.3 depicts

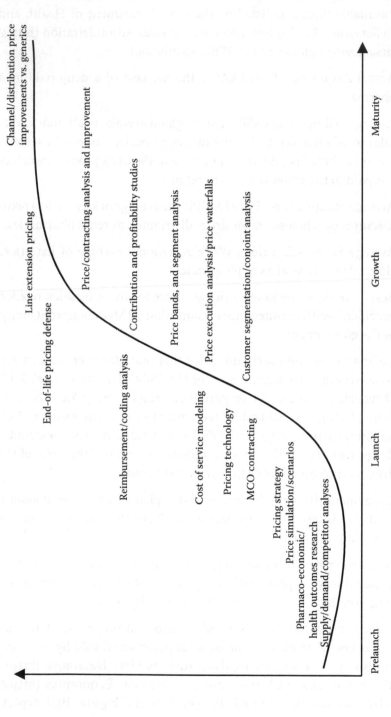

FIGURE 10.3 Pricing decisions over the product life cycle. (Adapted from Deloitte, Pricing and reimbursement strategies for the pharmaceutical and biotechnology industry, Deloitte Consulting LLP, New York, 2008.)

the complex pricing decisions often considered over a biopharmaceutical product's life cycle.

DEMAND ANALYSIS

Understanding the dynamics of prescription use is of critical importance to developing an optimal pricing strategy. Across different countries and physician types, the propensity to use a particular therapy and, as a result, the willingness to pay for a therapy, vary greatly. Biopharma companies explore a number of critical questions: What is the price sensitivity of physicians, payers, and health authorities? What are patient opinions regarding co-payment? How can pharmaceutical companies best avoid the negative impact of cost-containment measures? How can pharmaceutical companies best influence key stakeholders in healthcare systems?

The biopharmaceutical purchase decision-making factors for payers, prescribers, and payments are summarized in Table 10.7.

Price Sensitivities

According to Rankin et al. (2003), key decision makers might be price insensitive, depending on the regulatory structure of the market. Some countries, such as Japan, have regulatory systems that provide economic incentives for physicians to use certain therapies. Some European markets

TABLE 10.7   Biopharmaceutical Purchase Decision Making

Payer/gatekeeper	"Should I reimburse this product/add product to formulary?"	Disease priority/unmet need
		Clinical innovation
		Budget impact
		Quality of evidence
		Health economics
		Political motives
		Level of physician demand
		Level of patient demand/advocacy
Prescriber	"Should I prescribe this product?"	Expected clinical improvement
		Patient financial impact
		Personal financial impact
Patient	"Should I accept this prescription/fill this prescription?"	Prescriber recommendation
		Co-pays/out-of-pocket
		QoL impact

Source: Gregson, N. et al., *Nat. Rev. Drug Discov.*, 4, 121, February 2005, Posted at: http://faculty.fuqua.duke.edu/~willm/Classes/Pharma/Pharma2006/Materials/03_Pricing/Readings/OnLine/Gregson–Mauskopf-Paul-price-2005.pdf. With permission.

discourage physicians from higher-priced therapies by establishing physician budgets for prescriptions. Similarly, countries vary greatly in the degree to which patient price sensitivity is encouraged or structured in local regulations. Pharmaceutical managers should have a firm understanding of the local dynamics among these three parties when establishing a launch strategy. Integrating the results of these analyses would reinforce a tailored approach to maximize returns. Important disease and biopharmaceutical drivers of price sensitivity are summarized in Table 10.8.

Pricing Market Research

As mentioned above, demand analysis must focus on all three decision makers, namely, regulators, prescribers, and patients. In general, market research should evaluate the share response to changes in the status of competing products; the share response to clinical attributes, indications, efficacy, and patient profiles; price responsiveness; physician response to financial incentives and disincentives for prescribing; and patient awareness and willingness to pay.

TABLE 10.8   Disease and Product Drivers of Price Sensitivity

Disease or Product Characteristics	Degree of Price Sensitivity	
	Higher Sensitivity (Lower Price)	Lower Sensitivity (Higher Price)
Disease/patient characteristics		
Chronic/acute	Chronic	Acute
Prevalence	High	Low
Perceived disease severity	Low	High
Unmet need	Low	High
Asymptomatic/symptomatic	Asymptomatic	Symptomatic
Patient severity	Mild	Severe
Patient age	Old	Young
Product characteristics		
Product influence on unmet need	Low	High
Mode of administration	Oral	Parenteral
Formulation	Chemical	Biological
Offsetting cost savings	Low	High
Effect on patient's life	Enhancing	Extending
Differentiation from competitors	Small and unclear	Clear and large

Source: Gregson, N. et al., *Nat. Rev. Drug Discov.*, 4, 121, February 2005, Posted at: http://faculty.fuqua.duke.edu/~willm/Classes/Pharma/Pharma2006/Materials/03_Pricing/Readings/OnLine/Gregson–Mauskopf-Paul-price-2005.pdf. With permission.

TABLE 10.9   What Kind of Pricing Research Is Required for a New Biopharmaceutical Price Setting?

#	Type	Description
1	R&D costing	Resources invested to date, future patent royalties, regulatory approvals secured, new chemical entity, time remaining on patent
2	Manufacturing costing	Fixed manufacturing costs, variable manufacturing costs, contract manufacturing requirements, price per batch, price per kg, price per vial, distribution and storage costs
3	Prescriber choice	Unmet need, product and competitor rating scenarios, patient reaction scenarios, patient willingness-to-pay scenarios, payer willingness-to-pay scenarios, marketing exposure
4	Patient willingness to pay	Unmet need, disease severity, QoL improvement, alternative therapies, ease of use, co-payment percentage and value scenarios, marketing exposure
5	Government price controls	Effect of price controls, profit controls, and dispensing limitations imposed by local governments in target markets
6	Payer willingness to pay	Type of purchasing (volumes, values, frequency, tendering), cost effectiveness, reimbursement scenarios, formulary inclusion scenarios, product differentiation, added value requirements, payment terms, lobbying
7	Wholesaler and pharmacy willingness to stock	Distribution cost, storage costs, packaging size and standardization, minimum stocks required, price per unit scenarios
8	Marketing investment required	Audiences, channels, activities, timetables, and costs required across the biopharmaceutical product's life cycle
9	Price sensitivity on sales	Effect of price sensitivities of individual targets estimated above are incorporated into a master model predicting the price sensitivity of the biopharmaceutical on future sales, sales of competitors, market shares, markets entered, pricing achieved, pricing reduced, markets reimbursed, markets saturated
10	Product profitability	Based on the above, profitability estimates for the biopharmaceutical product over its life cycle

Table 10.9 summarizes the types of pricing research required for a new biopharmaceutical price setting, while Table 10.10 provides an example of determining the prescriber value of biopharmaceutical products.

Pricing Segmentation

A fundamental first step in determining an optimal price is to prioritize the opportunities available from those who might purchase or use the therapy, including patients, physicians and payers. Not all purchasers

TABLE 10.10   How Do You Determine the Customer Value of Biopharmaceutical Products?

Product	Your Prescribers		Competitor A		Competitor B	
Attribute	Importance	Value	Importance	Value	Importance	Value
Efficacy						
Safety						
Tolerability						
Adv. events						
Onset						
Other						

Source: Dogramatzis, D., *Pharmaceutical Marketing: A Practical Guide*, IHS Health Group, Englewood, CO, 2001. With permission.

will have the same sensitivity to price, and not all will purchase similar volumes. The goal of an optimal pricing strategy is to accurately predict the price sensitivity, willingness to pay, and expected purchase volumes of customer groups. Effective segmentation analysis will answer your questions across the global customer population: (1) Which segments of the market are price sensitive? (2) How price sensitive are these segments? (3) What percentage of the total market do price-sensitive segments represent? (4) How will competitor responses vary by segment?

Segments can be defined using a number of criteria, such as cost-sharing liability, disease status, physician type; acute/chronic disease type, payer size, and predisposition to generic use, among others (see Chapter 8). Once these categories of purchasers have been defined, prelaunch efforts and strategic focus should obviously be directed to those segments of the highest priority, typically those segments that exhibit the greatest profit potential.

PRICE NEGOTIATIONS, REFERENCE PRICING, AND PRICE BANDS

Price Negotiations

At the beginning of this chapter, we had mentioned several biopharmaceutical price and profit control mechanisms utilized by national governments in their quest for healthcare cost containment. These cost-containment mechanisms are especially evident in Europe, where biopharmas are often obliged to enter protracted price negotiations with pricing regulators. In some EU countries, the negotiations focus on the absolute selling price, while in others focus on the reimbursement percentage or the reimbursement price (reference price). In addition to prices and reimbursement, the industry's profitability may also need to agree.

There is a plethora of influencing factors that the biopharmaceutical industry needs to consider when entering these negotiations: (1) Price level approved, especially when this level is referenced by additional countries. (2) Price level reimbursed, leading to reduced patient potential within this market. (3) Product sales capped, leading to market prioritization. (4) Company profitability capped, leading to considerations about the local organizational structure. (5) Approved price differentials among countries, leading to parallel exports. (6) Possibility of other biopharma concessions toward the governments, instead of price discounting, for example, free products, local clinical trials, local investments, and local manufacturing. (7) Importance of lobbying at a national or EU level. (8) Importance of patient advocacy in demanding a biopharmaceutical approved and highly reimbursed. (9) Length of negotiations, leading to loss of product sales under patent protection. (10) Possibility to initially negotiate with the government a high price in a smaller patient subsegment (e.g., only non responders or high disease severity), and later renegotiating the approval and reimbursement of additional indications and usages.

Reference Pricing

Under a reference pricing framework the price of a pharmaceutical therapy is affected by the price of a reference drug. The reference product might be another drug in the same therapeutic class; it might be a drug with the same clinical indications; and it may or may not be available in the country of interest. Canada, for example, sets drug prices by comparing with prices charged for that drug in the United States and several European countries. Australia exercises firm reference pricing with reimbursements capped at the reference price.

Biopharmaceutical manufacturers have two strategic choices affected by reference pricing, assuming that the necessary clinical and regulatory information is available. First, manufacturers can choose a limited number of countries in which they would like to commercialize their product. The second strategic option available to manufacturers is to craft a globally consistent price negotiation strategy. The most commonly cited example of such a strategy involves the use of price bands.

For a reference pricing example see: IMS Health Forecasts 4.5–5.5 Percent Growth for Global Pharmaceutical Market in 2009, Exceeding

$820 Billion, Norwalk, CT, 2008a, IMS Health Press Release, October 29, 2008. http://www.imshealth.com.

Price Bands

According to Rankin et al. (2003), price bands define the allowable difference in prices across global markets. The narrowest price band is a single price charged in all markets. Such a price eliminates the concern of reference pricing, but also restricts a manufacturer from realizing the highest global profit levels. Alternatively, wide price bands allow some differences in prices across countries. Such price differences might allow for some negative effects due to parallel trade or reference pricing, but they also provide additional latitude to reach the profit-maximizing price in more markets.

BIOPHARMACEUTICAL THERAPY COSTS IN NUMBERS

The biopharmaceutical industry is relatively unaffected by changes in general economic activity. Demand for medicine in the United States is tied to the population's health, which has remained relatively constant over the years. In addition, drug demand is relatively unresponsive to price changes, reflecting the absence of alternate therapies for most diseases and the reimbursement of the bulk of drug costs by third-party insurance payers. New biopharmaceuticals are typically very lucrative, and manufacturers usually have wide discretion in pricing them. Many factors go into the pricing decision, as previously discussed.

Rising Pricing Pressures

In the United States, managed care describes a variety of techniques intended to reduce the cost of providing health benefits and improve the quality of care for organizations that use those techniques or provide them as services to other organizations ("managed care organization" or MCO). An HMO is a type of MCO that provides a form of healthcare coverage that is fulfilled through hospitals, doctors, and other providers with which the HMO has a contract. The Health Maintenance Organization Act of 1973 required employers with 25 or more employees to offer federally certified HMO options. Drug prices in recent years have come under pressure from the increased influence of managed care providers. Fixed-revenue customers like HMOs are strongly motivated to hold down costs, because excess expenses translate into losses. MCOs typically try to restrict pharmaceutical reimbursement to select "formularies," or lists, of approved drugs; these lists usually include the more cost-efficient drugs in each therapeutic category.

While not immune to these pricing pressures, biotech drugs do have advantages over traditional pharmaceuticals, because biotech drugs tend to be used in critical situations in which patients face a high risk of dying. As a result, the cost-benefit equation for these drugs is materially affected by the high value that society places on human life. In addition, a lack of alternative therapies for some conditions may leave doctors little choice in deciding what to prescribe. Tables 10.11 and 10.12 provide disease prevalence, annual treatment costs and biopharmaceutical candidates for select specialty health conditions.

ACHIEVING REIMBURSEMENT
What Is Biopharmaceutical Reimbursement?
Biopharmaceutical reimbursement refers to the share of medicine costs paid by the state through a compulsory social security system or by health insurance funds, according to the statutory national system. In most European countries, only prescribed products are reimbursed, although arrangements differ widely from country to country. Not all medicines are reimbursed, and few are reimbursed in full (except, in most countries, when they are dispensed in hospitals). Some countries limit reimbursement to a proportion of the price of the prescribed medicine while others reimburse a flat-rate amount according to packaging or prescription. Most countries operate a co-payment system, which requires patients to meet part of the cost of their prescribed treatment.

The Importance of Reimbursement for Biopharmaceuticals
Biotechnology is moving rapidly from the bench to the bedside. That superimposes additional challenges on healthcare providers already tested by declining reimbursements and increasing competition for scarce resources. The provider setting must begin strategically thinking about the future influences of biotechnology as personalized medicine, advances in molecular imaging, costly new devices and complex therapy regimens continue to grow.

TABLE 10.11   Prevalence, Cost and Products for Select Specialty Health Conditions and Therapies

Condition/ Therapy	Approximate U.S. Population Affected	Average Annual Specialty Drug Cost per Patient	Notable Specialty Products
Biologic response modifiers	Crohn's disease: 5,000,004 Psoriasis: 5.8 to 7.5 million Psoriatic arthritis: 10% to 30% with psoriasis Rheumatoid arthritis: 1.3 mil Ulcerative colitis: 5,000,008	$12,000 to $78,000	Amevive, Cimzia, Enbrel, Humira, Kineret, Orencia, Remicade, Rituxan Simponi TM
Bleeding disorders	Hemophilia A: 1 in 5,000 male births; Hemophilia B: 1 in 25,000 male births; von Willebrand disease: 1% to 2% of population	$150,000+	Advate, Alphanate, BeneFIX®, Humate-P, NovoSeven RT, Xyntha
Hepatitis C	3.2 million chronically infected	$23,000 (for interferon alone). $33,000 (combination therapy with interferon and ribavirin)	Infergen, Pegasys, Pegintron, ribavirin
HIV/AIDS	1.1 million13	$26,000	Atripla, Isentress, Kaletra, Norvir, Prezista, Reyataz, Selzentry, Sustiva, Truvada
Infertility	2.1 million females	$15,000 (based on three cycles)	Bravelle, Cetrotide, Follistim AQ, Ganirelix, Gonal-F, Gonal-F RFF, human chorionic gonadotropin, Luveris, Menopur, Ovidrel, Repronex

(continued)

TABLE 10.11 (continued)   Prevalence, Cost and Products for Select Specialty Health
Conditions and Therapies

Condition/ Therapy	Approximate U.S. Population Affected	Average Annual Specialty Drug Cost per Patient	Notable Specialty Products
Multiple sclerosis	400,000	$36,000	Avonex, Betaseron, Copaxone, Rebif, Tysabri
Oral chemotherapy	1.4 million new cancer cases per year	$42,000 to $130,000 Varies by type of cancer	Gleevec, Nexavar, Revlimid®, Sprycel, Sutent, Tarceva, Tasigna, Temodar, Thalomid, Tykerb, Xeloda
Respiratory syncytial virus	75,000 to 125,000 infants hospitalized per year	$6,000 to $12,000 based on variations in weight-based dosing	Synagis
Transplant	>163,000 persons living with a functioning organ transplant	$16,000	CellCept, Neoral, Prograf, Rapamune

Source: Courtesy of Walgreens Specialty Pharmacy—Outlook—State of the industry report 2009, Dallas, TX.

TABLE 10.12   Top 20 Biologics (2006) and Approximate Annual Treatment Costs in USD

Enbrel	20,000	Lantus	1,300
Aranesp	5,300	Humira	12,700
Rituxan	32,500	NovoLog	2,000
Remicade	22,450	Neo-recormon	4,500
Procrit	5,500	Avonex	19,900
Herceptin	36,000	Rebif	22,200
Epogen	5,500	Neupogen	11,000
Neulasta	17,500	Humalog	1,900
Novolin	1,100	Betaseron	21,100
Avastin	28,500	Pegasys	15,700

Source: Adapted from Purvis, L. and Rucker, L., Top 20 biologics (2006 ranking) and approximate annual treatment costs, AARP Public Policy Institute, Washington, DC, May 2007.

In the United States, healthcare providers, including doctors, hospitals and other healthcare professionals and facilities, are reimbursed for their services by the government through Medicare and other forms of public health insurance and private insurers, which are funded primarily through the payment of premiums from individuals, businesses, government, and taxes from individuals and businesses. Public and private components of this multi-payer system are described below.

Medicare and Other Forms of Public Health Insurance

Medicare is a social security program administered by the U.S. government, namely, the U.S. Department of Health and Human Services (HHS; http://www.hhs.gov/), through its Centers for Medicare & Medicaid Services (CMS; http://www.cms.gov/). Medicare was established with the signing of the Social Security Act of 1965 by President Lyndon B. Johnson. All persons aged 65 or older, who have been legal residents of the United States for at least 5 years are eligible for Medicare, provided that they have been paying relevant taxes. If no Medicare taxes have been paid for a minimum of 10 years, then Medicare enrollment requires a monthly premium, which, however, is waived for people disabled, those with end-stage renal disease, or those suffering from amyotrophic lateral sclerosis (ALS).

Medicare has four parts: Part A is hospital insurance. Part B is medical insurance. Medicare Part D covers prescription drugs. Medicare advantage plans, also known as Medicare Part C, are another way for beneficiaries to receive their Part A, B, and D benefits. Parts B and D are relevant for the coverage of physician-related expenses and prescription coverage for biopharmaceuticals.

Medicaid is a health program for low-income or disabled U.S. citizens and even resident aliens. Medicaid is a joint federal-state program that provides health coverage or nursing home coverage to certain categories of low-asset individuals, including children, pregnant women, parents of eligible children, people with disabilities, and elderly needing nursing-home care.

Some individuals are eligible for both Medicaid and Medicare (also known as Medicare dual eligibles).

Private Health Insurance

Employer-sponsored insurance represents the main avenue by which Americans receive private health insurance. Many employers provide health insurance as part of the benefits package for employees.

For a compact overview of private health insurance in the U.S. see relevant chapter in: AMGEN Annual Report 2008, Thousand Oaks, CA, http://www.amgen.com

For a patient assistance program example see: Amgen Reimbursement Connection, http://www.reimbursementconnection.com

INNOVATIVE APPROACHES TO PRICING

According to the Organization for Economic Cooperation and Development (OECD), spending on pharmaceuticals across OECD countries has increased by close to 50% in real terms since 1998. Growth in spending has been driven to a large extent by newer and more expensive drugs replacing older therapies. As a consequence, public and private payers are considering whether to (conditionally) reimburse newer and (usually) more expensive drugs. Effectively, payers are imposing a fourth hurdle that biopharmaceutical firms must clear in order to attain widespread market access, the first three being safety, efficacy, and quality of manufacturing practices.

Biopharmaceuticals: The Four "Hurdles"

The establishment of a fourth hurdle originated in Australia in the 1990s (Cohen, 2009), and has spread to other pharmaceutical markets, particularly in Europe (e.g., United Kingdom and Germany), while in the United States recent federal regulations allow cost and clinical evidence to be considered in outpatient drug reimbursement decisions affecting Medicare beneficiaries. In addition, CMS (http://www.cms.hhs.gov/) have stated that FDA authorization is insufficient to support reimbursement decisions for certain physician-administered biopharmaceuticals, and the Academy of Managed Care Pharmacy (AMCP; http://www.amcp.org) has issued guidelines specifying the parameters to be included by drug sponsors in the formulary dossiers they submit to payers for reimbursement.

Table 10.13 summarizes several strategies used by U.S. Health Plans and Pharmacy Benefit Management companies to manage biologics.

Contracting in the United States

According to IMS (2008b), industry-led proposals for contracting were traditionally based on unit price. Contracting strategies allow companies

TABLE 10.13   Strategies Used by U.S. Health Plans and Pharmacy Benefit
Management Companies to Manage Biologics, 2008–2009

Strategies	2008 (%)	Use in 2009 (%)
Limit coverage for any biologic agent to its FDA-approved indication(s)	39.0	23.0
Apply reference-based pricing to biologic agents	26.0	19.0
Require evidence of therapeutic efficacy through reports of specific patient outcomes once coverage is approved for a specific indication	22.0	26.0
Institute a new individualized case-management program for a condition treated with biologics	20.0	24.0
Provide cost-of-regimen information to providers related to a biologic intervention	18.0	27.0
Provide comparative prescribing practice data regarding any biologic therapies to network providers	17.0	26.0
Provide a new treatment algorithm/protocol to plan providers for a condition treated with biologics	16.0	23.0
Institute information technology upgrades that help better monitor use of biologic therapies	13.0	35.0

Source: Bristol-Myers Squibb, *2009 Biotechnology Monitor & Survey™: Market-place Policies, Practices, and Perspectives*, New York, 2009, Posted at: http://www.biotechmonitor.com/Publication.asp. With permission.

to move away from list price and uniform discount models. Under such arrangements, a manufacturer might contract for a 60% market share in exchange for a 10% rebate. Over the last few years, however, we have witnessed the advent of "innovative" pricing and contracting, with some companies focusing on reimbursement agreements, while other manufacturers have focused on "creative" pricing.

Contracting in Europe

According to IMS Health (2008b), in response to market pressures, European payers have implemented a number of cost containment measures. As a result, biopharma companies are facing significant external and internal pressures when working to secure optimal pricing and market access in today's market. Recent years have seen the emergence of innovative pricing and contracting solutions, with some companies focusing on reimbursement agreements, while others concentrate on more creative pricing strategies (Tables 10.14 and 10.15).

TABLE 10.14   Innovative Pricing in Europe

Product	Issue	Innovative Manufacturer Strategy
NEXAVAR	Refusal to reimburse products for broad range of patients in Italy	Performance risk-sharing agreements
TAXOTERE	Canadian provincial formulary authorities were concerned about efficacy and cost of Taxotere for oncology	Efficacy Guarantee
VELCADE	Product not covered in United Kingdom	Performance risk-sharing agreements—proposed
AVASTIN	Negative publicity on high overall cost of therapy in United States	Price Cap

Source: Courtesy of IMS Health, Pricing & Market Access Review 2007–08, Norwalk, CT, 2008b, Posted at: http://www.imshealth.com/deployedfiles/imshealth/Global/Content/StaticFile/Pricing_and_Contracting_Nwe_Times_New_Solutions.pdf

TABLE 10.15   Patient Access to Selected Biologics Restricted or Denied by NICE

Drug	Indication	Company	Patient Access
Tysabri (natalizumab)	MS	Biogen-Idec/Elan	Restricted
Humira (adalimumab)	Psoriatic arthritis	Abbott	Restricted
Rituxan/MabThera (rituximab)	RA	Genentech/ Biogen-Idec	Restricted
Fludara (fludarabine)	CLL	Bayer	Denied
Gemzar (gemcitabine)	Breast cancer	Lilly	Restricted
Avastin (bevacizumab)	Colorectal cancer	Genentech	Denied
Erbitux (cetuximab)	Colorectal cancer	ImClone Systems	Denied

Source: Burrill, G.S., Biochemistry 241y, Winter 2010, January 4 to March 15, Mondays, 4:00–6:00 pm, Genentech Hall, N 106, Mission Bay Campus, UCSF, BioCentury, San Carlos, CA, 2010. With permission.

QUESTIONS

1. What is the distinction between price-regulated and unregulated biopharmaceutical markets?
2. What kind of price regulation policies do biopharmaceutical companies face from national governments around the world?
3. How do various governments utilize international price comparisons when setting biopharmaceutical prices?

4. How do international governments attempt to contain healthcare-related costs by imposing controls on physicians and pharmacists?
5. What is meant by value-based pricing?
6. What are the launch pricing options for a biopharmaceutical? Can you identify actual biopharmaceutical examples?
7. Which are the international biopharmaceutical launch price strategy steps?
8. Define the following terms: actual acquisition cost (AAC), average selling price (ASP), average manufacturer price (AMP), average wholesale price (AWP), best price (BP), ceiling price, co-payment, and dispensing fee.
9. What is the importance of reimbursement for biopharmaceuticals?
10. What are the "four hurdles" for biopharmaceuticals around the world?

EXERCISES

1. Biopharmaceutical industry critics often charge that "free-pricing" leads to unjustified product prices. Choose either side and present your arguments in a debate.
2. There are various national biopharmaceutical price regulation barriers. Which are the arguments of the national governments versus those of the industry? Defend either side in debate.
3. By using publicly available web resources, identify any given pharmaceutical formulary, and present two cases of biopharmaceuticals that have either been included or excluded form the formulary. Explain the reasoning of the formulary creators.
4. You are a biopharmaceutical company executive liaising with international medical prescribers facing government-imposed control on their prescribing practices. What services and tools can you offer them so that your company's products are not severely affected? Be mindful of ethical requirements.
5. You are a civil servant working at an international health department (ministry). Your prime minister has requested an immediate pharmaceutical cost control, and you must recommend some tough new measures. Where do you start, and what objections do you anticipate from various stakeholders?
6. Your biopharmaceutical employer is preparing to launch a new product tentatively priced at an annual treatment cost of US$ 30,000 per patient. How do you demonstrate the product's value to the different stakeholders involved?

7. You are about to launch a new biopharmaceutical across the EU markets. What kind of pricing research do you need before setting the optimal launch prices across the member states?

8. Identify five different prescription assistance programs put in place for biopharmaceutical products in the U.S. market. Compare their services and rate them on a scale of one (worst) to ten (best).

9. How have biopharmas reacted to usage restrictions imposed on their biopharmaceuticals in the U.K. market by NICE?

10. Biopharmas have used various innovative pricing strategies in Europe. Which are the main advantages and disadvantages of these approaches?

REFERENCES

Bristol-Myers Squibb, 2009. *2009 Biotechnology Monitor & Survey™: Marketplace Policies, Practices, and Perspectives.* Posted at: http://www.biotechmonitor. com/Publication.asp

Burrill, G.S., 2010. Biochemistry 241y, Winter 2010, January 4 to March 15, Mondays, 4:00–6:00 pm, Genentech Hall, N 106, Mission Bay Campus, UCSF. Posted at: http://cbe.ucsf.edu/cbe/9212-DSY/version/default/part/ AttachmentData/data

Cohen, J., 2009. Market access in the wake of NICE: BioPharma's friend or foe? *European BioPharmaceutical Review* 48: 8–12, Summer 2009. Posted at: http://www.samedanltd.com/magazine/12/issue/114/article/2408

Deloitte, 2008. Pricing and reimbursement strategies for the pharmaceutical and biotechnology industry. Deloitte Consulting LLP, New York.

Dogramatzis, D., 2001, *Pharmaceutical Marketing: A Practical Guide.* Englewood, CO: IHS Health Group.

EUROPEAN COMMISSION—COMMISSION OF THE EUROPEAN COMMUNITIES, 2009. Pharmaceutical sector inquiry final report. Brussels, Belgium: EC, SEC(2009) 952, 8.7.2009. Posted at: http://ec.europa. eu/competition/sectors/pharmaceuticals/inquiry/communication_en.pdf

Gregson, N., Sparrowhawk, K., Mauskopf, J., and Paul, J., 2005. Pricing medicines: Theory and practice, challenges and opportunities. *Nature Reviews—Drug Discovery* 4: 121–130, February 2005. Posted at: http://faculty.fuqua.duke. edu/~willm/Classes/ Pharma/Pharma2006/Materials/03_Pricing/Readings/ OnLine/Gregson–Mauskopf-Paul-price-2005.pdf

IMS Health, 2008a. IMS Health forecasts 4.5–5.5 percent growth for global pharmaceutical market in 2009, exceeding $820 billion. IMS Health, Norwalk, CT, Press Release, October 29, 2008. Posted at: http://www.imshealth.com

IMS Health, 2008b. Pricing & market access review 2007–08. IMS Health, Norwalk, CT. Posted at: http://www.imshealth.com/deployedfiles/imshealth/ Global/Content/StaticFile/Pricing_and_Contracting_Nwe_Times_New_ Solutions.pdf

National Association of Chain Drug Stores, 2009. Industry facts at a glance. Posted at: http://www.nacds.org/wmspage.cfm?parm1=6536 (accessed on February 6, 2010).

OECD—DIRECTORATE FOR FINANCIAL, FISCAL AND ENTERPRISE AFFAIRS COMMITTEE ON COMPETITION LAW AND POLICY, 2001. Competition and regulation issues in the pharmaceutical industry, February 6, 2001, http://www.oecd.org/dataoecd/35/35/1920540.pdf

OECD, 2008. *OECD Health Data 2008*. Paris, France: OECD.

Pharmaceutical Research and Manufacturers of America, 2009. *Pharmaceutical Industry Profile 2009*. Washington, DC: PhRMA.

Purvis, L. and Rucker, L., 2007. AARP Public Policy Institute, Top 20 biologics (2006 ranking) and approximate annual treatment costs, May 2007.

Rankin, P.J., Bell, G.K., and Wilsdon, T., 2003. Global pricing strategies for pharmaceutical product launches. In *The Pharmaceutical Pricing Compendium. A Practical Guide to the Pricing and Reimbursement of Medicines*, Chap. 2. London, U.K.: URCH Publishing, March 2003, http://www.pharmaceutical-pricing.com

United Kingdom Department of Health—Department for Business Innovations and Skills, 2010. Life sciences in the U.K.—Economic analysis and evidence for "Life sciences 2010: Delivering the blueprint." DH: January 2010. Posted at: http://www.berr.gov.uk/files/file54303.pdf

United Kingdom NHS—National Institute for Health and Clinical Excellence (NICE), 2004. Final guidance on tacrolimus and pimecrolimus for atopic eczema (TA82), August 25, 2004. Posted at: http://guidance.nice.org.uk/TA82/Guidance

U.S. Centers for Medicare and Medicaid Services, 2009. Office of the Actuary, National Health Statistics Group, National health expenditure data. Posted at: http://www.cms.hhs.gov/NationalHealthExpendData/ (accessed September 2009).

U.S. Department of Health and Human Services—Health Resources and Services Administration, 2010. Pharmaceutical prices glossary. Posted at: http://www.hrsa.gov/opa/glossary.htm

Walgreens Specialty Pharmacy, 2009. Outlook—State of the industry report, Dallas, TX.

## CHAPTER 11

Biosupply Chain

Independent pharmacy in the United States is an $84 billion marketplace. Of those sales, $78 billion are prescription sales, originating from 1.4 billion prescriptions annually.

Source: Courtesy of National Community Pharmacists Association (NCPA), Alexandria, VA.

THE BIOPHARMACEUTICAL SUPPLY CHAIN or logistics network is any sequence of processes that is involved in the manufacturing, distribution, and sale of biopharmaceutical products. A supply chain is thus composed of organizations, individuals, technology, activities, resources, and information involved in the supply chain processes. As Figure 11.1 depicts, a biopharma supply chain typically consists of all biomanufacturing suppliers (e.g., raw materials, culture media, reagents, chemicals, bioreactors, purification tools), the process of purchasing the planned biomanufacturing quantities, the biomanufacturing processes themselves (upstream and downstream, fill and finish; see Chapter 7), physical distribution of the biopharmaceuticals to the wholesale distributors, and finally distribution of these goods to their final customers, for example, hospital and retail pharmacies, mail-order intermediaries, and the patients themselves.

A biopharmaceutical supply chain may include hundreds of interconnected providers and intermediaries, who rely on the products and services of other supply chain members, but may be located on opposite sides of the globe and may not even have direct knowledge of the others' contribution into this complex, and highly sophisticated healthcare-provision supply chain.

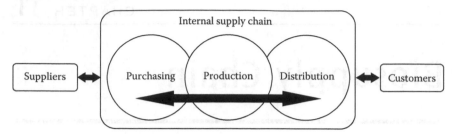

FIGURE 11.1   A supply chain schematic.

THE U.S. COMMERCIAL PHARMACEUTICAL SUPPLY CHAIN

The main participants of the U.S. commercial biopharmaceutical supply chain are depicted in Figure 11.2. We will study their individual role in detail.

Pharmaceutical Manufacturers

Manufacturers of pharmaceutical and biopharmaceutical products are involved in research and development, regulatory approval, manufacturing, as well as sales and marketing of these products to the public. There are various distinctions of pharmaceutical manufacturers, using a variety of criteria we will discuss next. *Pharmaceutical manufacturers* are responsible for the R&D, manufacturing, and selling of chemical-based medicines (also called traditional or small molecules), which have been produced for centuries, and originated as a specialized branch of the chemical industry. Their industry body in the United States is the Pharmaceutical Research and Manufacturers of America (PhRMA; http://www.phrma.org), which has previously reported that its member companies have had total global sales of $288 billion, while they have invested $50 billion to R&D during 2008 (PhRMA Profile 2009).

Biopharmaceutical manufacturers have originated during the 1970s, as a further specialization of the pharmaceutical industry, and they are responsible for R&D, manufacturing and selling of biopharmaceuticals (also called biosynthetic, biochemical, biological, recombinant, or large molecules). Their industry body is the Biotechnology Industry Organization (BIO; http://www.bio.org). According to Ernst Young's *Beyond Borders: Global Biotechnology Report*, global sales revenues of U.S. biotechnology was $66 billion, of which $25 was reinvested in R&D, with an annual net income of $417 million, and 128 thousand employees during 2008.

An additional distinction of pharmaceutical manufacturers is the manufacturers of *branded pharmaceuticals* (also called original or patent protected or ethical) who are involved in the actual discovery, research, and development of these products and their eventual commercialization under

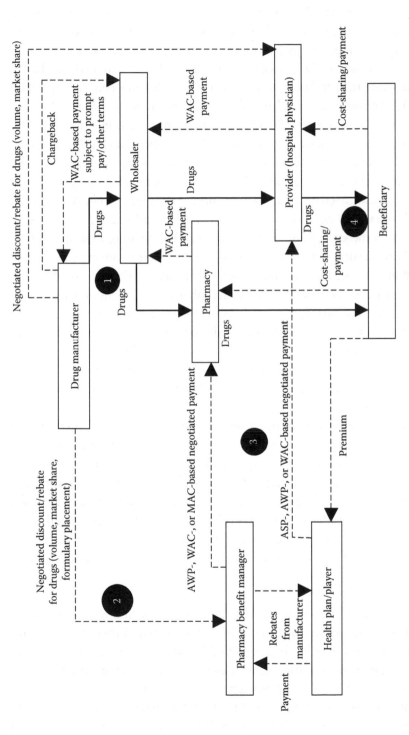

FIGURE 11.2 Flow of goods and financial transactions among players in the U.S. commercial pharmaceutical supply chain. (Courtesy of The Kaiser Family Foundation, Menlo Park, CA, 2005.)

patent protection. On the other side of the spectrum, *generic pharmaceutical manufacturers* are involved in the abbreviated development of therapeutically equivalent generic products, which are commercialized only after the patent protection of the respective original medicines has expired. In the United States, their industry body is the Generic Pharmaceutical Association (GphA; http://www.gphaonline.org), who have reported that total U.S. generic sales amounted to $59 billion, while generic medicines accounted for 69% of all prescriptions dispensed in the United States during 2007. A more recent distinction between the generic pharmaceutical manufacturers are those involved in generic copies of biopharmaceuticals, which are just coming off-patent (also called biogenerics or biosimilars or follow-on biologicals), the so-called *generic biomanufacturers* that will be further discussed in Chapter 14.

As far as the supply chain processes are concerned, biopharmaceutical and pharmaceutical manufacturers distribute their products to a variety of customers, that include large distribution intermediaries called wholesalers (see below), or directly to hospital pharmacies, retail pharmacies, or U.S. government purchasers, such as the Department of Veterans Affairs (VA, http://www.va.gov), which provides patient care and federal benefits to veterans and their families. The pharmaceutical wholesalers are the biggest purchasers of biopharmaceutical and pharmaceutical products for the manufacturers. Table 11.1 lists the top pharmaceutical manufacturers by U.S. sales, during 2004–2008.

Biopharmaceutical manufacturers are obliged to procure the required raw material quantities, to produce their products by methods and facilities that have previously been approved by regulators, to dependably manufacture safe and effective biopharmaceuticals (as per previously approved specifications), to package them in a patient-friendly and tamper-resistant manner, to distribute these products in a controlled, secure, expeditious, and on-demand basis, and to make them available to all distribution intermediaries or final customers in order to fully satisfy customer demand.

Wholesale Distributors

As mentioned above, wholesale distributors are distribution intermediaries between the biopharmaceutical manufacturers and their final customers. Wholesalers may be distinguished by whether they carry the entire product line of the manufactures (*full-line wholesalers*), or selected product items only (*short-line wholesalers*), in search of specialization, economies of scale, identical storage and transportation technologies, and more. Wholesalers may even be distinguished by the spectrum of final customer

TABLE 11.1   Top Pharmaceutical Manufacturers by U.S. Sales, 2004–2008
(in $ Billion)

#	Total U.S. Prescription-Bound Market	2004	2005	2006	2007	2008
	Prescription-Bound Market	**239.9**	**253.9**	**276.5**	**287.6**	**291.5**
1	Pfizer	31.1	27.3	26.8	23.6	20.5
2	GlaxoSmithKline	19.1	20.2	22.2	20.7	18.4
3	AstraZeneca	11.5	12.7	14.7	15.5	16.3
4	Johnson & Johnson	16.7	16.0	16.1	16.3	16.0
5	Merck & Co.	15.3	15.4	16.7	17.6	15.5
6	Amgen	9.6	11.9	14.5	14.3	13.4
7	Hoffmann-LaRoche (Incl. Genentech)	6.2	8.2	10.4	12.4	13.1
8	Novartis	11.5	12.9	13.9	13.9	12.4
9	Lilly	8.2	8.7	9.2	10.3	11.4
10	SanofiAventis	10.2	11.2	11.0	10.9	11.0
11	Abbott	8.0	8.7	9.5	9.7	10.0
12	Teva Pharma USA	4.7	5.7	7.4	7.9	9.2
13	Bristol-Myers Squibb	9.1	8.3	6.4	6.9	8.0
14	Takeda	6.2	6.6	7.2	7.7	8.0
15	Wyeth	8.1	8.1	8.2	8.6	7.6

Source: Courtesy of IMS National Sales Perspectives, http://www.imshealth.com

services, for example, hospitals, retail locations, mail-order, specialized clinics, physicians, or a selection of those.

In addition, wholesalers may specialize in the distribution of certain biopharmaceuticals with given characteristics (e.g., *specialty* injectables for severe and chronic diseases—see sub-chapter below). Furthermore, wholesalers may even be distinguished according to the specialized services they provide, apart from physical storage and transportation. These services may even not be considered as core, but are deemed as value added. For example, a *specialized wholesaler* may provide the manufacturers with services such as home delivery, product recalls, patient reimbursement support (claims processing), distribution of educational and promotional materials, repackaging (breaking a carton of 100 syringes into packages of 4—1 per patient per week), patient web order delivery, and more.

The U.S. industry body of the healthcare distributors is the Healthcare Distribution Management Association (HDMA; http://www.healthcare-distribution.org/). According to the Center for Healthcare Supply Chain Research, the research foundation of the HDMA (September 25, 2009), in 2008, $253 billion in prescription drug sales were completed through primary healthcare distributors, representing nearly 85% of the entire market. On an average business day in 2008, HDMA distributor members delivered a total of 9.4 million products to more than 165,000 pharmacies, hospitals, clinics, nursing homes and other outlets across all 50 states. Distributors reported an order fill rate in excess of 95% while keeping profit margins modest at an average of 1.8%.

Source: Courtesy of HDMA Press Release, Arlington, VA, September 25, 2009, Posted at: http://www.hcsupplychainresearch.org/press/20090925_factbook.asp

According to the Kaiser Family Foundation (2005), the wholesale distribution industry has gone through significant change and consolidation in the last 30 years, due in part to the increasing pressures to lower costs, and currently numbering fewer than 50 distributors. The top three wholesale distributors, McKesson, Cardinal Health, and Amerisource-Bergen, account for almost 90% of the entire wholesale drug market. This consolidation has forced the industry to change its revenue model, evolving its core distribution business into a low-margin enterprise that makes money by maximizing economies of scale, creating physical efficiencies in the distribution system (such as "just-in-time" deliveries to customers), and realizing financial efficiencies (such as retaining discounts for prompt payment). The industry has also extended and augmented its business model by moving into specialty pharmacy and disease-management services. Table 11.2 details the U.S. Pharmaceutical distributor sales of all products (both Rx and Non-Rx) by customer category: 2007–2008.

Pharmaceutical Wholesaler Example: McKesson Corporation
$107 billion in revenues in FY09. #1 in pharmaceutical distribution in United States, Canada, and Mexico—#1 generics distributor—#2 in rapidly growing specialty distribution & services market—#1 in medical-surgical distribution to alternate care sites. 2000 + Health Mart retail pharmacy franchisees. Comprehensive retail information systems and automation offerings. More than 32,000 employees. $15 billion market cap. Founded 1833, headquartered in San Francisco.

Source: Courtesy of McKesson Corporate Presentation, San Francisco, CA, 2009.

Pharmacies

Before a prescribed biopharmaceutical can reach its final customer (i.e., the patient), it is first purchased, received, inventoried, dispensed, explained to the patient, and relevant prescription information is collected, verified,

TABLE 11.2   U.S. Pharmaceutical Distributor Sales of All Products
(Both Rx and Non-Rx) by Customer Category: 2007–2008

	2007 Sales (USD Billion)	2007 Weighted Average (%)	2008 Sales (USD Billion)	2008 Weighted Average (%)
Chain drug stores	44.43	18.46	44.41	17.53
Mass merchandisers and food stores	11.70	4.86	11.58	4.57
Chain warehouse sales	63.37	26.33	62.62	24.72
Chain sales total	119.50	49.65	118.60	46.82
Independent drug stores	39.16	16.27	39.49	15.59
Hospitals and HMOs	43.85	18.22	42.89	16.93
Specialty pharmacies	0.05	0.02	0.05	0.02
Clinics and nursing homes	20.07	8.34	29.28	11.56
Mail order	15.40	6.40	20.42	8.06
Other distributors	0.34	0.14	0.38	0.15
Government sales	1.73	0.72	NA	NA
Physicians/physicians' offices	0.10	0.04	0.13	0.05
Other customers	2.21	0.92	2.08	0.82
Total sales	240.69		253.31	

Source: Center for Healthcare Supply Chain Research, *2009–2010 HDMA Factbook*, Arlington, VA. With permission.

Notes: (1) 2007 data has been restated. (2) Rounding differences may result in slight calculation variations. NA = not applicable.

and processed by pharmacists. Registered pharmacists (the author is one) and their assistants are the final interface between the biopharmaceutical manufacturer and prescribing physician with their patient-customers and fill a vital role in patient education, patient adherence to treatment, collection of co-payments, claims processing, and even validation of the prescription versus a variety of applicable laws and regulations (e.g., reimbursement coverage, formulary inclusion, dosage appropriateness, side effect management, controlled substances dispensing).

The pharmacy services can be distinguished as *front office* and *back office*. The former refers to directly liaising with the customer, checking their credentials, explaining the therapy, and managing their adherence, while the latter refers to services away from the patient's attention, happening in the background, for example, receiving the biomedicine supplies, storing them in controlled conditions, dispensing them as per instructions, labeling them with special information, handling the prescription claims, submitting information back to prescribers, pharmacy benefit managers (PBMs), insurance providers, and more.

TABLE 11.3   U.S. Retail Prescription Sales in 2007–2008 ($ Billion)

	Number of Pharmacies	Rx Sales 2008	% of Total	Rx Sales 2007	2008 vs. 2007
Traditional chain	20,884	104.14	41.1	101.19	2.9
Mass market	6,970	24.77	9.8	23.60	5.0
Supermarket	8,864	25.77	10.2	27.29	−5.6
Total chain	36,738	154.75	61.0	152.08	1.0
Independents	16,920	43.70	17.2	44.62	−2.1
Mail order		55.13	21.7	52.49	5.0
Total sales		253.58		249.19	1.8

Source: Material pulled from NACDS website http://www.nacds.org (February 15, 2010). NACDS shall not be liable for any errors or omissions in content. © 2010 National Association of Chain Drug Stores, Inc. ("NACDS"). Used with permission. All rights reserved.

There is a variety of different pharmacy settings. For example, they are located at hospitals, specialized clinics, nursing facilities, retail locations, employer locations, or mail-order settings. In addition, they may also be *full-service,* or *specialty-oriented,* for example, catering to biopharmaceuticals used for chronic and severe diseases, usually in injectable form. Pharmacy trade associations in the United States include, among others, the American Society of Health-System Pharmacists (ASHP; http://www.ashp.prg), the National Association of Chain Drug Stores (ÑACDS; http://www.nacds.org), and the National Community Pharmacists Association (NCPA; http://www.ncpanet.org). Table 11.3 provides the U.S. retail prescription sales in 2007–2008.

Pharmacist Association Example: The U.S. National Association of Chain Drug Stores

Nationwide, there are more than 39,000 pharmacies operated by traditional chain pharmacy companies, supermarkets, and mass merchants. In addition, there are another 20,000 independent pharmacies. In recent years, the retail prescription drug industry has grown dramatically. The number of retail prescriptions dispensed each year increased from 2.0 billion in 1992 to 2.6 billion in 1997. This represents a 23 percent increase in just five years. In 1998, this number reached 2.73 billion. The chain pharmacy is the leading component of this industry. It dispenses more than 60 percent of these prescriptions, which equals 1.6 billion prescriptions a year or 4 million each day.

According to data from the April 2000 DHHS ASPE report, Prescription Drug Coverage, Spending, Utilization, and Prices: Over the past few years, the wholesale drug industry has become quite concentrated. While there are still a number of wholesalers in operation, the top five wholesalers account for 90 percent of the entire wholesale drug market. In 1998, the net sales of prescription drugs by wholesalers were $57 billion. Mail order pharmacy accounts for about 12 percent of the total retail prescription market. Between 1997 and 1998 mail service pharmacy grew by 19 percent. This compares to the total prescription market, which grew by 18.5 percent. It is interesting to note that Internet pharmacies use mail order to distribute their products and are members of the mail order pharmacies' professional organization.

Source: National Association of Chain Drug Stores, Inc. ("NACDS"). Posted at: http://www.nacds.org (accessed on February 15, 2010). With permission.

Pharmacy Chain Example: Walgreens Store Base (as of December 31, 2009)
Total locations: 7,651. Total drugstores: 7,149 in all 50 states, the District of Columbia and Puerto Rico. Drugstores with drive-thru pharmacies: 6,223. Locations with one-hour photofinishing: 6,931. Locations open 24 hours: 1,596.

Employee Count 2009: 238,000.

Total Prescriptions Filled 2009: 651 million. Number of Customers Served Daily Chainwide: 5.6 million

A Typical Store: Total size: 14,500 square feet. Sales area: 11,000 square feet. Items for sale: 20,000. Employees: 25-30. Annual sales: $8.9 million.

Source: Courtesy of Walgreens. http://news.walgreens.com/article_ display.cfm?article_id=1047

Pharmacy Benefit Managers

In the U.S. pharmaceutical market, more than 200 million citizens rely on their health insurance to cover all or part of the healthcare services and pharmaceuticals they receive. Healthcare coverage is provided from three distinct sources: (1) government insurance (public health programs), (2) employer insurance (programs relying on employer/worker contributions), and (3) private insurance (individuals choose their private coverage by paying an agreed monthly fee. All three of these healthcare coverage categories have a vested interest in properly managing the healthcare services and pharmaceutical consumption of their members. They do so by either safeguarding the medical rationale for their treatment, or by monitoring the per patient consumption and adherence to recommended treatments, or by evaluating the efficacy, safety, and cost-effectiveness of the administered pharmaceuticals, or by containing the costs of therapy, so that the insurance coverage schemes remain viable and self-sustainable.

The role of safeguarding these four basic qualities of reimbursed healthcare coverage is increasingly played by independent, for-profit organizations, which are collectively called *PBMs*, represented by the Pharmaceutical Care Management Association (PCMA; http://www.pcmanet.org), and responsible for administering prescription drug plans for more than 210 million Americans.

The way by which PBMs assist in managing third-party health plans (state-, private-, and employer-based) is by defining the pharmaceuticals that can be used by their members and the degree of reimbursement coverage affecting the patients' co-payment, by educating their members in better managing their disease and adhering to recommended treatments, by substituting prescribed pharmaceuticals with therapeutically equivalent medicines, and by collecting, managing, and acting on huge patient data that may lead to new and improved treatment guidelines and recommendations. As far as the enrolled member is concerned, PBMs may provide them with treatment formularies, reimbursement levels, recommended healthcare providers, participating pharmacies, mail-order services, informational hotlines, educational materials, and more.

PBMs are basing their effectiveness in managing pharmacy benefits on using their significant bargaining power (see Porter's five forces in Chapter 8) in negotiating either lesser fees for purchased products or services (supply side), or imposing usage limitations and adherence to treatment guidelines (demand side). In other words, every single player under the PBMs' sphere of influence is influenced toward concessions in order to be included. Let us study some of their tools.

- *Pharmaceutical formularies*: selection of the most cost-effective biopharmaceuticals and incentives for the patients to use therapeutically equivalent and cheaper alternatives.

- *Product rebates*: biomanufacturers are asked to offer volume discounts, while insurance providers are incentivized to use the more economical alternatives.

- *Pharmacy providers*: they are asked to provide lower dispensing fees and free services to referred PBM members in exchange for the PBM's large population under coverage. An additional component is incentives to members to use the cheaper pharmacy networks, often mail-order ones, that can guarantee home delivery of biopharmaceuticals at significant economies of scale.

- *Claims processing*: a huge IT infrastructure where all insurance providers, participating product and service providers, and consumers are online, so that treatment guidelines, formulary categories, treatment adherence, therapeutic substitution, dosage recommendations, refill frequencies, and fees charged and received are automatically checked, verified, and approved where needed.

- *Generic and therapeutic substitution*: generic substitution promotes the shift from brand to chemically equivalent generic drugs as a cost-saving device. Therapeutic interchange programs promote the use of preferred drugs (i.e., drugs on a plan's formulary) that are determined to be clinically similar.

- *Quality-focused programs*: PBMs develop programs that provide disease management, compliance strategies, and other clinical expertise promoting the safe, educated use of prescription drugs.

Table 11.4 lists the top 12 pharmacy benefit management companies and market share by membership, as of 2009.

For a PBM example see: Medco Health Solutions, Inc., http://www.medcohealth.com/medco/corporate/home.jsp

THE ROLE OF PHYSICIANS, EMPLOYERS, AND HEALTH PLANS IN THE U.S. SUPPLY CHAIN

Physicians

Physicians are involved in maintaining and restoring human health, through the study, prevention, diagnosis, and treatment of disease. They directly liaise with their patients, either as *general practitioners* or family physicians, or as *specialized physicians* after referral from the family physicians (gatekeepers). More specifically, a patient feeling a disease symptom(s) seeks the advice of a physician, who in turn makes a diagnosis, chooses the appropriate pharmacological treatment, the proper dosage and formulation, and the future mode of disease monitoring and

TABLE 11.4   Top 12 Pharmacy Benefit Management Companies and Market Share
by Membership, as of First Quarter 2009

Company	Rx Covered Lives	Market Share (%)
CVS/Caremark Rx, Inc.	82,000,000	12.02
Walgreens-OptionCare	75,000,000	10.99
ICORE Healthcare, Inc.	60,000,000	8.79
Medco Health Solutions, Inc.	60,000,000	8.79
Express Scripts/CuraScript	55,000,000	8.06
NovoLogix (formerly Ancillary Care Management)	40,000,000	5.86
WellPoint NextRx	35,049,000	5.14
Argus Health Systems, Inc.	28,600,000	4.19
MedImpact Healthcare Systems, Inc.	27,000,000	3.96
HealthTrans	15,300,000	2.24
Prime Therapeutics, LLC	14,700,000	2.15
Provider Synergies, LLC	14,000,000	2.05

Source: Reprinted from Atlantic Information Services, Inc., *2000–2009 Survey Results, Pharmacy Benefit Trends and Data: Costs, Benefit Design, Utilization PBM Market Share*, Washington, DC, http://www. AISHealth.com. With permission.

follow-up. Over the long term, physicians also follow the patient's adherence to treatment, other recommended life changes (e.g., diet and exercise), and disease progression or cure. In many cases, a patient may be seen and treated for various lifetime ailments by the same family physician.

As far as the biopharmaceutical industry is concerned, the most important physician activity is the prescription decision, which is influenced by a variety of factors we have previously discussed in Chapter 9. Based on the importance of the prescribing decision, biopharmaceutical marketers direct a major portion of their promotional activities toward the physician, in a "push strategy." In addition, because of the rise of internet communications, patient education, and patient advocacy, biopharma marketers also target the patients with a variety of informational, educational, and promotional activities, in a "pull strategy." Following diagnosis and prescription writing, patients refer to retail pharmacies or web pharmacies, to have their prescription "filled" and "refilled" by licensed pharmacy personnel. As far as the biopharmaceutical supply chain is concerned, physicians may also be called at home by patients to assist them with drug administration or management of their disease, while patients can have the medicines administered to them at the physician's office, when the drug characteristics require direct medical attention (e.g., injectable anticancer medicines). Table 11.5 describes the multiple medical specialties and their respective physician numbers in the United States in 2006.

TABLE 11.5   American Physicians by Specialty in 2006 (Thousands)

Activity	Total	Office Based
Doctors of medicine, total	921.9	560.4
U.S. medical graduates	685.2	423.3
International medical graduates	236.7	137.1
Male	665.6	407.9
Female	256.3	152.5
Allergy/immunology	4.2	3.3
Anesthesiology	41.2	31.7
Cardiovascular diseases	22.4	17.5
Child psychiatry	7.3	5.3
Dermatology	10.7	8.9
Diagnostic radiology	24.6	17.6
Emergency medicine	30.0	20.1
Family practice	82.9	66.0
Gastroenterology	12.3	9.9
General practice	10.5	8.9
General surgery	37.7	25.7
Internal medicine	155.7	107.3
Neurological surgery	5.4	4.1
Neurology	14.6	10.4
Obstetrics and gynecology	42.3	34.2
Ophthalmology	18.1	15.8
Orthopedic surgery	24.3	19.2
Otolaryngology	10.0	8.2
Pathology	19.8	11.9
Pediatrics	75.1	53.1
Physical med./rehab.	7.7	5.6
Plastic surgery	7.1	6.0
Psychiatry	41.4	27.4
Pulmonary diseases	10.2	7.4
Radiology	8.9	7.0
Urological surgery	10.5	8.9
Unspecified	7.5	4.0
Not classified	46.3	(X)
Other categories	108.8	(X)

Source: American Medical Association (AMA), Chicago, IL, http://www.ama-assn.org. With permission. Copyright 2006. American Medical Association. All rights reserved.

Large Employers

Employers, large or small, in several countries choose to offer health benefits to their employees as an added work incentive, and also to positively influence employee retention, work-related health problems, work absenteeism, and more. In most cases, the employer agrees to match the employee's health contribution with their own contribution (can be higher), in order to cover for a given degree of coverage, for as long as the employee remains with the company. Employer plans may range in their coverage levels, and usually include physician, nurse, and pharmacy services, mental health plans, a network of collaborating specialty centers (heart disease, cancer, transplantation, etc.), as well as disease management (information, education, and services) aimed at better managing one's disease.

Employers often do not have the specialized personnel or expertise to manage their employee's health plans internally, so they outsource these plans to managed care organizations (MCOs) or PBMs, who in turn oversee their employees' health plans. MCOs attract a large number of employers and their employees, and are thus able to exert significant bargaining power toward manufacturers or healthcare providers for discounts, rebates, or other special offers. MCOs are either reimbursed by participating employers on a per employee basis, or by keeping a portion of the provider-offered discounts for themselves. The employer–MCO collaboration is set by detailed contracts, describing the offered healthcare services, their levels of coverage, the upper limits of covered health expenses, the nature of procedures and medicines used, etc.

Health Plans

Health insurance is based on the management of a group's collective health risk by predicting the long-term financial costs of providing health insurance, and subsequently spreading these costs to every single covered member of the group for specified insurance fee (co-payment) over a specified period of time. Health insurance may be offered by one's government, an employer, or the individual opting to pay for private insurance. In the United States, private insurance (employer or individual) is the major contributor of health coverage, while government-provided insurance is usually targeted at lower-income households. Until early 2010, there were also a large number of Americans without health insurance, an issue that is being addressed by the recent Affordable Care Act, signed into law by president Obama on March 23, 2010 (see http://www.healthcare.gov/law/introduction/index.html.)

Health plans manage their members' health coverage by negotiating discounts and rebates for all healthcare product and service providers involved.

These providers are pressured to provide discounts in order to be included in mandatory treatment guidelines, preferred provider lists, medicinal formulary lists, recommended procedures, and more. As far as the biopharmaceutical supply chain is concerned, manufacturers need to provide pharmacoeconomic data and significant discounts in order to be included, prescribing physicians are obliged to follow formularies or are incentivized to prescribe more cost-effective medications, retail pharmacies are required to lower their dispensing fees and offer value-added services to patients, while the patients are asked to see only approved providers and have their prescriptions filled at approved locations or via the Internet.

THE EUROPEAN BIOPHARMACEUTICAL SUPPLY CHAIN

The European biopharmaceutical supply chain is similar, but not identical, to the United States. Major differences involve the compartmentalization of the European side, the greater presence of national healthcare coverage of the population, the presence of both price-regulated and unregulated EU countries, the lack of MCOs, the lack of large retail pharmacy chains (with the exception of the United Kingdom), the parallel trade phenomenon, and the relatively smaller patient advocacy and Internet penetration than those seen in the U.S. biopharmaceutical marketplace.

On the European supply side, we observe the same role of biopharmaceutical manufacturers or their subsidiaries. Other important players include the wholesalers, pharmacies, and parallel traders. Pharmaceutical wholesalers are active throughout Europe, although showing greater fragmentation than the concentration seen in the United States.

Wholesalers

European full-line wholesalers play the same role with their U.S. counterparts, while this supply chain sector is undergoing massive changes and recent consolidation. Full-line wholesalers provide a plethora of front-office and back-office services, several of which are adding value to the supply chain, for example, product recalls, patient claims processing, and educational material distribution. The final result of the wholesale distribution is the availability of biopharmaceuticals at a variety of settings (hospital, retail, mail-order), in a safe and timely manner, and in every remote location of the European continent.

The *European Association of Pharmaceutical Full-Line Wholesalers* (GIRP; http://www.girp.eu) is the umbrella organization of pharmaceutical full-line wholesalers in Europe. It represents the national associations of over 600 pharmaceutical full-line wholesalers serving 31 European countries, including major facilities who distribute €100 billion worth of medicines every year. Between them, their members number more than 140,000 staff and supply products from over 3,500 manufacturers to more than 133,000 pharmacies across Europe. According to GIRP, direct sales now account for 17% of the retail pharmaceutical market in Germany. In the United Kingdom, 24% of the retail market is direct to pharmacies. In Italy, hospital distribution accounts for 30% of the market.

The wholesaler is the intermediary between the manufacturer and the pharmacy. In general terms, the wholesale sector comprises so-called *full-line* wholesalers and *short-line* wholesalers. Full-line wholesalers carry and distribute a range of products suitable to meet the needs of those with whom they conduct business (normally pharmacies). They are also able to deliver all medicines used in their geographical area within a short period of time. In addition, full-line wholesalers generally carry full stock-holding responsibility and usually hold a minimum stock level of 2 weeks' supplies. In a number of Member States, in addition to the full-line wholesalers, short-line wholesalers exist. These companies supply a more restricted range of prescription medicines, focusing on the distribution of high-value and high-volume products. In the European Union, there is no obligation for manufacturers to distribute medicines via wholesalers. Forms of *direct distribution* include direct sales, sales through agents (e.g., in smaller EU Member States) and direct to pharmacy (DTP) distribution.

For a European wholesaler example see: AAH Pharmaceuticals, Coventry, United Kingdom, http://www.aah.co.uk/aah-home/about-us.aspx

Pharmacies

Retailers of prescription medicines are typically community pharmacies. Further channels of supply include self-dispensing doctors, hospital pharmacies, and, for nonprescription products, pharmacy outlets, medicine stores, herbal shops, and even supermarkets and fuel stations. On July 8, 2009, the European Commission adopted the Final Report on its competition inquiry (http://ec.europa.eu/competition/sectors/pharmaceuticals/inquiry/index.html) into the pharmaceutical sector. According to information received in the course of the sector inquiry, there are in total approximately 140,000 community pharmacies in the EU, and approximately 21,000 hospital pharmacists employed in pharmacies located inside hospitals mainly dispensing to in-patients.

Most pharmacies in the European Union are SMEs or single-unit oper-ators. The pharmacy sector is also highly regulated and some member states (e.g., Germany, Italy, Spain, and France) prohibit horizontal or ver-tical integration of pharmacies or ownership by non-pharmacists. Other member states establish rules on the distance between pharmacies and number of inhabitants per pharmacy in order to control the distribution of pharmacies in their territory. This is, for example, the case in Spain, Austria, Italy, Greece, and France. Table 11.6 showcases the number of retail pharmacies in major European markets and number of inhabitants per retail pharmacy in 2004.

The *Pharmaceutical Group of the European Union* (PGEU; http://www. pgeu.org) is the European association representing community phar-macists. PGEU's members are the national associations and professional bodies of community pharmacists in 29 European countries including EU Member States, EU candidate countries and EFTA members. Through its members, PGEU represents around 400,000 community pharmacists con-tributing to the health of over 500 million people throughout Europe. It is estimated that over 46 million people visit the community pharmacies in the EU member states every day.

In addition to dispensing medicines, pharmacists provide advice on nonprescription medicines (OTC medicines). With respect to prescription medicines, pharmacists are obliged to dispense the medicines prescribed by the doctor and, therefore, do not determine the medicine that is given to the patient. However, in some member states, the pharmacist is allowed or even required by law to either substitute an originator medicine with

TABLE 11.6   Number of Retail Pharmacies in Major European Markets and Number of Inhabitants per Retail Pharmacy in 2004

	Number of Retail Pharmacies	Number of Inhabitants per Retail Pharmacy
France	23,380	2542
Germany	20,760	3970
Spain	20,495	2108
Italy	16,808	3448
United Kingdom	12,467	4820
Netherlands	1,732	9407
Austria	1,172	6952

Source: Courtesy of European Association of Pharmaceutical Full-Line Wholesalers (GIRP), Brussels, Belgium, http://www.girp.eu

a cheaper generic version (if available), or prescriptions are issued on the basis of an active substance (INN) rather than a brand, in which case the pharmacist can or must select an appropriate generic product (if available) at the lowest price.

Parallel Traders

Price differentials between member states create the opportunity for arbitrage, that is, the purchase of pharmaceutical products in low-price member states and subsequent resale in high-price areas. It is from this price differential that parallel traders derive their profits. According to the 2009 EU competition inquiry into the pharmaceutical sector, the turnover of parallel traders is approximately €3.5 billion—€5 billion in Europe, which is between 2% and 3% of the overall market. There are approximately 100 companies engaged in parallel trade in the European Union employing in total between 10,000 and 15,000 people. The *European Association of Euro-Pharmaceutical Companies* (EAEPC; http://www.eaepc.org/welcome/index.php) is the professional and representative voice of pharmaceutical parallel trade in Europe. Through national associations and individual company membership, it encompasses over 70 firms from 16 countries in the European Economic Area (EEA).

Some studies indicate direct and indirect savings in importing member states as a result of parallel trade. Other studies contest these savings or at least the level of savings achieved and point to other effects of parallel trade. Leading companies have taken steps to improve supply management, for example, direct distribution for one product or differential pricing across Europe. On October 6, 2009, however, the EC Court of Justice determined that dual pricing is anticompetitive and violates the EC Treaty.

The Demand Side

The demand side of the pharmaceutical sector is characterized by a complex interrelationship between patients, doctors, hospitals, insurance providers, and reimbursement systems. Both insurance providers and reimbursement systems have been already discussed in this book. For prescription medicines, the ultimate consumer (i.e., the patient) systematically differs from the decision maker (generally the prescribing doctor) and very often also from the bearer of the costs (generally the health system). As a consequence, price sensitivity is rather limited for the decision makers and patients.

Physicians

The special relationship between patients and their physicians, as well as the factors influencing the prescribing decision have been previously discussed. Table 11.7 provides relative European healthcare indicators (per 100,000 inhabitants). On average, the number of physicians (outpatient doctors) per 100,000 inhabitants in the European Union has increased slightly during the last decade to over 300.

Unlike other markets, the patient is normally not in a position to choose directly which product he or she wishes to use. The relationship between patient and doctor is characterized by an information asymmetry where the patient generally must rely on the doctor's expertise. Doctors are therefore decisive for the choice of pharmaceutical products (type and volume).

The relationship between pharmaceutical companies and doctors is the subject of controversy, given the potential for a conflict of interest between the business objectives of the industry and the duty of the doctor to prescribe the most appropriate medicines. Several guidelines exist within the European Union on the physician–industry relationship. For example, the Prescription Medicines Code of Practice Authority (PMCPA) is responsible for administering the Association of the British Pharmaceutical Industry's (ABPI) Code of Practice for the Pharmaceutical Industry at arm's length from the ABPI. The Code incorporates the principles set out in

- The International Federation of Pharmaceutical Manufacturers and Associations' (IFPMA; http://www.ifpma.org) Code of Pharmaceutical Marketing Practices

- The European Federation of Pharmaceutical Industries and Associations' (EFPIA; http://www.efpia.org) Code on the Promotion of Prescription-Only Medicines to, and Interactions with Healthcare Professionals

- The EFPIA Code of Practice on Relationships between the Pharmaceutical Industry and Patient Organizations

- Directive 2001/83/EC on the Community Code relating to medicinal products for human use, as amended by Directive 2004/27/EC

- The World Health Organization's ethical criteria for medicinal drug promotion

TABLE 11.7   European Healthcare Indicators (per 100,000 Inhabitants)

	Practicing Physicians		Hospital Beds	
	1996	2006	1996	2006
EU-27	—	—	694.8	590.4
Belgium	360.3	404.7	798.3	672.3
Bulgaria	354.8	366.1	1049.6	621.4
Czech Republic	298.6	355.7	886.9	817.0
Denmark	252.3	308.4	459.8	—
Germany	310.8	345.5	957.8	829.1
Estonia	317.0	328.9	795.5	565.3
Ireland	208.5	282.4	673.7	524.7
Greece	386.3	499.4	517.3	473.8
Spain	290.2	368.3	389.1	334.1
France	324.4	338.2	853.8	707.5
Italy	409.9	366.6	655.0	395.2
Cyprus	246.9	250.4	498.7	373.7
Latvia	282.1	286.1	1038.3	755.4
Lithuania	373.2	364.8	1092.0	801.0
Luxembourg	212.6	327.7	1079.9	—
Hungary	304.3	303.7	903.0	792.1
Malta	—	332.8	576.8	237.8
Netherlands	189.9	—	522.2	438.2
Austria	280.6	375.7	746.3	770.9
Poland	235.1	218.0	766.3	647.5
Portugal	262.3	267.8	399.3	365.1
Romania	—	215.8	757.0	658.6
Slovenia	—	235.8	566.6	477.5
Slovakia	257.1	315.9	832.7	671.4
Finland	213.7	244.5	803.0	695.6
Sweden	289.0	356.6	559.8	287.7
United Kingdom	—	235.6	433.4	388.7
Croatia	219.9	—	618.5	545.0
FYR of Macedonia	226.4	245.2	523.0	470.2
Turkey	—	—	248.5	241.2
Iceland	310.9	364.0	—	—
Norway	283.1	377.7	400.6	402.7
Switzerland	180.0	—	665.9	555.6

Source: Eurostat, *Europe in Figures—Eurostat Yearbook 2009*, Posted at: http://
epp.eurostat.ec.europa.eu/portal/page/portal/publications/eurostat_
yearbook. With permission.

Hospitals

In the European Union, both public and private providers operate in the hospital sector. Typically hospitals buy directly from manufacturers and prices may be determined, as well as providers selected, via public tenders. At times, medicines are also supplied by wholesalers. Suppliers have generally more freedom to decide the price of their medicines than when selling to the retail segment. According to the European Commission's 2009 Final Report on its competition inquiry into the pharmaceutical sector, "competition between originator and generic companies in the hospital segment can be strong, especially because originator companies believe that outpatient doctors will continue to prescribe the product patients have received for treatment in hospital."

Founded in 1970, the *European Association of Hospital Managers* (EAHM; http://www.hospital.be) is the umbrella association for 27 leading hospital management associations in 25 European countries, representing over 16,000 individual members. EAHM is the world's largest hospital management association, representing over 90% of all hospital beds across the entire European continent (including CEE countries), and serving a population of over 450 million.

Patients

Patients are individuals who receive medical attention, care, or treatment for illness or an injury. An outpatient is a patient who is not hospitalized overnight but who visits a hospital, clinic, or associated facility for diagnosis or treatment. Treatment provided in this fashion is called *ambulatory care*. An inpatient, on the other hand, is "admitted" to the hospital and stays overnight or for an indeterminate time. Patients are the ultimate consumers of medicines.

Per European citizen, on an average, over €430 is spent on pharmaceutical products per year, obviously with significant differences over time and patients, mainly through public or third party funding. Since most prescription medicines are provided under public health (insurance) schemes, the overwhelming majority of European patients do not directly pay the price of the prescription medicines they receive. They may, however, make a direct contribution to the price, for example, in the form of a "co-payment" representing a fraction of the full price, or other forms such as a flat fee contribution.

Social Security/Health Insurers

According to European Commission's Pharmaceutical Sector Inquiry Final Report (2009), "patients do not pay directly the (full) costs of prescription medicines, and consequently health systems must organize the reimbursement to patients and/or distributors of relevant costs. This may be done through state agencies (e.g., the National Health Service in the United Kingdom) or through relatively autonomous social insurers, as in Germany. However, there appears to be a trend for health insurers to directly negotiate prices and rebates with the manufacturers.

The level of reimbursement is often the subject of controversy between health insurers and pharmaceutical companies. High co-payments can discourage certain patients from buying the pharmaceutical products concerned. In order to find a solution to controversial reimbursement decisions, member states tend to delegate the cost benefit assessment of medicines to independent experts such as the National Institute for Health and Clinical Excellence (NICE) in the United Kingdom and the Institute for Quality and Efficiency in Health Care (IQWIG) in Germany. These institutions assess medicinal products or treatments on two criteria: the effectiveness of a medicine in providing therapeutic benefits and the effectiveness of a product or treatment in relation to its cost and alternative products, as a measure of the (relative) efficiency of the medicinal product or treatment."

DISTRIBUTION MODELS FOR BIOPHARMACEUTICALS

Drug distribution is gradually transforming. The "traditional" distribution model—aggressive forward buying by wholesalers and a lack of transparency—has vanished. *Fee-for-service (FFS)* agreements have taken hold, but fees do not fully reflect the value to either the manufacturer or the wholesaler. A second generation of FFS models is emerging, as described below.

There are currently four different distribution systems for biopharmaceuticals in operation:

- *Wholesaler model*: This cost-effective distribution alternative for the majority of pharmaceutical products allows wholesalers to provide logistical efficiencies across manufacturers and focus on demand fulfillment and provide a high level of service to end customers.

- *Managed distribution model*: A model that requires the manufacturer to approve each distributor or dispenser of the product; generally contains a single point of reference.

- *Limited distribution model*: By limiting wholesaler relationships, manufacturers hope to improve inventory management, reduce costs, and mitigate concerns about product and supply chain integrity.

- *Direct distribution model*: Direct distribution by manufacturers has emerged as a viable distribution model, particularly for high-priced biologics with a limited provider base and direct-bulk shipments to customers with their own central distribution warehouse. Table 11.8 provides a comparison of four biopharmaceutical distribution models.

SPECIALTY PHARMACY

In a traditional pharmaceutical supply chain setting, a physician writes a prescription, which the patient then takes to a retail pharmacy location, has it filled, and then takes the prescribed medicine home for oral administration in order to treat a common ailment, for example, back pain. Since the advent of biotechnology, however, this picture has slowly been changing. Let us notice the differences. Advanced biopharmaceuticals have gained marketing authorizations to treat chronic and severe diseases, for example, cancer, rheumatoid arthritis, and multiple sclerosis. These new biomedicines have become available in more sophisticated formulations (intramuscular or even intravenous injectables), which require a cold distribution chain (storage at 2°C–8°C, throughout) have commanded a significant price (some in excess of $10,000 per patient per year), and also require significant healthcare personnel supervision, patient education, and increased patient adherence.

Based on their new sophisticated characteristics and prerequisites, the traditional pharmaceutical distribution model had to slowly evolve. How so? Injectables required either a medical setting for administration (usually out-patient) or a nurse assisting the patient at his or her home. The cold chain required different distribution facilities, different transportation fleets, additional training for their handling, and new technology (e.g., portable temperature monitors). The higher price demanded new distribution agreements between manufacturers and distributors, for example, instead of a traditional percentage of wholesale prices (for a 5%, the distribution of a single yearly patient supply would be priced at $1,000 for a

TABLE 11.8   Comparisons of Four Biopharmaceutical Distribution Models

	Open Distribution	**Managed Distribution**
Description	Product is available via wholesale channel to any state-approved dispenser	A model that requires the manufacturer to approve each distributor or dispenser of the product; generally contains a single point of reference
Positives	A cost effective and efficient model for reaching all channels within the U.S. healthcare system for a typical pharmaceutical product	Excellent date, flexible, strong stakeholder cooperation, excellent compliance and persistency programs and superb data
Risks	Inefficient data, compliance challenges, adherence challenges, reverse logistics, presents possible product pricing challenges	Network can become too large, active management by the manufacturers needed
	Limited distribution with registry	Sole distribution
Description	A model that requires an official patient and/or physician registration prior to the release of the drug	Generally small volume orphan drugs. Available via one distributorship only either drop ship or non-drop ship (direct)
Positives	Excellent for product shortages, comprehensive clinical issues, recall functionality, prevents inappropriate prescribing, packaging issues or manufacturing problems	Excellent for product shortages, comprehensive clinical management, packaging issues or manufacturing problems
Risks	Possible competitive disadvantage, payer cooperation, program cost, Physician/VA/DOD/FEP adoption, significant training and certification	Possible competitive liability, payer cooperation, cost, Physician/VA/DOD/FEP adoption and significant training

Source: Furgal, P., Distribution models for biopharmaceutical products, McKesson Specialty, San Francisco, CA, 2009, PowerPoint presentation posted at: http://www.nacdsfoundation.org/user-assets/Documents/PDF/Biopharmaceuticals%20Presentations/Furgal.pdf. With permission.

wholesale cost of $20,000), a more logical fee-for-service. Furthermore, the new biomedicine would demand homecare services at the patient's home, additional information and education, patient adherence training, better self-identification of disease symptoms, and treatment of side effects, and more.

The special characteristics of this new breed of biomedicines have given rise to a new pharmaceutical service: *specialty pharmacy*. Specialty pharmacy is defined as the family of services aimed to manage the special service requirements of specialty pharmaceuticals. These requirements encompass every single aspect of their physical distribution, their storage conditions, their administration conditions, as well as every other aspect of patient assistance, including home delivery, home training, nurse support, psychological support, patient monitoring, patient adherence training, frequent visits to or from a physician, prescription claims handling, formulary authorizations, prescription processing, and more.

Let us be clear. Specialty pharmacy is aimed at the patients receiving specialty pharmaceuticals, but it does not only satisfy their needs alone. It also serves the increased needs of the biomanufacturers (safe, secure, fast, cost-efficient, and according to strict specifications transportation and handling), and the needs of the healthcare provider (physician, nurse, psychologist) who need to coordinate their efforts and share information and services. In addition, the needs of insurance providers to maintain treatment costs, and those of PBMs who need to supervise and manage the whole process according to specifications and strict limitations agreed in common with the insurance providers.

The specialty pharmacy model itself, has evolved over the last 25 years. As the biopharmaceutical pipeline grew, their market penetration was increased; more patients and new indications were added. This led to a gradual transformation of the pharmaceutical supply chain, first to accommodate the "brave" new biopharmaceuticals who demanded "special" attention, and later to create new facilities, new services, and new "treatment paradigms" that were custom created for them.

Specialty Pharmacy Services

As mentioned above, specialty pharmacy is aimed at patients suffering from chronic and severe diseases who receive specialty biopharmaceuticals requiring special transportation, storage, administration, and more. The list of specialty services has gradually progressed and today includes claims processing; homecare services (physician, nursing, psychological support); logistics, inventory, and administrative services; monitored infusion settings; nuclear pharmacy; patient and family education; patient home delivery; patient monitoring; patient transportation to and from

TABLE 11.9   Key Distinctions between Specialty Pharmacy and Community Pharmacy

Management of Specialty Pharmaceuticals	Management of Community Pharmaceuticals
High level of patient training required and enlightenment regarding usage and proper handling	Patient training required and enlightenment regarding usage and proper handling other than traditional counseling
High and continued patient interactions beyond the initial dispensing process	Generally a one-time patient counseling session on first fill and availability to respond to questions as needed
Drug therapy may result in a higher frequency of side effects that are potentially more severe	Potential drug therapy side effects are less frequent and not as potentially debilitating
Dosage administration, side effects, storage condition, and other factors may require altering daily patterns	Drug therapy generally does not require significant alteration to patient's daily patterns
Patient noncompliance has potential for significant impact on expected improvements from therapy and can increase related costs	Lack of patient compliance may have modest impact and may likely be a progressive rather than immediate negative consequence
Rigorous patient education is required, often provided by nursing or pharmacist staff together with monitoring to ensure optimal outcomes	Patient compliance education is generally limited to counseling and labeling of the product and distribution of Consumer Medicine Information (CMI)

Source: Steiber, D. and Erhardt, D.P., Specialty Pharmacy in Community Pharmacy: The Time is Now—and How!, 2006, VCG & Associates, Holliston, MA. With permission.

diagnostic facilities; prescription assistance; prior authorizations; storage methods and conditions; transportation methods and conditions; Web and telephone support, and Web pharmacy services.

Table 11.9 lists some of the key distinctions between specialty pharmacy and community pharmacy.

The following is a list of some of the large, higher-volume providers: Accredo Health Inc. (Medco), AdvancePCS (Caremark Rx Inc.), Pharmacare, a subsidiary of Massachusetts-based CVS Corp., Priority Healthcare Corp. and CuraScript Pharmacy Inc. (Express Scripts), U.S. Bioservices Corp. (AmerisourceBergen Corp.), and Walgreens Health Initiatives.

Specialty Pharmaceuticals

Specialty pharmaceuticals are defined as medicines used to treat chronic and severe disease, that due to disease and product characteristics require special storage, handling, administration, and monitoring, as well as a variety of additional services for better treatment outcomes that are cost-efficient and affordable. Let us take a look at some of the special characteristics that define this product category: (1) complex reimbursement support, (2) frequent dosage adjustments, (3) higher costs than "traditional" products ($10,000–$100,000 annually), (4) increased potential to slow disease progression of chronic/severe disease and improve the patient quality of life, (5) more severe side effects than traditional drugs, (6) narrow therapeutic range, (7) patient compliance management, (8) patient registration, (9) patient training and clinical call center, (10) periodic laboratory or diagnostic testing, (11) small numbers of targeted patients (5,000–100,000), (12) special storage, handling and/or administration, and (13) supervised dosage administration of injectables and infusibles.

Specialty pharmaceuticals can be broken down into four distinct categories and are commonly defined and/or classified by the method of administration: (1) office-administered injectable products, (2) self-administered injectable products, (3) clinic-/office-administered infusible products, and (4) select oral agents. Table 11.10 lists some of the key medications in the specialty pipeline during 2009.

According to CAREMARK's 2006 Focus on Specialty Pharmacy, while the specialty segment currently accounts for about 15% of pharmaceutical spending in the United States, the specialty pipeline is approaching parity in terms of the number of potential new products. The pipeline is expanding in scope as well as volume. An increasing number of products are aimed at chronic conditions—RA, psoriasis, asthma—with higher incidence rates than the "orphan" diseases that first dominated the specialty sector.

For a specialty pharmacy provider example see the corporate profile of CVS Caremark, Posted at: http://info.cvscaremark.com/our-company/cvs-caremark-facts.

DISEASE MANAGEMENT SERVICES OFFERED BY SPECIALTY MANUFACTURERS

Disease management has evolved from managed care, specialty capitation, and health service demand management, and refers to the processes and people concerned with improving or maintaining health in large populations. It is concerned with common chronic illnesses, and the reduction of future complications associated with those diseases. Illnesses that disease management would focus on would include

TABLE 11.10   Key Medications in the Specialty Pipeline

Therapeutic Use	Brand Name (Generic Name)/Manufacturer	Route of Administration	Status
Bone loss	Prolia™ (denosumab)/ Amgen	SC injection	Under FDA review
Cystic fibrosis	NA (denufosol)/Inspire Pharmaceuticals	Inhalation	In phase III studies
Hepatitis C	Albuferon® (albinterferon alfa-2b)/Human Genome Sciences and Novartis	Injection	In phase III studies
HIV/AIDS	NA (vicriviroc)/ Schering-Plough	Oral	In phase III studies
Infertility	NA (corifollitropin alfa)/ Schering-Plough	SC injection	In phase III studies
Inflammatory diseases	Actemra® (tocilizumab)/ Roche	IV infusion	Under FDA review
	Stelara® (ustekinumab)/ Centocor	SC injection	Under FDA review
Multiple sclerosis	NA (dirucotide, MBP8298)/ Eli Lilly and BioMS Medical	IV infusion	In phase III studies
	NA (fingolimod, FTY720)/ Novartis	Oral	In phase III studies
Oncology	Provenge® (sipuleucel-T)/ Dendreon	IV infusion	Under FDA review
	Zactima® (vandetanib)/ AstraZeneca	Oral	In phase III studies

Source: Courtesy of Walgreens Specialty Pharmacy—Outlook—State of the industry report, Dallas, TX, 2009.

coronary heart disease, chronic obstructive pulmonary disease (COPD), kidney failure, hypertension, heart failure, obesity, diabetes mellitus, asthma, cancer, arthritis, clinical depression, osteoporosis, and other common ailments.

SPECIALTY PHARMACY IN NUMBERS

The high cost of the medications and the duration of therapy are just two of the reasons why expenditures for specialty drugs increased faster than any other sector of healthcare in 2008 and—with growth forecasted at 18.1% in 2009—are projected to continue outpacing growth in other areas of healthcare. The pipeline for specialty drugs is robust, with more than 600 specialty medications currently under development for a market expected to top $98 billion by 2011.

According to IMS Health, three specialty therapeutic classes were among the top 10 therapeutic classes by U.S. sales in 2008. The specialty classes, which ranked seventh, eighth, and ninth, respectively, include certain cancer drugs known as antineoplastic monoclonal antibodies; erythropoietins, which stimulate red blood cell production in the bone marrow; and biologic response modifiers (BRMs), which are used in the treatment of conditions such as RA, psoriasis, psoriatic arthritis, and Crohn's disease. BRM sales rose 131% between 2004 and 2008, increasing from $2.6 billion to $6.0 billion. This growth is attributable in part to new indications that expand BRM use.

Table 11.11 lists the top 10 specialty categories globally during 2008.

Finally, according to the WALGREENS SPECIALTY PHARMACY—Outlook 2009 (Walgreens 2009, With permission), three of the top 10 products in 2008—Enbrel®, Neulasta®, and Epogen®—are specialty drugs. Sales of Enbrel, a BRM, increased 70% between 2004 and 2008; Neulasta sales increased 72% during the same period. (Neulasta is prescribed to

TABLE 11.11   Top 10 Specialty Categories Globally, 2008

	% m.s.	% Growth, $	% CAGR, 03–07
Specialty pharmaceuticals	100.0	11.4	13.9
Oncologics (e.g., Avastin, Erbitux, Herceptin, Rituxan, Xeloda)	35.7	11.9	18.1
HIV antivirals (e.g., Atripla, Kaletra, Truvada)	9.1	11.9	12.5
Immunosuppressants (e.g., Prograf, Cellcept, Rapamune)	9.1	17.9	13.8
Erythropoetins (e.g., Aranesp, Procrit)	8.5	−14.0	4.5
Specific Antirheumatics (e.g., Enbrel, Humira, Remicade, Kineret)	8.2	18.2	35.5
Immunostimulants (excl. Interferons; e.g., Neulasta, Neupogen)	6.6	6.0	14.2
Interferons (e.g., Roferon, Avonex, Betaseron)	4.2	8.1	7.6
Immunoglobulins (e.g., Gamimmune, Gamunex, Octagam)	3.7	11.5	12.0
Blood coagulation (e.g., Helixate FS, Koate)	3.0	8.6	11.7
Antivirals (Hepatitis B&C) (e.g., Rebetol, Copegus, Baraclude)	2.9	6.2	5.1
Total others	9.0	9.8	11.4

Source: Courtesy of IMS MIDAS, *IMS Specialty Market Dynamics*, December 2008.
CAGR: Compound annual growth rate.

maintain white blood cell count in some chemotherapy patients.) At $3.1 billion in 2008, Epogen sales remained below their 2006 high of $3.3 billion as safety concerns continued to affect utilization of this drug along with other erythropoietins.

BIOSUPPLY CHAIN MANAGEMENT

What Is Supply Chain Management?

Supply chain management (SCM) is the management of a network of interconnected businesses involved in the ultimate provision of product and service packages required by end customers. SCM spans all movement and storage of raw materials, work-in-process inventory, and finished goods from the point of origin to the point of consumption (supply chain). The definition one American professional association put forward is that SCM encompasses the planning and management of all activities involved in sourcing, procurement, conversion, and logistics management activities. Importantly, it also includes coordination and collaboration with channel partners, which can be suppliers, intermediaries, third-party service providers, and customers. In essence, SCM integrates supply and demand management within and across companies. Table 11.12 explains the main objectives of a biopharmaceutical supply chain function.

TABLE 11.12   What Are the Main Objectives of a Biopharmaceutical Supply Chain Function?

1	2	3	4	5
Profitable Growth	Cost Minimization	Tax Minimization	Fixed Capital Efficiency	Working Capital Efficiency
New product development	Process cost reductions	Asset location	Return on assets	Cash-to-cash cycle time
Global reach	Shared services	Sales location	Capacity management/ throughput	Accounts receivable (DSO)
After-sales service	Outsourcing	Transfer prices	Network optimization	Inventory turns
Perfect orders		Customs duties	Outsourcing	Accounts payable (DPO)
		Commissionaire structure		

Source: Courtesy of The Kaiser Family Foundation, Menlo Park, CA, 2005.

SCM is a cross-functional approach to manage the movement of raw materials into an organization, certain aspects of the internal processing of materials into finished goods, and then the movement of finished goods out of the organization toward the end consumer. As organizations strive to focus on core competencies and becoming more flexible, they have reduced their ownership of raw materials sources and distribution channels. These functions are increasingly being outsourced to other entities that can perform the activities better or more cost effectively.

The purpose of SCM is to improve trust and collaboration among supply chain partners, thus improving inventory visibility and velocity. Several models have been proposed for understanding the activities required to manage material movements across organizational and functional boundaries. Supply chain operations reference (SCOR) is a SCM model promoted by the Supply Chain Management Council (http://www.supply-chain.org/). Another model is the SCM Model proposed by the Global Supply Chain Forum (GSCF; http://www.gsb.stanford.edu/scforum/).

Supply Chain Management Activities and Functions

The key supply chain processes are customer relationship management, customer service management, demand management, order fulfillment, manufacturing flow management, supplier relationship management, product development and commercialization, and returns management. One could suggest other key critical supply business processes combining these processes: customer service management, procurement, product development and commercialization, manufacturing flow management/support, physical distribution, and outsourcing/partnerships. The SCM activities and functions can be distinguished as strategic, tactical, and operational, examples of which are indentified below.

Strategic

Strategic network optimization, including the number, location, and size of warehouses, distribution centers, and facilities. Strategic partnership with suppliers, distributors, and customers, creating communication channels for critical information and operational improvements such as cross-docking, direct shipping, and third-party logistics. Product design coordination, so that new and existing products can be optimally integrated into the supply chain, load management. Information Technology infrastructure, to support supply chain operations. Where-to-make and what-to-make-or-buy decisions. Aligning overall organizational strategy with supply strategy.

Tactical

Sourcing contracts and other purchasing decisions. Production decisions, including contracting, scheduling, and planning process definition. Inventory decisions, including quantity, location, and quality of inventory. Transportation strategy, including frequency, routes, and contracting. Benchmarking of all operations against competitors and implementation of best practices throughout the enterprise.

Operational

Daily production and distribution planning, including all nodes in the supply chain. Production scheduling for each manufacturing facility in the supply chain (minute by minute). Demand planning and forecasting, coordinating the demand forecast of all customers and sharing the forecast with all suppliers. Sourcing planning, including current inventory and forecast demand, in collaboration with all suppliers. Inbound operations, including transportation from suppliers and receiving inventory. Production operations, including the consumption of materials and flow of finished goods. Outbound operations, including all fulfillment activities and transportation to customers.

Now let us take a look at some very useful templates used in biopharmaceutical SCM. Table 11.13 describes how you can compare potential specialty service providers for the distribution of a new biopharmaceutical, while Table 11.14 describes how you compare costs between an existing internal distribution versus an outsourced specialty distribution for a given biopharmaceutical.

Furthermore, Table 11.15 presents what a service specification document between a biopharmaceutical company and a specialty pharmacy services provider contains.

The biopharmaceutical SCM presents a plethora of challenges, some of which are presented below. Supply chain execution is managing and coordinating the movement of materials, information, and funds across the supply chain. The flow is bidirectional. Table 11.16 explains some of the critical processes with which a biopharmaceutical company manages its supply chain.

TABLE 11.13   How Do You Compare Potential Specialty Services Providers
for the Distribution of a New Biopharmaceutical?

#	Characteristic	Provider 1	Provider 2	Provider 3
1	Additional comments			
2	Advance notice on discontinuation of collaboration			
3	Advance notice on start of collaboration			
4	Air freight used			
5	Biopharma-to-specialty provider payment terms			
6	Checks performed on incoming goods			
7	Cold chain			
8	Competitive biopharmaceuticals delivered			
9	Computer enterprise system			
10	Delivery service levels			
11	Financial stability			
12	Focus and fit with biopharma's business			
13	Image on biopharma's business			
14	Innovation and development			
15	Key personnel			
16	One-time costs, e.g., travel, inspections, problem handling			
17	Order entry			
18	Ordering customer credit control			
19	Other biopharmaceuticals delivered			
20	Patient compensation claims handling			
21	Pick and pack operation			
22	Premises and security			
23	Premises locations			
24	Quality control on goods released			
25	Query handling			
26	Reporting			
27	Returns procedure			
28	Service costs (absolute and as % of net sales)			
29	Specialty provider image among our therapeutic area			
30	Stock control			
31	Storage			
32	Transition planning			
33	Truck fleet used			

TABLE 11.14 How Do You Compare Costs between an Existing Internal Distribution versus an Outsourced Specialty Distribution for a Given Biopharmaceutical?

| | Year −3 | Year −2 | Year −1 | Launch | Year +1 | Year +2 | Year +3 |
	2008	2009	2010	2011	2012	2013	2014
Switch costs							
Additional one month accounts receivables							
Customer notification							
Invoicing materials							
IT modifications							
License amendments							
Packaging materials							
Redundancy/retention							
Stock transfer							
Training							
Travel (setup)							
Internal cost savings							
Customer service							
Accounts receivable							
Storage							
Net impact (switch − cost savings)							
Annual internal distribution costs							
Internal costs as % of sales							
Annual specialty pharmacy distribution costs							
Specialty distribution costs as % of sales							
Net annual savings							

TABLE 11.15   What Does a Service Specification Document
between a Biopharmaceutical Company and a Specialty Pharmacy Services
Provider Describe?

#	Part Title	Description	Spec	Bio
1	Background	What is the collaboration for		
2	Objective	Document contents		
3	Scope	Biopharma, specialty provider, brand, territory		
4	Patient services			
4.1		Service branding, e.g., trucks, personnel, packaging, disposables, waste, forms, correspondence		
4.2		Patient enrolment process, e.g., prescription, authorizations, insurance, database checks		
4.3		Home nursing support, e.g., training, support, advice, emergency contacts		
4.4		Patient services, e.g., toll-free hotline, specialist on call, ambulance transfers, patient Web sites		
4.5		Product home delivery, e.g., therapy initiation, refills, emergency replacements, after-hour service		
4.6		Prescription handling, e.g., origin, authorizations, discrepancies, problem reporting		
4.7		Reimbursement, e.g., document collection, submission, approval, and notification of patients and biopharma		
4.8		Non-reimbursed item payment, e.g., psychotherapy, unscheduled visits, after-hours delivery		
4.9		Waste collection and disposal		
4.10		Complaint handling, e.g., cold chain disturbed, products leaked, broken syringes, lack of professionalism, lack of confidentiality		
5	Inventory management	Ordering frequency, safety stock, reporting		
6	Rejections	When product arrives defective from biopharma factory to specialty provider storage facility		
7	Recalls	When biopharma decides to recall the product on safety concerns		

(continued)

TABLE 11.15 (continued)   What Does a Service Specification Document between a Biopharmaceutical Company and a Specialty Pharmacy Services Provider Describe?

#	Part Title	Description	Spec	Bio
8	Returns	When patient does not accept a shipment, e.g., due to storage temperature concerns		
9	Management reporting	Stock, sales volume, sales value, free-of-charge items, complaints, contact reports, delivery performance, under all applicable patient data confidentiality regulations		
10	Clinical reporting	To prescribing physicians, hospital authorities, insurance companies, state agencies		
11	New products	Handling and training for new formulations, dosages, storage conditions, administration devices		
12	Training and development	Biopharma to specialty provider, provider to all its personnel, SOPs applicable		
13	Sales support	Biopharma marketing activities, key account planning, special promotions, tendering requirements		
14	Service monitoring	By both Biopharma and specialty provider, technical tests, queries		
15	Service development	Patient feedback, family feedback, nurses suggestions, specialty personnel observations, new product and service suggestions, materials, training, new sales opportunities		
16	Communication	Daily, weekly, monthly, quarterly, and yearly reports, paper/electronic, contacts on either side		
17	Confidentiality	Authorized personnel only, patient confidentiality, local, national and international laws and regulations		
18	Payment for services	Frequency, method, reporting, authorizations, and approvals		
19	Dispute resolution	Combined task force, executive committees, external arbitration, local courts of law		

TABLE 11.16 How Does a Biopharmaceutical Company Manage Its Supply Chain?

Demand management	Sales and operational planning	Production planning and scheduling	Procurement	Production	Customer order management	Distribution
Sales forecasting	Sales, production and inventory planning	Demand management	Strategic purchasing	Production	Order processing	Supply planning
Collect market intelligence	Operating plans	Schedule maintenance	Purchase order management	Materials handling	Price file management	Product reservation
Determine R&D requirements	Reporting and follow-up	Reporting and control	Vendor management	Production reporting	Billing	Physical distribution
Manufacturing financial forecasting	Manage co-marketing alliances	Capacity planning and control	Payment processing	Costing	Accounts receivables	Internal customer service
	Subcontracting and outsourcing	Manage assets		Quality assurance	Return management	Intercompany trading
		Manage facilities			Inquiry and complaint management	Warehousing
					Recall management	

QUESTIONS

1. What is the flow of goods and financial transactions among players in the U.S. commercial pharmaceutical supply chain?
2. How can wholesale pharmaceutical distributors be distinguished among themselves?
3. What is the role of PBMs in the U.S. pharmaceutical market?
4. How do health plans manage their members' health benefits within the U.S. healthcare market?
5. What is the distinction between full- and short-line pharmaceutical wholesalers in the European pharmaceutical market?
6. Which are the main functions of pharmacists within the pharmaceutical market?
7. What is the action of parallel traders within the European pharmaceutical market?
8. Describe the four main distribution models for biopharmaceuticals that exist around the world.
9. How does the management of specialty pharmaceuticals differ from that for community pharmaceuticals?
10. Describe some of the most common disease management services offered by specialty pharmacy.

EXERCISES

1. Pharmaceutical, biopharmaceutical, and generic manufacturers have their own USPs (unique selling points) when promoting their services to their stakeholders. Find out what they are, respectively, and how do they see each other?
2. You are a young pharmacy graduate, embarking on a retail career in the United States. You are not sure who to select between traditional chain, mass market, supermarket, or independent pharmacy as an employer. By visiting publicly available web resources how do you compare their working environments and their remuneration packages? The latter is often posted in classifieds.
3. You are based in the United States and trying to evaluate the top pharmacy benefit management companies? How do they compare, and which are their unique advantages, if any?
4. Parallel trade between the EU member states has been a factor for some time, fully protected by EU law. On the other side of the

Atlantic, parallel trade between the United States and Canada is still a hotly contested issue. What are the two sides of the parallel trade debate in the U.S. market?

5. You are the GM of a U.K.-based biopharmaceutical subsidiary. What measures are you suggesting to the American HQ for limiting the extent of parallel trade into the United Kingdom, responsible for lower national sales out of your subsidiary?

6. Why do most biopharmaceuticals require specialty services for their successful commercialization?

7. You are a biopharmaceutical executive trying to secure the services of a specialty pharmacy distributor in the U.S. market. What services do you go after, and how do you present your case to your board of directors for approval?

8. Your company's growth hormone has just been approved for pediatric use in Europe. How would you design a dedicated disease management program to support its commercial introduction? What services are essential to this DM program?

9. You are a junior biopharmaceutical supply chain manager and you have been tasked to evaluate your main competitors' supply chain operations, including their strategies, facilities, and tactics. Choosing three of the top global biopharmas, attempt to summarize and present your findings to your superiors.

10. There have been several global supply chain models proposed by experts over the recent years. Identify three of the best known attempts and describe their advantages and disadvantages.

REFERENCES

AAH Pharmaceuticals, Coventry, United Kingdom, http://www.aah.co.uk/aah-home/about-us.aspx

Atlantic Information Services, Inc., *2000–2009 Survey Results, Pharmacy Benefit Trends and Data: Costs, Benefit Design, Utilization PBM Market Share*, Washington, DC, http://www.AISHealth.com

CVS Caremark, Minneapolis, MN, http://info.cvscaremark.com/our-company/cvs-caremark-facts

CVS Caremark, Minneapolis, MN, 2006, Focus on Specialty Pharmacy. Posted at: http://www.caremark. com/portal/asset/2006_SpecialtyPharmacy.pdf

Ernst & Young, 2009. Beyond borders: The global biotechnology report 2009. Boston, MA: E&Y.

European Association of Pharmaceutical Full-Line Wholesalers (GIRP), http://www.girp.eu

EUROPEAN COMMISSION—COMMISSION OF THE EUROPEAN COMMUNITIES, 2009. Pharmaceutical Sector Inquiry Final Report. Brussels, Belgium: EC, SEC(2009) 952, 8.7.2009. Posted at: http://ec.europa.eu/competition/sectors/pharmaceuticals/inquiry/communication_en.pdf

Eurostat, 2009. *Europe in Figures—Eurostat Yearbook 2009*. Posted at: http://epp.eurostat.ec.europa.eu/portal/page/portal/publications/eurostat_yearbook

Furgal, P., 2009. Distribution models for biopharmaceutical products. McKesson Specialty, San Francisco, CA. PowerPoint presentation posted at: http://www.nacdsfoundation.org/user-assets/Documents/PDF/Biopharmaceuticals%20Presentations/Furgal.pdf

Healthcare Distribution Management Association (HDMA), Arlington, VA: 2009. *2009–2010 HDMA Factbook: Facts, Figures & Trends in Healthcare*. The Center for Healthcare Supply Chain Research.

HDMA Press Release, Arlington, VA, September 25, 2009. Posted at: http://www.hcsupplychainresearch.org/press/20090925_factbook.asp

IMS MIDAS, *IMS Specialty Market Dynamics*, December 2008.

IMS National Sales Perspectives, Norwalk, CT, http://www.imshealth.com

McKesson Corporate Presentation, San Francisco, CA, 2009.

Medco Health Solutions, Inc., http://www.medcohealth.com/medco/corporate/home.jsp

Pharmaceutical Research and Manufacturers of America, 2009. *Pharmaceutical Industry Profile 2009*. Washington, DC: PhRMA.

Pharmacy Benefit Trends and Data: Costs, Benefit Design, Utilization PBM Market Share, 2000–2009 Survey Results, Atlantic Information Services, Inc. http://www.AISHealth.com

Steiber, D. and Erhardt, D.P., 2006. Specialty pharmacy in community pharmacy: The time is now—and how! VCG & Associates, Holliston, MA.

The Kaiser Family Foundation, 2005. Follow the pill: Understanding the U.S. commercial pharmaceutical supply chain. The Health Strategies Consultancy LLC for The Kaiser Family Foundation, Menlo Park, CA, March 2005. Posted at: http://www.kff.org/rxdrugs/upload/Follow-The-Pill-Understanding-the-U-S-Commercial-Pharmaceutical-Supply-Chain-Report.pdf

The National Association of Chain Drug Stores (NACDS), 2010. Industry facts, NACDS, Alexandria, VA. Posted at: http://www.nacds.org

Walgreens Specialty Pharmacy, 2009. Outlook—State of the industry report, Dallas, TX.

## CHAPTER 12

Biobrand Life Cycle Management

Global generic pharmaceutical manufacturer sales were $83 billion during the twelve-month period ending with September 2009. The top four global generics manufacturers—Teva, Sandoz, Mylan and Watson—also accounted for 47% of the US market as of 2009.

Source: Courtesy of IMS Health, IMS National Sales Perspective, Norwalk, CT, MAT Sep 2009.

IN CHAPTERS 4, 5, 8, THROUGH 10, we have discussed how a biopharmaceutical product is tested, developed, approved, priced, promoted, and distributed. What happens though, after a product is commercially launched? Do its sales and profits rise continuously? Does it need continuous sales and marketing support from its manufacturer? Will it ever be withdrawn from the marketplace to pave the way for a successor molecule? These are dilemmas faced by biopharmaceutical marketers who have described several distinct phases in a product's evolution. In fact, every single biopharmaceutical has a life cycle of its own.

In general, a product's life begins early even before patent protection; it then spends an average of 10 years to become commercially available, and it races to capture the commercial sales and profits required to cover its large R&D costs over the remaining 10 years on patent protection. Immediately after loss of patent protection, a plethora of generic competitors rush to take away its significant sales and profit streams, until the biopharma manufacturer decides that it no longer pays to promote and sell this old product, and it would be wiser to replace it with a newer, more effective and innovative biomedicine.

It thus becomes apparent that all biomedicines have a finite life cycle; most of these life cycles resemble each other in exhibiting distinct phases, their sales and profits rise and fall over their lifetime, and they also require different strategies for their manufacturers in order to succeed and remain competitive in a fierce marketplace battleground. We will study the characteristics of the biopharmaceutical life cycle in this chapter.

THE PRODUCT LIFE CYCLE

The Different Stages in a Biopharmaceutical Life Cycle

Each biopharmaceutical has a finite life cycle, which can be divided in distinct stages with common characteristics, as shown in Table 12.1. In general, we can distinguish five distinct phases: introduction, growth, turbulence, maturity, and decline. During the biopharmaceutical product *introductory phase*, the biopharma manufacturer deploys a limited sales force that targets a gradually expanding prescriber base. Among these limited prescribers targeted, it is anticipated that a select few, namely, the innovators who keep abreast of all the latest scientific developments and are willing to try a new therapeutic alternative, will try the new biomolecule first on a small number of their patients. Respectively, the biopharmaceutical's sales are limited, and rarely surpass the significant promotional expenses undertaken by the biopharma, leading to a negative or negligible profitability. The product mix refers to a very basic model, for example, a single formulation of a prefilled syringe, value-adding product benefits, for example, free homecare services, are lacking, and the advertising objective is either to inform the patients about seeking treatment for their disease symptoms, or informing the prescribers that a new medication is now available.

During the *growth phase*, the prescriber and patient bases are increasing, raising the product sales and boosting its profitability. Suddenly, new competitors are either being launched or appearing over the horizon. Driven by the increased competition and the growing user demands, the biopharma manufacturer is expanding the line, either by adding additional product formulations (e.g., self-injector devices), or by adding new benefits (e.g., free hotline support or home delivery). Product prices are starting to recede, while advertising turns to persuasive, that is, "why use

TABLE 12.1 Characteristics and Marketing Objectives of the Different PLC Stages

Characteristics	Introduction	Growth	Turbulence	Maturity	Decline
Revenues	Small	Moderate	Large	Large	Moderate
Sales growth	Slow	Rapid	Slow	None	Negative
Costs	High fixed—High variable	Moderate fixed costs	Low fixed—Low variable	Low fixed—Low variable	Rising fixed costs
Profits	Negative	Increasing	Maximum	High	Decreasing
Customers	Innovators	Early adopters	Early majority	Late majority	Laggards
Competitors	0–2	Many	Fewer than before	3–4	Fewer than before
Marketing objectives	Introduction	Growth	Turbulence	Maturity	Decline
Information needs	Positioning, targeting, profiling	Life cycle management		Life cycle management	Life cycle management
Overall strategy	Attract opinion leaders	Expand distribution	Product extensions, service	Maintain advantages	Harvest/terminate
Product mix	Basic model	Expand line		Full line	Best sellers
Product changes	A few	Many	Insignificant	Insignificant	Insignificant
Product offerings	Basic benefits	Major features	Major features	Secondary characteristics	Basic benefits
Pricing objective	Penetration/skimming	Fight competition	Protect position	Maximize profits	Maximize profits
Price	Stable	Declining	Declining	Stable	Declining
Distribution	Stable	Increasing	Decreasing	Stable	Decreasing
Advertising	Informative	Persuasive		Competitive	Informative
Sales force	Large—targeted	Large—wide-focused		Key account management	Reduced

Source: Dogramatzis, D., *Pharmaceutical Marketing: A Practical Guide*, IHS Health Group, Englewood, CO, 2001. With permission.

our product versus theirs?" Sales forces are also growing, as their target audience grows significantly, and new prescriber groups or specializations are now being focused on.

During the product's *maturity phase*, sales revenues are large and stabilizing, new prescribers are hard to find, and they tend to be the so-called late adopters, those who prefer to wait until a large pool of knowledge becomes available, before they try it on their patients. The overall biopharma's strategy is to maintain the product's advantages versus the competition, and the product mix has grown to a complete line encompassing a full range of strengths, formulations, and dosages aimed at various indications. Pricing and distribution remain stable, while the sales force is slowly turning away from the mass number of prescribers, and is focusing more on select key accounts possessing either opinion leader status or a heavy prescribing base.

Here, experts often observe a preceding phase called the *turbulence period*. During this period, a variety of environmental changes lead the manufacturer to successive (turbulent) adaptations of its marketing messages, pricing, distribution, and advertising approaches. In other occasions, the turbulence period is not easily distinguished from the fast-ensuing maturity phase. Finally, during *product decline*, patent protection has been lost or is fast approaching, sales are rapidly decreasing, it is hard to capture any new prescribers and patients, pricing is decreasing, while the biopharma is focused on maximizing sales profits by reducing the sales and marketing efforts and planning the biomolecule's successor that will ultimately dictate the market withdrawal of its presently available product offering. The product life cycle example (Table 12.2) summarizes the product status of Genzyme's biopharmaceutical pipeline.

TABLE 12.2   Genzyme's Product PLC Status

Late-Stage Development	Launch	Growth	Mature
Clolar adult AML	Mozobil	Thyrogen	Cerezyme
GENZ-112638	Synvisc-One	Seprafilm	Renagel
Lumizyme	Renvela	Fabrazyme	
Alemtuzumab-MS	Myozyme	Aldurazyme	
Prochymal—GvHD		Thymoglobulin	
Prochymal—Crohn's		Campath	
Ataluren-DMD		Synvisc	
Mipomersen HoFH			

Source: Courtesy of Genzyme Corporation, Genzyme Annual Report 2008, Cambridge, MA, 2008, 2009.

RESEARCH AND DEVELOPMENT PHASE

The biopharmaceutical research and development phase is a long, arduous, and risky stage. On average it takes 10 years to gain a marketing authorization approval, it costs in excess of $1 billion, and it leaves the newly approved biopharmaceutical with an additional 10 years of commercial sales under patent protection, during which the significant R&D costs need to be recuperated and a profit to be made. During the R&D phase each biopharmaceutical enterprise is faced with two critical dilemmas. First, how can an unmet clinical need be identified, leading to potentially higher therapeutic advantages for the molecules selected. Second, how a marketable biopharmaceutical product can be selected, maximizing its potential for regulatory approval, maximizing its commercial sales potential, and minimizing its risks. We will start by focusing on unmet medical needs.

IDENTIFYING UNMET MEDICAL NEEDS

An unmet medical need has been the biopharmaceutical industry's holy grail ever since its very creation during the seventies. It specifically refers to patients suffering from a disease (usually chronic and severe) for which the existing treatment alternatives are not ideal to either the patient's or their treating physician's eyes. In other words, the patient or his or her physician feels that the efficacy, safety, or tolerability of the available treatments can be further improved, and that the patient's quality of life can thus be improved in the process.

It therefore becomes obvious that a given unmet need may have various degrees, ranging from the easily improvable formulation, to the vast side effects the existing therapy may cause. In summary, the degree of an unmet medical need is associated to (1) the severity and chronicity of the disease and (2) the effectiveness of the best available treatment, often labeled the "gold-standard." The first parameter is closely associated with disease morbidity, the patient's quality of life and mortality. Respectively, the second parameter is associated with the treatment's efficacy, safety, tolerability, onset of action, frequency of administration, contraindications, interactions, special warnings ("black-box"), and others. Table 12.3 describes the unmet clinical need criteria.

Using the unmet clinical need criteria listed above, biopharmaceutical companies of all sizes and shapes embark on an extensive effort of identifying diseases with significant unmet needs. These diseases are then prioritized with the use of additional criteria, for example, the disease incidence and prevalence, their respective pharmaceutical market size, the degree

TABLE 12.3   Unmet Clinical Need Criteria

How Serious Is the Disease?		Disease Severity–Weighted Unmet Clinical Need	How Effective Is the Gold-Standard Therapy?
Disease Severity		Unmet Medical Need	
Morbidity	Mortality	Efficacy	Compound Attributes
Disability		Effect on mortality	Side effects minor—significant
Hospitalization		Effect on disability	Drug interactions
Potential for complications		Effect on hospitalization	Contraindications
Pain		Effect on potential for hospitalizations	Dosage form
Non-pain symptoms		Effect on pain	Dosing frequency
		Overall response	Onset of action
		Complete response	
		Effect on non-pain syndromes	
		Overall response	
		Complete response	

Source: Decision Resources, Market research to drive (and focus) R&D innovation, PBIRG 2002, Workshop 4, PowerPoint presentation, Posted at: http://www.pbirg.com/new/docs/2002AGM/Interact_wrksp/workshop4.ppt, 2002. With permission.

of patient compliance, the number of available pharmaceutical competitors, the characteristics of the available treatments, and their respective gaps for the "ideal treatment." When all these criteria are put in place, the preeminent diseases emerge with the highest unmet needs. Focusing on these indications, biopharma professionals identify the missing product characteristics and predict the respective difficulty in achieving (e.g., turning a short-acting lyophilized powder for injection to a long-acting depot injection contained in a prefilled syringe). Later, depending on the emerging competitive advantages, a price premium over the gold-standard treatment is quantified, the product reimbursability and formulary inclusion is debated, and the expected sales potential of the target biopharmaceutical is carefully forecasted.

By definition, healthcare biotechnology companies have targeted chronic and severe diseases with high unmet needs, compared with their big pharma competitors. As the U.S. Biotechnology Industry Organization (BIO) reports (2008), since 1982 hundreds of millions of people worldwide have been helped by more than 230 biotechnology drugs and vaccines.

There are more than 400 biotech drug products and vaccines currently in clinical trials targeting more than 200 diseases, including various cancers, Alzheimer's disease, heart disease, diabetes, and arthritis. Biotechnology is one of the most research-intensive industries in the world, spending $22.9 billion on research and development in 2006.

CRITERIA FOR IDENTIFYING A MARKETABLE PRODUCT

We have just seen how an unmet clinical need is identified, compared, and rated, until it becomes a solid target for a given biopharma. The next critical step is the identification of a biopharmaceutical pipeline product suitable to be approved and commercially marketed. The process followed by an innovative biopharma is described below.

Focused on the indication rating with the highest unmet clinical needs, biopharmaceutical R&D professionals set about to create an extensive network of contacts, advisors, internal and external experts, opinion leaders, clinical investigators, patients and their families, patient organizations, regulatory professionals, and reimbursement experts who can guide them throughout the arduous process of biopharma R&D development. Armed with this collective knowledge and expertise, they set upon shifting through their expansive pipeline in search for the next "best thing" that closely resembles the unmet clinical needs profile. If their own molecules in pipeline are not deemed close enough to the required properties, or if one of their best candidates could acquire such properties only by a specialized modification, the necessary "freedom-to-operate" is sought. When this is secured, the R&D process continues, until the next "freedom-to-operate" gap. Eventually, multiple gaps are overcome, and the new candidate molecule enters clinical trials that will ultimately prove its merits. When all stakeholders are satisfied with the emerging clinical trials profile, the new biopharmaceutical is submitted for regulatory approval and, if successful, is commercially launched with unique advantages that closely resemble the unmet clinical needs profile upon which it was originally designed. But let us step back into this process' building blocks, by starting with the research project selection that comes at an early R&D stage.

Research Project Selection

Having identified a suitable indication, biopharma researchers shift through their extensive in-house pipeline that targets this indication. The latest biochemical insights from this indication refer to a few distinct pathways. In addition, some of these targetable pathways are successfully modulated by pipeline molecules in vitro. These original findings form the biopharma's valuable "proof of concept."

The next development steps involve several directions: (1) What are the physicochemical properties of the biopharmaceutical in question and can they be improved so that a suitable pharmacological dose be created? (2) Are there available animal models for this indication available in house? (3) What is the optimal process for manufacturing this molecule? Specialized teams are assigned to follow each direction and they work parallely to each other. When skill gaps are identified, additional personnel are employed, and when "freedom-to-operate" gaps are foreseen, the business development team seeks to bridge them. Eventually, all obstacles are overcome, and a unique prospect is identified. At this point, a detailed feasibility analysis for each molecular lead is conducted. An example of such an analysis is provided in Table 12.4.

Here, R&D, marketing, regulatory, legal, and financial colleagues collaborate to create a clear and realistic feasibility plan for the molecule in question, that is, assessing the therapeutic category acceptance and penetration, the forecasted development costs and product sales, the predicted product profitability, potential competitive reactions, and more. The completed feasibility analyses are then presented to the biopharma's new product development task force, which may decide to present it to the board of directors for a final "go" decision, or postpone its presentation until further development and testing.

Target Product Profile

Following the approval of the research project by the biopharma board of directors a critical new process is set in place. A multifunctional company team embarks on the creation of the new molecule's target product profile (TPP), an example of which is provided in Table 12.5. The TPP is a short document describing all the important details of the lead molecule, in a future state, that is, when it eventually becomes commercially available. It is a target profile, meaning that not all of the characteristics listed on the TPP may be achievable today, but give, nevertheless, guidance to the R&D teams to pool their resources and stretch their capabilities until finally they meet all of the TPP's mandates.

As the example indicates, the TPP is a wish-list, combining presently achieved and still sought product characteristics. It describes what the molecule treats, how effective and safe it is, what does it achieve versus the competition, its dosage, formulation and administration route, its patent strength, regulatory and reimbursement plan, cost of goods, anticipated

TABLE 12.4   New Product Feasibility Analysis

Parameter	Question	Data Sources
Disease epidemiology	What is the disease incidence and prevalence? Is there a seasonal disease manifestation? Are there any geographical area irregularities?	WHO, OECD, International Scientific Associations, National Medical Asns, Medical Journals
Market size and growth	What is the market size (in patients, treatment cycles, units, and values) and evolution?	IMS Trade publications
Satisfaction with existing therapies	Are prescribers, patients, patient families, and health personnel satisfied with existing therapies?	Opinion leader input, market research, Web site feedback, press, sales force feedback
Competition	Who are the prescription, generic, and OTC competitors? What are their number, size, and specialization?	Marker research, management consultants, financial analysts, suppliers, sales force
Ther. category acceptance and penetration	What is the acceptance of this therapy among prescribers and patients? Which is the life cycle stage and penetration rate of the treatment?	Customer feedback, market research, Web site feedback
Development costs	How much will it cost to develop 10 preclinical/4 clinical leads? Do we have the know-how and resources? Do we possess the necessary technologies?	R&D department, management consultants, CRO organizations
Expected sales	How can we forecast our future sales (units and values)? What was the market penetration rate of previous competitive launches?	IMS Managed care/ government hospital data
Category expertise of company	How many years have we been active? What is our product portfolio depth? How many NCEs have we introduced in the category?	Internal data (R&D, marketing, past sales)
Company image	How do our stakeholders perceive our company and our products? How do we rate in customer satisfaction, patient quality of life improvement focus, animal testing, environmental sensitivity, and community relations?	Market research Customer service department feedback Sales department feedback Web site feedback

Source: Dogramatzis, D., *Pharmaceutical Marketing: A Practical Guide*, IHS Health Group, Englewood, CO, 2001. With permission.

TABLE 12.5   Target Product Profile for a Fictitious Product to Treat Osteoarthritis

Key Attributes	Target Product Profile
Disease to be treated	Osteoarthritis
Route of administration	Oral
Efficacy	Analgesic and anti-inflammatory activity better than "gold standard"
Safety/tolerability	No GI side effects No interactions with other agents
Competitive advantages	The first ever select pathway inhibitor, without significant side effects, that is indicated for first-line, long-term monotherapy
Competitive offerings	"Gold therapy" is currently a chemical macromolecule, available in sachets for daily administration. Competitor X plans to introduce an injectable depot biopharmaceutical, to be administered every other day, with significant local list reactions and antibody formation
Pharmacoeconomics	Reduced healthcare costs by preventing disease progression
Dosage/presentation (type/size)	Immediate release tablet No more than two strengths
Dose and dose frequency	Once daily
Pack design/type	Blister calendar pack with moisture barrier. Must be able to be opened by patient. Tamper evident
Process	Use standard processing equipment for tablets
Aesthetic aspects (color, flavours, taste, etc.)	Color to differentiate tablet strengths Taste masked to reduce bitterness
Patent strength	Our product was exclusively licensed from the University of Texas Medical Branch at Galveston, and a key pharmacologist is now in our team providing the additional "trade secrets" needed for its biosynthesis. Our patents are pending with the USPTO, EPO, and JPO, and will start expiring in June 2028
Regulatory plan	IND applications to be submitted to FDA, EMEA, and JMHLW by early 2012
Reimbursement plan	To become fully reimbursed and included in important formularies within the top 10 pharmaceutical markets in the world
Commercial synergy	Our molecule will be assigned to our emerging Rheumatology/orthopaedics team, and will provide synergies to our RA molecule in development
Territories to be marketed	United States, Europe, Japan
Cost of goods	No more than 10% of commercial price
Commercial price	Equivalent or less than "gold standard"

Source: Adapted from Gibson, M. (ed.), *Pharmaceutical Preformulation and Formulation*, Interpharm/CRC, Boca Raton, FL, 2004. With permission.

sales, and more. A TPP template is given in Table 12.6, while a fictitious example is provided in Table 12.5.

As previously mentioned, the TPP is a biopharmaceutical pipeline product's wish list. Here are some other basic characteristics of it:

1. Even though it is a wish list, it needs to be realistic and achievable.

2. It follows the molecule throughout its development life and beyond, that is, it describes its patent strength, its development timetable, its regulatory and reimbursement plan, etc.

3. It encompasses the input and desires of all stakeholders involved, for example, the unmet clinical needs as expressed by prescribers, patients, and their families; the development needs; the legal requirements; the regulatory aspects; the manufacturing details; the marketing conclusions, etc.

4. It is an all-encompassing summary document, but does not delve into technical details, detailed Gannt charts, or thorough NPV formulas—instead it should be easily understood by multiple functions.

5. It should ideally contain the ideal product characteristics, as well as the minimum required specifications before this molecule is submitted for regulatory approval.

6. It is a development blueprint that will guide the entire biopharma until it becomes commercially available as per the specifications set by the TPP.

Guiding Compounds through Development Example: Merck

- Project teams (Merck and joint with partners)—implement drug development; project teams are little companies within a large company

- Commercialization-type teams—are charged with assuring that all company areas are aligned to make the product candidate a success (clinical research/ manufacturing/regulatory/ marketing)

- Other Committees—cross-divisional Senior Management oversight and approvals

- Large Clinical Outcomes Studies—Demonstrate the Value of Merck Products

Source: From Merck, Guiding compounds through development, Financing Forum, Whitehouse Station, NJ, May 15, 2002, Posted at: http://www.merck.com. With permission.

TABLE 12.6   A Target Product Profile

	Infants	Pediatrics	Adolescents	Adults	Elderly	Other (specify)	Both sexes	Men only	Women only	Race specific
Trade mark										
Generic name (INN)										
Project ID number										
Therapeutic area										
Pharmacological/chemical class										
Estimated market entry dates in targeted regions										
PLT leader										
SPB approval date										
Target indication										
Target indication extensions										
Target populations					Target profile					
Indication										
Positioning										
Dosage and administration										
Efficacy										
Tolerability/safety										
Pk, ease of use										
Price and reimbursement										
Time window										

Target positioning
Target geographies
Target price
IP situation
Patentability
Freedom to operate
Patent expiry date
Data exclusivity/
 protection
Trademark
Target dosage and
 administration
Pharm form(s)/size(s)
Administration route(s)
Administration with food
Dose(s)
Dosing schedule(s)/
 duration(s)
Packaging/storage

Note: One TPP to be completed per indication.

PRODUCT LAUNCH

The first biopharmaceutical companies created 30 years ago followed a progressive evolution model that is still in place today. In detail, the companies focused on making their product approvable by regulatory authorities, but outsourced it when approaching its marketing approval, so that they secured the significant funds required for continuing their R&D programs. When the received royalties reached a minimum level, they opted to offer the international commercial rights of their newer product interactions to global big pharma organizations, while keeping the rights for their domestic markets themselves. In a third evolutionary step, the first biopharmas became well capitalized and secure, to launch their latest products on their own into the global marketplace.

The brief paragraph describing their evolution is only a huge understatement of the obstacles, risks, and dilemmas they have faced until becoming the select few biopharma powerhouses we admire today. Over the process, they were forced to create multiple regulatory strategies and dossiers, they liaised with numerous international pricing and reimbursement authorities, they had to learn the individual market and therapy area characteristics from the bottom up, they established local government and prescriber relationships over the years, while they also dealt with unexpected market conditions (due to predispositions and different values), abrupt changes (e.g., government repricings), dubious practices in place (e.g., kickbacks), and more.

Launching a new biopharmaceutical in multiple global markets is a monumental task, of critical importance to not only the product in question, but to the entire biopharma organization's sustainability over the long run. It becomes imperative that all organizations need to put in place a robust, well-structured, strategic, and tactical operations plan, that can dependably be repeated with every commercial launch in every foreign pharmaceutical market. Primarily, each biopharma needs to devise a foreign market evaluation, rating, and prioritization process, the proper market entry strategies according to the market characteristics, the local stakeholders that need to be approached and influenced, the marketing and distribution strategies, the appropriability of local collaborators, and more.

In addition, the organization needs to create detailed plans that describe the timetables and budgets involved, the organizational structures and skills that need to be in place, the regulatory-reimbursement-marketing dossiers to be deployed, the decision-making and reporting lines needed, and more. Table 12.7 provides us with the main prelaunch strategies for a biopharmaceutical product.

Tables 12.8 and 12.9 provide two useful product-launch tools. Table 12.8 summarizes the prerequisites for preparing for a biopharmaceutical product launch, while Table 12.9 explains the prerequisites for a successful biopharmaceutical launch.

PLC Management Example: The ROCHE Life Cycle Teams (LCT)

According to ROCHE (2006), their Life Cycle Teams (LCT) are in charge from late stage development onward, comprising of 50–200+ members on the extended LCT. More specifically, a core team is comprised of an LC Leader, as well as Functional Leaders. Furthermore, the Extended Team includes members from: preclinical—technical, clinical, regulatory, and supply. Finally, there also exist major affiliate strategy teams, incorporating input from: economics, strategy, medical, and marketing.

Source: ROCHE Oncology Event, June 19, 2006, www.roche.com/irp060619soriot.pdf

Market Entry Strategy

The pioneering biopharmas originally outsourced their first biopharmaceuticals to larger big pharma organizations for them to commercialize all together, or later they kept their domestic markets for themselves, while outsourcing the global rights to their biopharmaceuticals to others. Over the last 10 years, however, multiple biopharmas have significantly grown in size and have selected to keep the global commercial rights for their newer innovations in-house.

The new market entry strategy has brought additional dilemmas associated with it. For example, first, biopharmas needed to identify, study, evaluate, and rate the potential foreign markets for entry. Second, they needed to prioritize their market entry sequence, and select the suitable entry strategy, that is, through a local intermediary or with their own fully owned subsidiary. Third, they had to select an organizational structure suitable for each foreign market, as well as its main office and branch locations. Finally, they had to implement a common strategy for attracting local talent, hiring it, training, and employing it with the common organizational philosophy that existed in all their locations around the world. In addition, biopharmas needed to select international or local IT tools, external consultants, opinion leader advisory boards, patient organization liaisons, government contacts, and more.

During my own corporate career, I had previously been asked to work out of home for as long as necessary, working for the preparation of a new

TABLE 12.7 Which Are the Main Prelaunch Strategies for a Biopharmaceutical Product?

	Preclinical	Phase I	Phase II	Phase III	Launch
Clinical	Access unmet medical needs	Dosage and safety (human volunteers)	Safety and efficacy (pts with disease)	Efficacy and safety in large studies	Physician monitoring attitude/acceptance
	Thought leader identification and input	Trial investigator recruitment (Phase II)	Opinion leader recruitment	Early access programs	Start Phase IV clinicals (new indications)
	Targets (indications, dosages)	Global advisory board	Phase II conference presentations	Phase IV planning	Continue publications
	Investigator recruitment (Phase I)	Leader development	Plan articles/shape labeling	Publications	
				Global CME	
Commercial	Competitive comparators	Global brand teams	Market needs: validate early insights	Forecast and financials	Marketing ROI analysis
	Preliminary pricing study	Early advocacy collaborations	Refine physician and patient segmentation	Patient/physician ad pretests	Access positioning
	Preclinical positioning/initial attribute mapping	Global payer assessment	Quantitative product profile	Advocacy program expansion	Monitor advertising effectiveness
	Pharmacoeconomics study		Comparative analysis	Final pricing/reimbursement	Monitor competitor response
	Early segmentation		ROI modeling	Labeling/monograph	Link with advocacy groups for Phase IV
	Develop product profile		Build communications	Sales training/complete communications	

TABLE 12.8 How Do You Prepare for a Biopharmaceutical Product Launch?

Shape the Product	Shape the Market		Shape the Company
Multiple indications	Docs	Opinion-leader capture	Resource allocation
Dosage/formulations		Physician education	Integrated brand teams
Speed to market (e-recruitment)	Payers	Reimbursement strategy	Speed to market (parallel R&D processes)
Price (first in class or comparator choice)		Pharmacoeconomics	Balance of central planning and local execution
Identify optimum product characteristics by patients		Disease awareness	Infrastructure for fast global rollout
Create ideal product profile		Links with patient community	
Create core values of the product	Patients		
Early positioning (data-driven differentiation)			
Financial analysis			
Create launch program			

TABLE 12.9 Prerequisites for a Successful Biopharmaceutical Launch

Product	Market	Payer
Target product profile	Epidemiology	Payer mix
Clinical proposition	Treatment patterns/goals	Value proposition
Branding and positioning	Drivers and success factors	Pricing and reimbursement
Promotion	Market development	Support programs
Life cycle		Distribution channel
Competition	**Physician**	**Patient**
Current barriers	Unmet needs	Unmet needs
Emerging competition	Concentration/targeting	Demographics
Approaches to treatment	Influence patterns	Attitudes and usage
	Attitudes and usage	Advocacy
	Engagement channels	Engagement channels
	Segmentation	Segmentation

Source: INCYTE, Corporate Presentation, *BAIRD 2009 Health Care Conference*, New York, September 2009, Posted at: http://investor.incyte.com/phoenix.zhtml?c=69764&p=irol-presentations. With permission.

biopharma subsidiary in the local market. Although the whole project was susceptible to local and international risks, as well as invisibility as per the corporate strategy months or years down the line, that very experience still remains one of my most challenging, exhilarating, and mentally rewarding career experiences that I have ever had. As per the strategic parameters that may serve as critical prerequisites for a successful bio-pharmaceutical launch, please see Table 12.9.

Market Prioritization

We have just mentioned that among a biopharma's market entry strategy, foreign market prioritization plays a critical role. This is due to the fact that each biopharma's financial resources are not only limited, but they must also be carefully assigned to different company functions that compete for the same finite amount of resources. For example, entering one more foreign market may not be financially wiser than constructing a new biomanufacturing plant, or even in-sourcing a new molecule in development. Second, each foreign market expansion entails significant risks, which need to be clearly identified, quantified, and rated within the market prioritization process. Third, local conditions and restrictions within a foreign market may reversely affect the biopharmaceutical's life cycle in other markets, for example, its reimbursability or pricing or formulary inclusions. Finally, different foreign markets may require different entry schemes, such as a fully owned subsidiary, a joint venture, or just a sales and distribution agreement with a local agent. Taking all these limitations in consideration, biopharmaceutical executives embark upon a careful foreign market prioritization process that is both extensive and time consuming.

The criteria for biopharmaceutical market prioritization are multiple. For example, the size of the overall pharmaceutical market, local disease characteristics and treatment, the rate of diagnosis and pharmacological treatment, the number of prescribers and patients, the marketing authorization, pricing and reimbursement conditions, the inclusion into local formularies, or the existence of additional hurdles, such as the pharmacoeconomic evaluation. Another important factor is the local IP enforcement environment, and the participation into international trading organizations, for example, TRIPPS, EU, and NAFTA. In addition, domestic and international competitors active in the local market, and the occasional existence of a local pharmaceutical powerhouse with an extremely strong penetration and contacts, may also dictate the market prioritization agenda. Furthermore, the existence of skilled local human resources, the availability of interested partners, the local distribution and IT infrastructures, as well as the attitudes and beliefs of medical opinion leaders, prescribers, and patients all play a critical role.

A commonly used market prioritization scheme is the global pharmaceutical market division into four main areas, following the existence of respective regulatory policies and procedures. In particular, these four groups belong to North America, Europe, Japan, and the so-called Rest-of-World (RoW). Based on their regulatory processes and trade agreements in place, it can be easily forecasted that these four groups would be in general homogeneous in their market structures, given the limited homogeneity of the RoW market. When it comes to the latter, further international subdivisions may be defined, the most usual of which are the following: South and Central America (LATAM), Eastern Europe (outside the European Union), Former Soviet Union (FSU), Middle East, North and South Africa, Asia, and Pacific and Oceania (Japan and Australia–New Zealand). Each of these multinational subdivisions share significant similarities and are often present in most global biopharmaceutical organizational structures. In fact, the biopharma work force abounds with senior managers with significant experience in one or more of these groups of national markets.

A biopharma can then decide on a truly global launch (across every single group of markets named above), or a less ambitious and risky cascade of market launches, starting from the highly regulated North American, European, and Japanese markets and later progressing into more markets, one at a time. The size and timing of the global biopharmaceutical launches are dictated by the size of the manufacturer, the availability of resources, the disease's unmet clinical needs, the product's competitive advantages, the competitive offerings, the anticipated product reimbursability and pricing, the availability of foreign market resources, contacts, and collaborators, and even more.

Distribution Strategy

The biopharmaceutical supply chain management essentials have been discussed in Chapter 11. As far as a biopharmaceutical product life cycle management is concerned, each biopharma needs to decide its product distribution policy well in advance of commercial availability, with special emphasis given in setting up international market distribution networks. When it comes to international markets, there are various distribution strategies available for consideration.

First, a biopharma may set up its own distribution network, complete with storage facilities, transportation vehicles, and dedicated personnel. Second, a local distribution partner may be selected for a given distribution fee, which usually ranges from 2% (for low-volume, high-price products) to 7% of ex-factory prices (for high-volume, low-priced products). In the second scenario, order taking is either done by the biopharma subsidiary or the distributor, the biopharma factory ships directly to the distributor's warehouse, who in turn distributes the products, and collects the customers' payments on behalf of the biomanufacturer. Under a third scenario, the local biopharma subsidiary stores the biopharmaceutical quantities, and only employs a third-party logistics provider (even a courier service provider) on a shipment-by-shipment basis.

Alternative distribution scenarios are more limited in penetration, including direct shipments from the manufacturer's factory to local wholesalers, or even direct shipments from the manufacturer to patients (where allowed by law, and especially for very high-priced specialty pharmaceuticals). The biopharma's distribution strategy does not end there, however. Order taking, repackaging, facility location and architecture, fleet design, vehicle selection, personnel training, areas serviced, complaint handling, and additional value-added services (e.g., training material distribution or patient home-delivery) are critical issues to be decided on a market-by-market basis, and pending on the local networks, skills, and laws in existence. The existing IT infrastructure and national telecommunications networks play an important role in setting up and effectively operating an efficient and profitable biopharmaceutical distribution network.

Commercial Strategy

When it comes to commercial strategy, every biopharma operates on the basis of a well-researched, realistic, and thorough business plan, which encompasses a detailed marketing plan. The function of the marketing plan is to guide the whole organization toward the achievement of common goals, which are spelled out in detail. Detailed timetables are attached, marketing objectives are defined, marketing messages are built around the product's unique selling points (USPs), and the allocated resources are described. Furthermore, the success of the marketing effort is described under the heading marketing audit, while potential upsides and downsides are also mentioned and rated. At the end of the annual marketing cycle process, which in general gets finalized in September of each year, the next year's targets, strategies, tactics, resources, and timelines are clearly and unequivocally agreed by all stakeholders involved. A brief biopharmaceutical marketing plan outline is provided in Appendix B, at the end of this book.

NEW PRODUCT FORECASTING

Throughout Chapters 3 and 6 through 11, we have repetitively described the creation of in-licensing, research and development, manufacturing, pricing, regulatory, reimbursement, marketing, and foreign market expansion plans based on a single and common prerequisite, namely, a thorough and realistic forecasting. The importance of these forecasts become increasingly apparent if we take into account some of the financial projections attached to various biopharmaceutical industry deals. For example, an in-licensing acquisition may be valued at $1 billion, a new biomanufacturing plan may require $100 million, a biopharma merger may cost $15 billion, while a new commercial product introduction may achieve blockbuster status, or lifetime sales in excess of $10 billion. Basing all these company activities on carefully constructed forecasts thus becomes immediately apparent, while the outcome of false forecasts may even bring about the financial ruin and eventual demise of an entire biopharma organization.

Looking at the art and science behind biopharmaceutical forecasting, one may easily distinguish various approaches, methodologies, and constructs. First, forecasting is usually more challenging when attempting to estimate the future sales evolution of a new biopharmaceutical molecule, and especially those that belong to new biological entities (NBEs), or a new therapeutic class of their own. New product forecasting will be further elaborated in the following paragraphs.

In addition to new product sales forecasting, biopharma executives are often called to come up with forecasts on a global (total world), or regional (EU), or country (Canada), or business unit (neurology), or indication (Alzheimer's disease) basis. Furthermore, forecasts may be required by various biopharma functions, each demanding their own degree of detail and specificity. Forecasts may also span varying time durations, spanning from the ever-present biopharmaceutical quarter, to a 20 year long company mission forecast. In addition, forecasts may be read by only financial professionals, who are usually after revenues and profits, while marketing forecasts may need to spell out forecasted patients, treatment cycles, product vials, product milligrams, packages, and dollar sales.

Each of the forecasts mentioned above require their own specificity, inputs, outputs, and related methodology. Junior biopharmaceutical managers usually start with volumes (i.e., number of product packages sold), values (i.e., amount of product sales in local currency), or profitability (i.e., as a percentage of ex-factory pricing). More advanced forecasts may be used by other functions, in search of a number of culture bottles, bioreactors, or media required for biomanufacturing, or test animals, laboratory supplies, and test runs required for research purposes.

Forecasting Challenges

Before we embark on actual biopharmaceutical forecasting methodology, we have to mention certain challenges facing this very complex and time-consuming methodology. First, every single assumption made by any function must be clearly described, validated by external experts—if possible—and agreed upon by the other biopharma functions. Second, a top-down company-wide sales forecast needs to be disseminated into multiple functions and they, in turn, need to consolidate their functional forecasts into a self-validating bottom-up construct. Third, multiyear forecasts need to be carefully broken down into yearly and quarterly forecasts, taking into consideration the potentially changing market conditions, the product sales seasonalities, as well as the smooth continuation from one forecasting period to the next. Fourth, forecasts often need to come into alternative realistic, pessimistic, and optimistic scenarios, and the respective influencing downsides or upsides need to follow immediately after the forecast as accompanying notes. Fifth, forecasts need to be constantly updated and reevaluated, especially those spanning longer time periods (e.g., more than 3 years). Finally, forecasts need to take into account the input of various stakeholders, such as prescribers, patients, and regulators, if a biopharma organization is serious about its future forecasting efforts.

There exist various forecasting methodologies. For example, a time-series approach attempts to forecast future performance by looking at historical performance, as is described by Table 12.10. In plain words, if 2008 product sales were $500 million, 2009 sales were $600 million, and 2010 sales were $700 million, then 2011 sales can be easily forecasted at $800 million. On the other hand, rolling forecasts do not simply extrapolate long-term historical data, since the recent market events may indicate to a different picture in the near future. In plain words, recent events influence the future forecast more than in their respective time-series approximation.

Causal/Econometric and Judgmental Methods

Most biopharmaceutical forecasting approaches rely on the assumption that it is possible to forecast future events if the underlying factors influencing the forecasted variable are thoroughly identified and studied. For example, as far as future biopharmaceutical product sales are concerned, here is a series of influencing factors that may have an impact on future

TABLE 12.10 How Do You Forecast Volume, Value, and Market Share Data for a Biopharmaceutical Launch?

	Year −3	Year −2	Year −1	Launch	Year +1	Year +2	Year +3	Year +4	Year +5
	2008	2009	2010	2011	2012	2013	2014	2015	2016
Bioproduct market potential									
Total population									
Disease prevalence									
Disease patients									
Diagnosed patients									
Patients on treatment									
Patients on reference pharmaceutical									
Patients on biopharmaceuticals									
Bioproduct sales data									
Volume (units)									
Growth (absolute)									
% growth									
Value									
Average unit price (ASP)									
Growth (absolute)									
% growth									
Net sales									
% growth									
Bioproduct market share data									
% Volume market share									
% Value market share									
Market position									
Leading competitor's market share									

sales: total population, male versus female population, population target age groups, disease prevalence, disease incidence, patient percentage symptomatic, patient percentage seeing a physician, diagnosis rate, treatment rate, compliance rate, treatment duration, product dosage, product packages per treatment cycle, number of pharmacological alternatives, and competitive advantages of available medicines. As an example, Table 12.11 provides a template for forecasting biopharmaceutical product shares using internal attributes. As far as the most commonly used data tools in new product forecasting are concerned, Table 12.12 gives us a brief insight.

Alternative forecasting methods can be judgmental, for example, relying on the judgment of company executives, prescribers, nurses, patients, and others. For example, by directly asking a sample physician group "what percentage of your patients would you prescribe the new biopharmaceutical for?" or a group of patients "which biopharmaceutical would you prefer given their respective product attributes described below, and how compliant would you be toward your chosen treatment?" detailed

TABLE 12.11   Product Shares Using Internal Attributes

Attribute	Weight (%)	Drug	Drug 2	Drug 3	New Product
Speed of action	65	15	12	8	17
Efficacy (defined)	90	18	15	16	20
Drug interactions	45	7	8	11	15
Price	65	20	20	20	15
Overall drug score		42.1	37.9	37.6	45.6
Relative score		100	90	89.3	108
Current share		45	35	20	
Final market share		41.2	29.2	16.5	13.1

TABLE 12.12   What Are Some of the Most Commonly Used Data Tools in New Product Forecasting?

1	Primary research	IMS Consulting, Dun and Breadstreet, various market research agencies
2	Proprietary data tools	IMS, GPI, Pharmadynamics
3	Market reports	Ernst & Young, Burrill & Company, PwC Moneytree report, Datamonitor, Decision Resources, company reports and announcements, financial analyst reports
4	Medical and pharmaceutical literature	Medical World Review, Scrips, medical literature, pharmaceutical and biotechnology journals, statistical agency reports
5	Web sites	Decisionstrategies.com, real-options.com, royaltysource.com, recap.com, autm.net, hoovers.com

product forecasts may be constructed and extrapolated to the total prescriber/patient population.

Additional methods are based on simulation, for example, under a Phase III "crossover-design," patients receiving a new biopharmaceutical are switched to a reference medication, and vice versa, until their compliance is measured, or a new biopharmaceutical's sales are forecasted based on a similar product introduction in the same market over the recent years.

Defining the Market—Epidemiology Approach

Now let us review a forecasting example of how a biopharmaceutical market size can be approximated by using the disease epidemiology approach.

Country market total population, male population versus female population, population age groups influenced by the disease, disease prevalence, disease incidence, patient percentage symptomatic, patient percentage seeing a physician, diagnosis rate, treatment rate, compliance rate, treatment duration, product dosage, and product packages per treatment cycle.

Total packages required   +
Number of pharmacological alternatives and competitive advantages of available medicines

----

Product market shares estimated   +
Patients on each medication, product packages sold, and product pricing

----

Product value sales forecasted

Defining the Market—Patient Flow Approach

An alternative biopharmaceutical forecasting method is the use of a patient flow model. By using this approach, a forecaster starts by carefully mapping every single step in the patient journey (patient flow), from the moment the patient feels the first disease symptoms, later deciding to visit a physician, who may decide to refer the patient to a specialist. The patient may then be taken through a series of tests, eventually assisting the specialist in reaching a medical diagnosis. The specialist may then only recommend lifestyle and diet changes, or put the patient on a pharmacological treatment. The duration of such a treatment depends on either the existing disease treatment guidelines, or the specialist's recommendations, and the patient's compliance to the treatment prescribed. Depending on the treatment's efficacy, safety, and visible improvements, the patient may either continue on the treatment, or drop out, or switch medications. When on a new medication, the same patient process is anticipated, until finally the patient decides to stay on a given biopharmaceutical.

As seen in the illustrative Figure 12.1, a patient suffering from a severe and chronic disease may proceed through numerous steps, in search of a significantly improved quality of life while on the medication, as compared with no treatment or alternative therapies in the past. For the biopharmaceutical forecasting to be completed, the forecaster has to then collect all available epidemiology and treatment information and statistics, as well as inquire with respected medical experts, as well as patients and their families, in search of percentage allocations at every single patient step. When the patient flow model is complete with all potential treatment steps and their corresponding probabilities, a precise biopharmaceutical usage forecast can be constructed, which becomes an invaluable input for biopharmaceutical strategy decisions in the future.

WHAT ARE SUSTAINABLE BIOBRANDS?

Having succeeded in launching a biopharmaceutical product, all biopharmas are actively engaged in maximizing their commercial success, either by capturing increased market shares or prolonging their commercial growth stages, or discovering and launching an improved, successor molecule. As far as commercial success maximization is concerned, biopharmas may focus on either capturing market share from their competitors (chemical or biochemical), or creating new market potential, by increasing the approved indications, by launching higher doses, or by approving a more frequent dosage scheme.

According to Simon and Kotler (2003), in addition to creating new market space, biopharmas must also be engaged in creating and managing sustainable biobrands. This strategy depends on three separate activities: (1) balancing their biopharmaceutical portfolio, (2) growing their franchises, and (3) growing their brands. The combination of these three activities lead to sustainable biobrands with significant blockbuster potential, which are capable of not only defeating their competition while under patent protection, but also prolonging their lives by carefully building a program of future successor molecules with their own blockbuster and patent-protection attributes.

For a commercialization example see: GENENTECH, San Francisco, CA, http://www.gene.com

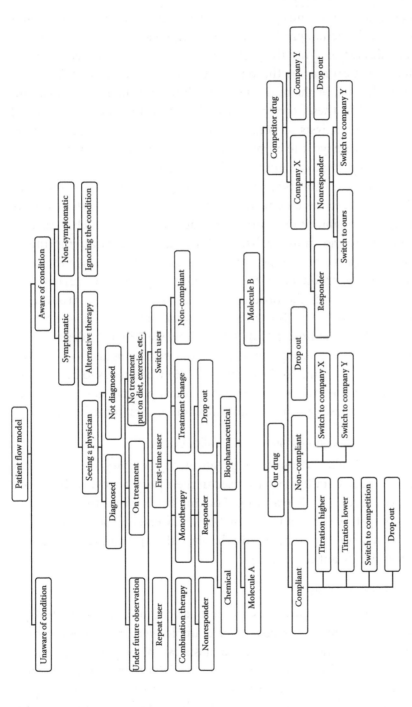

FIGURE 12.1 A patient flow model. (From Dogramatzis, D., *Pharmaceutical Marketing: A Practical Guide*, IHS Health Group, Englewood, CO, 2001. With permission.)

PRODUCT RELAUNCH

Quite often during the life cycle of a biopharmaceutical, the manufacturer realizes that the actual product sales are lagging significantly behind the original sales targets. And the problems do not stop here. In fact, the new biopharmaceutical may be the very first product commercially launched by the biopharma, or the only "next best thing" for many years to come. In situations like these, the biopharma board of directors is soon faced by the financial analysts responsible for the company's rating, and under their strong challenge, the biopharma is forced to issue a profit warning, immediately leading to a significant drop in their share price.

Before, however, the biopharmaceutical product's sales reach such a critical shortage, the biopharma's marketing and sales executives are debating the possibility for a product relaunch. The relaunch is usually constructed around more realistic sales targets, and is attempting to reverse the negative market performance and hopefully revive the commercial life of the product over the next planning period. The turnaround strategy that precedes the product relaunch is constructed around the following objectives: (1) Did we have a sound segmentation-targeting-positioning (S-T-P) approach? (2) Did we go after a realistic sales forecast? (3) Have we planned the appropriate sales and marketing tactics? (4) Have we performed according to the above plan? (5) what needs to be changed and how do we relaunch our biopharmaceutical product going forward?

Let us study these critical turnaround components in further detail.

Segmentation-Targeting-Positioning Validation

Going back to Chapter 8, our team of Advanced Therapies' marketers may reassess the segmentation criteria used in their plan, or revisit the targeting process used in their planning. Looking further into their product's unique competitive advantages, new USPs may emerge, necessitating the creation of a new positioning within the given therapeutic area, and versus their most significant competitors.

Forecast Reevaluation

When it comes to the product's forecast, several aspects, both strategic and tactical, need to be reassessed. For example, were the epidemiological statistics valid, or was the disease diagnosis rate as originally estimated? Furthermore, are physicians following the available therapeutic guidelines or are they more conservative versus our new therapeutic modality? What about the patients' compliance rate or switching rate among medications?

The new product's forecast is also associated with the competitor products' attributes. For example, are competitive products gaining or losing patients due to switching as originally anticipated? Are these products used only within their approved indications, or are they being prescribed off label too (e.g., strictly in the disease's relapsing phase and not in the progressive phase)? Furthermore, are the original product attribute ratings by our prescriber and patient target groups valid, or were they subjective and biased?

In addition to the above, what about our forecasting method? Was the patient flow approach a valid approximation, or were there too many assumptions influencing the final estimate? Have we taken into account every single stakeholder, or have we ignored the input of secondary stakeholders, for example, formulary committees, or healthcare personnel other that treating physicians? Can we reevaluate our forecasts, or possibly eliminate erroneous parameters skewing our results?

Marketing Tactics Reassessment

The turnaround team is often involved in an in-depth reassessment of the sales and marketing tactics used. For example, was it appropriate to invite the given foreign opinion leader to the launch symposium? Were the promotional materials clearly communicating the product's USPs? Did all the materials have the collective clearance from the company's R&D, medical marketing, sales, marketing, and legal departments? Have the product's teasing and direct-to-consumer campaigns worked to their fullest potential? And have the sales professionals communicated the USPs clearly and effectively to their intended recipients?

Sales and Marketing Performance Benchmarking

During the performance evaluation process, the marketing and sales professionals need to reassess every single aspect of their launch efforts. Critical to these assessments are the opinions of every single stakeholder originally targeted. What do the disease experts think, and what is the opinion of individual prescribers, other healthcare professionals, administrators, insurance funds, formulary committees, the patients and their carers, or the general public? Have the biopharma's messages been communicated clearly? Do the stakeholders remember the USPs originally planned for them? Have they been approached by the company's efforts as often as necessary (often called the biopharma's "share of voice")? What were their reactions and/or objections, and how have these customer reactions been handled by the biopharma?

Also, were more senior biopharma executives available to the customers' requests for information? Was there a large volume of corroborating R&D literature available to the stakeholders who requested it? Was it communicated freely, objectively, and swiftly? Were adjustments made after the biopharma faced customer opposition or doubts? Overall, how has the whole organization reacted to its marketplace demands?

In addition, was the sales organization as effective as it should have been, given the sophisticated nature of the stakeholders involved, or the characteristics of the competitive sales forces? Was the deployed sales force properly sized, trained, incentivized, deployed, and targeted? Have they been using the proper messages and sales tactics? Were they relaying all customer reactions back to the sales and marketing command center? Have there been unrealistic sales targets, strong hierarchical pressure, and bad management of low performance or depressed morale? Were the signs and symptoms of an underperforming sales organization properly identified and managed?

Salvaging the Impending Biopharmaceutical Wreck

When all the above evaluations have been thoroughly and objectively completed, experienced biopharma sales and marketing managers need to take the situation into their hands. New targets need to be set, new tactics created, new messages crafted, new approaches tried, and new problem-handling procedures need to be implemented. The whole effort needs to be clearly communicated to every single person involved, complete with realistic targets, milestones, and timelines. In most cases, one turnaround attempt will be the last available tool in stopping the biopharmaceutical product's demise and withdrawal. Furthermore, given the very nature of the healthcare biotechnology industry, a single product will often be the sole achievement of an entire biopharma organization after more than 15 years in the making. Such a gargantuan effort is only for the brave few.

For a biopharmaceutical relaunch example see: AMITIZA. In: Sucampo Board of Directors Issues Statement Regarding Sales Performance by Takeda Pharamaceuticals North America for AMITIZA, Sucampo Pharmaceuticals Press Release, Bethesda, MD, May 28, 2009, http://www.sucampo.com

PATENT EXPIRATION

As discussed in Chapter 2, a biopharmaceutical patent is a legal title conferred by the relevant Patent Office, which protects the inventor's right to prevent others from manufacturing, promoting, selling, distributing or out-licensing the given biopharmaceutical invention covered by the patent. Thus, the original inventor is usually a scientist involved in its creation, while the patent holder is usually a biopharma organization, which is either employing the inventing scientist, or has licensed the exclusive rights to its commercialization from the inventor. In other words, the patent confers commercial exclusivity over the given biopharmaceutical, which lasts for a limited period of time, usually 20 years from filling the invention with the Patent Office.

Generic Entry

In a typical biopharmaceutical industry scenario, the biopharma organization spends in excess of $1 billion over a minimum of 10 years of research and development efforts, before it is able to receive regulatory approval for its commercial launch in the relevant pharmaceutical market (United States, Europe, Japan, or RoW). At the time of its commercial launch, the biopharma is thus left with an additional 10 year period of commercial availability under patent protection, during which it attempts to recuperate the money involved and make a commercial profit. Eventually, the patent protection period expires, and the patent no longer confers commercial exclusivity to its holder. In most cases, pharmaceutical products with significant commercial sales revenues are quickly imitated by generic pharmaceutical manufacturers, which are soon launched in the market place with reduced prices, quickly capturing significant market shares from the original pharmaceutical patent holder.

The generic introduction of biopharmaceuticals losing their patent protection has recently become a reality, since the first biopharmaceutical introductions entered the global pharmaceutical markets during the Eighties. The expiration of a biopharmaceutical product's patent protection is a critical step in its entire life cycle, and will be further discussed below. As far as the issue of regulatory approval of biogeneric copies of biopharmaceutical medicines losing their patent protection, and their subsequent introduction into the major pharmaceutical markets are concerned, the drivers as well as the obstacles to their introduction will be further elaborated in Chapter 13.

We will start our post-patent expiration PLC discussion, by addressing the critical issue of market exclusivity of new biopharmaceuticals in the marketplace. According to data provided by the Tufts Center for the Study of Drug Development (Tufts CSDD, 2009, http://csdd.tufts.edu/), marketing exclusivity for first-in-class drugs has shortened to 2.5 years (see Table 12.13).

Table 12.14 presents several biopharmaceuticals going off patent during 2008–2010.

TABLE 12.13   Marketing Exclusivity for First-in-Class Drugs Has Shortened to 2.5 Years

Follow-on approvals underscore competitive nature of new drug development

Marketing exclusivity periods for first-in-class drugs have fallen dramatically in recent decades—from a median of 10.2 years in the 1970s to 2.5 years in the 2000–2003 period

Average time between first and second follow-on drugs fell even more rapidly—from a median of 16.1 years in the 1960s to 1.1 years in 2000–2003

Nearly one-third of all follow-on drugs have received a priority rating from the U.S. Food and Drug Administration (FDA)

Since the early 1990s, 90% of follow-on drugs had initial pharmacologic testing and 87% were in clinical studies somewhere in the world prior to the first-in-class drug approval

Patent filings for follow-on drugs often occur in advance of first-in-class patent filing

Source: Courtesy of Tufts Center for the Study of Drug Development, Impact Report 1(5), Boston, MA, September/October 2009.

TABLE 12.14   Biopharmaceuticals Going Off Patent during 2008–2010

Trade Name	Generic Name	Manufacturer	Expiration Date
Genotropin	Somatropin	Pfizer	2008
NovoSeven	Coagulation factor VIIa	Novo Nordisk	2008/2011
BeneFIX	Coagulation factor IX	Wyeth	2009
Infergen	Interferon alfacon-1	Valeant	2009
Humira	Adalimumab	Abbott	2010

Source: Courtesy of FDA Electronic Orange Book, Silver Spring, MD, http://www.fda.gov/cder/ob

Product Attributes Affect Its Off-Patent Share

A critical issue for the off-patent commercial performance of any given biopharmaceutical product is the retention (or not) of the majority of its on-patent sales, in the face of increasing generic competition on various fronts, for example, price, marketing, and value added. Although it is difficult to predict its off-patent performance, the most dependable method of estimating its share retention is to compare its competitive advantages to those of the emerging competition. In essence, this is similar to predicting its future sales upon its original commercial introduction, based on its unique characteristics versus the competition, as previously discussed earlier in this chapter.

The unique product characteristics of any given biopharmaceutical can be further elaborated in therapeutic class or product related. Let us see what these predictive product attributes may be. We will start with product characteristics or attributes related to the therapeutic class itself. In order to understand the influence of the therapeutic class, let us use a common example from the consumer goods industry. For example, when the moment of buying a new toothbrush comes to us, we may visit a single supermarket, and look for some basic product attributes, that is, the brush hair softness, its shape and color, the handle, and maybe even the price. In the hardest scenario, a 10 min search within a single store should suffice. Let us now jump over to the scenario of buying a new house. In this case, the potential buyer may visit two or three different real estate agent offices; consult with local newspaper classifieds; visit the Internet; conduct surveys among his or her relatives and friends; visit in excess of 80 potential houses; inquire about local schools, sports facilities, shops, and more; bargain for the price; and eventually decide on the house after a 12 month search.

A similar situation applies in the biopharmaceutical marketplace. The more chronic and severe the disease is, the more advanced the stage of the disease is presently, the more complicated the potential side effects and interactions are, and the largest unmet medical needs exist within the given therapeutic category, the hardest it is for a patient on a given branded biopharmaceutical to switch over to a new generic alternative. The same situation applies to the prescriber who is also having significant unsatisfied clinical needs, the regulator who is debating whether to include the new biopharmaceutical into a hospital formulary, the pharmacy benefit management organization that is evaluating the generic product for inclusion into its recommendations, as well as the patient's carers who will be involved in learning to administer and manage the side effects of the new alternative medication.

Now let us focus on the biopharmaceutical product's attributes per se. A significant product price, a narrow therapeutic index (i.e., the distance between its effective and toxic dosage), its degree of reimbursement, its route and frequency of administration, its potential side effects and product interactions, may also play a role in preventing a patient switching to an alternative generic equivalent, when the original product finally loses its patent protection. On the other hand, the generic manufacturer's degree of marketing efforts, or price discounting, or additional value-adding product characteristics would make the product switching easier.

In conclusion, based on both therapeutic class and product characteristics, all branded biopharmaceuticals may be compared and rated versus their emerging generic alternatives, and their eventual off-patent performance can be quite dependably predicted. The eventual off-patent sales forecast will then dictate the originator biopharma's marketing, sales, pricing, and distribution strategy versus the emerging competition. Table 12.15 lists some product and class attributes that are associated with higher post-expiration brand share.

TABLE 12.15 Prescription Retention Attributes Following Patent Expiration

Product Attributes	Class Attributes
Considered as "golden standard"	Disease difficult to titrate
Harder to manufacture	Health professionals specially trained on this class
In-frequent dosing (e.g., twice yearly)	Less subject to managed care control
Innovative (in a class of its own)	Media advocacy
Lacking a follow-on product	Part of a class with less new-brand activity
Less interchangeable with other brands (unique pharmacodynamics and/or pharmacokinetics)	Part of a class with many prior generics
Massive stocks in the marketplace	Patient advocacy
More potential for risk, adverse outcomes	Patient friendliness (e.g., anti-Alzheimer's patches)
Prescribed by few physicians (specialists only)	Significantly increased quality of life
Requires gradual discontinuation	Smaller category size (niche)

Sources: Tuttle, E. et al., Beyond lifecycle management—Optimizing performance following patent expiry. Analysis Group, Boston, MA, July 2004, Posted at: http://www.analysisgroup.com/uploadedFiles/Publishing/Articles/Patent_Expiry.pdf, 2004a; Tuttle, E. et al., Your patent is about to expire: What now?, *Pharmaceutical Executive*, November 2004. With permission.

LIFE CYCLE MANAGEMENT METHODS

Having completed a thorough evaluation of their own biopharmaceutical product's attributes versus those of the generic competition appearing over the horizon, originator biopharma company executives engage in elaborate life cycle management strategies aiming at a single strategy, that is, the prolongation of their product's life cycle, the maximization of its sales turnover and profitability, as well as the hopeful protection of their previous market share via the smooth switching of their prescriber and patient base to an improved, new generation replacement of their own aging and patent-losing original biopharmaceutical.

These strategies are of paramount importance to every single biopharmaceutical in the marketplace, given the following facts: (1) it takes a significant investment and a very long and arduous effort to develop and launch a new biopharmaceutical; (2) several biopharmas are often one-product companies, leading to significant sustainability risks following their product's patent expiration; (3) blockbuster pharmaceuticals have previously faced fierce generic competition leading to a very rapid erosion of their market shares post-patent expiration; and (4) it is more financially sound to launch an improved successor product than create a new molecular entity into a new therapeutic area from the ground up.

Figure 12.2 and Table 12.16 summarize the main PLC management strategies for a biopharmaceutical product.

Branding

We have previously mentioned the increased possibility for significant market share erosion for any biopharmaceutical upon losing its patent protection, due to fierce generic competition. Given this pessimistic possibility, most originator company marketers would be withdrawing most of their product marketing investments just before the loss of patent protection. However, given the therapeutic class, and product attributes mentioned above, it may be wiser to prevent the rapid share erosion by continuing the marketing investments toward the direction of a stronger branding of the product. For example, a branding campaign using the messages "We were the first," "We are the most commonly used," "We have successfully treated 10 million patients in 63 countries," or "Most prescribers recommend our product" may lead to a stronger branding base and longer product sales following its patent expiration.

Reduce Price

As previously mentioned, generic manufacturers may embark on significant price discounting in an attempt to quickly capture market shares away from the branded original biopharmaceuticals. It goes without saying that in price-sensitive markets (see Chapter 10), price discounting may go a long way in capturing market shares. Therefore, a common post-patent expiration strategy for originator biopharmas is to lower their own prices, making it less enticing for price-sensitive prescribers and patients to switch away to a new generic alternative.

This strategy has several consequences, however. First, it sends a negative branding message that the originator product is no better to the emerging generic. Second, it reduces the product's profitability at the end of its life cycle evolution. Third, it may escalate into a price war, with often unpredictable consequences, especially when the generic manufacturer is using lower production sites.

On the other hand, the price discounting may not work in a price-insensitive market (e.g., where the government is offering full reimbursement to this therapeutic class). Nevertheless, when the manufacturing costs of the generic itself are significant enough (see biogenerics in Chapter 13),

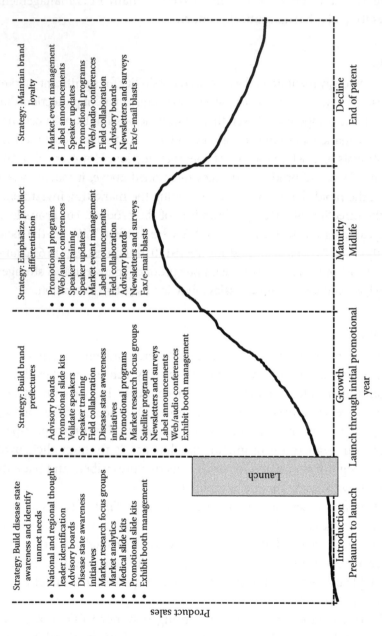

FIGURE 12.2 Successful life cycle management. (Courtesy of Genzyme Corporation, Genzyme Annual Report 2008, Cambridge, MA, 2008, 2009.)

TABLE 12.16   Which Are the Main PLC Management Strategies for a Biopharmaceutical?

	Prelaunch	Early Growth	Late Growth	Patent Expiry
Multiple indications	▓	▓	▓	▓
Multiple patents	▓	▓	▓	█
Market expansion (disease awareness)	▓	▓	▓	▓
Reformulations		▓	▓	▓
Successor products		▓	▓	▓
Repositioning/relaunch			▓	▓
Combination product			▓	▓
OTC/branded generic				▓

Note: Shaded areas indicate applicable areas.

or when the market is still price sensitive, price discounting may significantly delay the market penetration of a new generic.

Trade Relationships

A common practice among originator biopharmas facing the risk of patent expiration is the strengthening and capitalizing on their existing trade relationships, with various stakeholders of their biopharmaceutical supply chain. For example, existing prescribers may be asked to conduct an efficacy and safety "observational study" and present these results in an upcoming scientific publication or training session. Hospital pharmacists may be asked to increase their stock levels, due to an upcoming price increase just before the originator product's price erosion. PBM managers may be offered a significant volume discount, or other healthcare institutions may receive a tender offer too hard to resist. All the above originator biopharma activities are aimed at capitalizing on their existing trade relationships, raising the barriers to entry for their generic competitors, or blocking future potential sales for weeks and months to come following their patent expiration. Attention needs to be given in following all ethical guidelines, and avoiding "unfair competition" claims from the emerging generic competitors.

Provide More Value for the Money

Instead of lowering a biopharmaceutical's price upon patent expiration, originator biopharmas may opt to enhance the value offered by the product to the customer for the same price. For example, a biopharmaceutical may have been available in lyophilized vials for recomposition with a solvent just before its daily administration. Should this medicine become available in prefilled syringes, the added value offered to the patients and their carers may translate into higher market share retention following patent expiration, especially if the new formulation is covered by additional process patents still in effect.

In addition to new and improved formulations, branded biopharmaceuticals may become available with bundled offers and services. For example, every new patient may receive free homecare nursing visits or home delivery of the medication, every prescription refill may be accompanied with free coupons for products and services, while each switching away from the competition may come with free psychotherapy or diagnostic testing. In this way, the biopharmaceutical going off-patent may prolong its life cycle and fend-off generic competition, before the generic manufacturers offer their own value-added services in return.

Product Improvements

Instead of offering additional value-added services, biopharmaceutical manufacturers may opt to offer improved product versions of the biopharmaceutical medicine going off-patent. For example, new and improved formulations may include better-tasting syrups, pills instead of injectables, inhalation means instead of syringes, needle-free children-friendly self-injecting devices, long-acting depot injections, easy-to-apply-and-forget skin patches, and more. Every single product improvement, especially those still protected under additional patents, increase the patient-retention rate and raise further barriers to entry for the generic competitors. Product improvements follow several strategies (see Table 12.17).

TABLE 12.17   What Are the Most Common Biopharmaceutical Product Modification Strategies?

#	Strategy	Example
1	Product modification	A molecular structure change resulting in higher efficacy
2	New therapeutic areas	A new clinical trial indicating its efficacy in a different indication
3	New uses	An antibiotic now available in a pediatric form
4	New dosage strength	A halving of the previous strength allowing individualization
5	New formulation	An injection now available in tablets and nasal spray
6	Relaunch	New promotional drive for maturing product
7	Cost reduction	A temporary rebate or permanent price reduction
8	Rx to OTC switch	Switching to OTC status and selling it through grocery chains

Authorize Own Generic or Defend to the End of the World?

As the patent expiration deadline approaches for a branded biopharmaceutical, generic manufacturers prepare to launch their generic versions, first by copying the published portions of the soon-to-expire patent, second by conducting limited tests indicating the bioequivalence of their generic versions to the original product, and third by preparing to submit an abbreviated new drug application (ANDA) to the relevant regulatory authorities. The overall approach of the originator biopharma can be twofold, each strategy having its own merits. The originator biopharma may opt to defend its intellectual property assets in the relevant Courts, or actually authorize the commercial availability of a generic version of their own biopharmaceutical, even in collaboration with a generic manufacturer. Let us study the two approaches.

In the first strategy, the biopharma may decide to sue the generic manufacturer on various grounds, for example, infringing on additional process patents that may confer additional exclusivity to them, if the generic manufacturer cannot find an alternative way of manufacturing the product, losing its patent protection. This approach obviously delays the commercial availability of a generic, may lead to punitive damages collected from the infringer, and further prolongs the life cycle of the patented biopharmaceutical. The disadvantages to this approach are multiple. For example, the additional patents may not be enforceable on the methods chosen by the generic manufacturer, it costs a significant amount to defend the original patents, and the legal challenge may lead to not only additional expenses but also punitive damages payable to the challenger.

In the opposite strategy, the originator biopharma may even approach the leading generic competitor and offer them a win-win proposition. This approach is often called "flanking" or "authorized generic" approach. In this case, the originator authorizes the generic manufacturer to sell a single generic version of the product, manufactured by the originator, and offered for a commonly agreed manufacturing cost plus royalties to the generic marketer. The second approach often comes as a court resolution to patent infringement suits.

How should a branded manufacturer decide on the alternative strategy depends on the anticipated number of generic manufacturers able and willing to enter the marketplace soon after patent expiration of the original. For example, if competitive intelligence has revealed that there are 15 international manufacturers ready to launch their generics, the originator may opt to offer an authorized generic to a single competitor, in a

TABLE 12.18 How Do You Come Up with a Future Product Portfolio Plan?

	Liquid Cartridge	Multi-Injector Pen	New Refill Cartridge	Oral
Formulation				
Route of administration				
Dosage strengths				
Pack sizes				
Storage conditions				
Shelf life				
Approval date				
FDA				
EMEA				
Japan				
Indication				
Starting dose				
Pricing				

tactic planned to delay the additional fourteen alternatives. If, on the other hand, there are only two competitors ready to launch their versions of the biopharmaceutical, it may be better to defend the original product in the courts, for as long as it takes.

Table 12.18 describes how you come up with a future product portfolio plan.

Is It Time to Divest Our Sacred Biopharmaceutical?

As previously mentioned, a product attribute comparison between the original biopharmaceutical losing off its patent protection and the impending generic alternatives, will often suffice for the originator manufacturer to choose among one of the multiple life cycle management methods following patent expiration. Should the attribute analysis indicate that there are no unique competitive advantages to prevent market share erosion from generic competitors, the originator may opt to completely abandon its product upon patent expiration.

This method is called divesting, and it calls for the abrupt discontinuation of every single sales and marketing effort for the original brand upon its patent expiration. Furthermore, given the predicament that market share erosion will fast ensue from multiple generic alternatives, the originator biopharma may opt to even raise the selling price of its biopharmaceutical, in order to take advantage of the last dying market segment that still prefers the original product over its untested alternatives. The whole strategy leads to a significant loss of market share, loss of profitability, and eventual withdrawal from the marketplace. Table 12.19 presents the various methods by which a biopharma manufacturer can leverage its patents as in the Remicade example presented in Table 12.20.

TABLE 12.19   How Does a Biopharma Manufacturer Leverage Its Patents?

	Strategy	Advantages	Risks and Limitations
Develop	Develop broad patent portfolio	Value protection from substance, method of use, process, and other patents	Should be started in early development stage
Maximize	Obtain orphan drug status	Seven year extension (United States) maximum 10 years (European Union)	Applies only to rare diseases
	Obtain SPC (supplementary certificate)	Maximum 5 year extension in the United States to offset regulatory review delays	Applies only if regulatory delays can be proven
	Pediatric extension	Six month extension in the United States Fairly low cost of new clinicals, low filling costs	Does not apply to all diseases
	Submarine patent	Additional patents for elements of compound not previously covered	Under investigation by regulators
Defend Patents	Bioequivalence defense	Blocks generics due to non-bioequivalence	Applies to new drugs Alienates consumer groups
	Patent infringement defense	"Thirty month stay" in U.S. blocks generic entry during litigation	Litigation is unpredictable Pending legislation to eliminate multiple stays
	Citizen petition with FDA	Questioning safety or bioequivalence of generics can delay their approval	FDA has upheld only 4 of 51 citizen petitions since 1990
	Lobby government for legislation or addition to unrelated bill	May lead to a multiyear extension (to offset delays in approval process)	Increasingly ineffective

TABLE 12.20   Ever-Greening Example: Remicade Development

Phase III	Pediatric Ulcerative Colitis
2006	Chronic severe plaque psoriasis
2006	Psoriatic arthritis structural damage
2005	Ulcerative colitis
2005	Psoriatic arthritis signs and symptoms
2004	Ankylosing spondylitis signs and symptoms
2002	Rheumatoid arthritis physical function (MTX-failures)
2000	Rheumatoid arthritis structural damage (MTX-failures)
1999	Rheumatoid arthritis signs and symptoms (MTX-failures)
1998	Crohn's disease—luminal and fistulising

QUESTIONS

1. What are the characteristics and marketing objectives of the different biopharmaceutical product life cycle stages?
2. Describe the most important unmet clinical need criteria.
3. What are the main prelaunch strategies for a biopharmaceutical product?
4. What are the main requisites for a successful biopharmaceutical launch?
5. How do you create new market space for a biopharmaceutical product?
6. What role do biopharmaceutical product attributes play in affecting its off-patent market share?
7. What are the main biopharmaceutical life cycle management methods?
8. What are the most common biopharmaceutical product-modification strategies?
9. Describe the steps required for an Rx to over-the-counter (OTC) switching in the U.S. market.
10. What are the European Union supplementary protection certificates?

EXERCISES

1. You work in biopharmaceutical business development for a big pharma. A start-up biopharma proposes their lead biopharmaceutical as an in-licensing opportunity to your organization? How would you conduct a feasibility analysis to be presented to your board of directors?
2. Patient organization sites abound with patient testimonials about their treatments. Select any given diagnosis treatable by a commercially

available biopharmaceutical today, and try to design a TPP for the biopharmaceutical's successor molecule.

3. By using public Web sites dedicated to rheumatoid arthritis, can you draw an RA patient flow model?

4. What has happened to marketing exclusivity for first-in-class drugs over the last few years? What are the main reasons for any changes observed?

5. You are the EMEA (Europe, Middle East, and Africa) head for an American biopharma, getting ready to launch your new biopharmaceutical across these markets. How do you prioritize between them, and what company resources do you recommend employing in each subregion?

6. Choose one of the top biopharmaceuticals approved for the treatment of rheumatoid arthritis. By visiting the manufacturers' Web site and also epidemiology databases, try to construct a sales evolution table (patients available, diagnosed, and treated) over the last 5 years.

7. You are a biopharmaceutical consultant writing a report on multiple sclerosis. Name 20 different sources of information for disease treatments and the sales evolution of three treatments since their commercial introduction.

8. You are a biopharma head of R&D. How do you plan your company's R&D program for life cycle management of your diabetes product?

9. You are the marketing head of a biopharma selling a biopharmaceutical used in the treatment of Crohn's disease. Your product requires daily injections and is available in a lyophilized form. What product improvements will you ask your R&D colleagues to come up with? Present some of the actual competitive offerings today.

10. Is your biopharma employer ready to defend its valuable patents expiring soon? What strategies do you employ and what are their advantages and disadvantages?

REFERENCES

Biotechnology Industry Organization, 2008. Biotechnology industry facts. http://www.bio.org/speeches/pubs/er/statistics.asp

Decision Resources, 2002. Market research to drive (and focus) R&D innovation. PBIRG 2002, Workshop 4. PowerPoint presentation posted at: http://www.pbirg.com/new/docs/2002AGM/Interact_wrksp/workshop4.ppt

Dogramatzis, D., 2001. *Pharmaceutical Marketing: A Practical Guide*. Englewood, CO: IHS Health Group.

FDA Electronic Orange Book, Silver Spring, MD, http://www.fda.gov/cder/ob

Genentech, San Francisco, CA, http://www.gene.com

Genzyme Annual Report 2008, Cambridge, MA.

Gibson, M (ed.), 2004. *Pharmaceutical Preformulation and Formulation*. Boca Raton, FL: Interpharm/CRC.

IMS Health, IMS National Sales Perspective, Norwalk, CT, MAT Sep 2009.

INCYTE, 2009. Corporate presentation, *Baird 2009 Health Care Conference*, New York, September 9, 2009. Posted at: http://investor.incyte.com/phoenix. zhtml?c=69764&p=irol-presentations

MERCK, 2002. Guiding compounds through development. Merck, Financing Forum, Whitehouse Station, NJ, May 15, 2002. Posted at: http://www. merck.com

ROCHE Oncology Event, June 19, 2006. Posted at: http://www.roche.com/ irp060619 soriot.pdf

Simon, F. and Kotler, P., 2003. *Building Global Biobrands: Taking Biotechnology to Market*. New York: Free Press, August 12, 2003.

Sucampo Pharmaceuticals Press Release, Bethesda, MD, May 28, 2009, http:// www.sucampo.com

Tufts Center for the Study of Drug Development, 2009. Impact Report 1(5). Tufts University, Boston, MA, September/October 2009.

Tuttle, E., Parece, A., and Hector, A., 2004a. Beyond lifecycle management— Optimizing performance following patent expiry. Analysis Group, Boston, MA, July 2004. Posted at: http://www.analysisgroup.com/uploadedFiles/ Publishing/Articles/Patent_Expiry.pdf

Tuttle, E., Parece, A., and Hector, A., 2004b. Your patent is about to expire: What now? *Pharmaceutical Executive*, November 2004.

VI

Running the Business

## CHAPTER 13

Biobusiness Models

A total of 873 applications have been submitted to date for the designation of orphan medicines. The Committee for Orphan Medicinal Products (COMP) has adopted 598 positive opinions on orphan designation. A total of 569 medicines have been awarded orphan-designation status by the European Commission.

Source: European Medicines Agency's (EMEA) Committee for Orphan Medicinal Products (COMP), November 2008.

E VER SINCE THE DOTCOM era, the meaning of the term "business model" has been brought under the public eye. Today, there exist countless descriptions for what it means, and how important it is after all. But let us go back into the ages, for a moment. Somewhere in the plainfields of today's Silicon Valley, in the south of San Francisco, ancient people would have exchanged their captured (raw meat) and later cultivated goods (starch and corn) as a means of feeding themselves and, much closer to us, doing business. Back then, this basic method of producing something from the land and selling it for a profit would become the very first business model the world had ever known.

As the years progressed, and industrial production caught up with the now revered Silicon Valley, business models started to evolve. For example, aspiring entrepreneurs starting thinking that offering something for sale and waiting for customers to "catch the bait" would not suffice for their business ideas to take off. Instead, somebody must have thought of giving out black and white cameras for free, and expecting the customers to start buying photographic film in order to record their most precious moments. Later, others must have thought of selling color inkjet printers at a loss, and start making profits by selling their color ink refills.

Now wait till you hear about the web business models! How about setting up a web search engine, and making money from sponsored links? Or, what about the idea of comparing net prices and getting paid by the web page clicks you refer to other Web sites? And finally, what about bringing people together looking for auction bargains, and getting paid on a commission basis?

Now, let's fast-forward to the healthcare biotechnology world. Pioneering biopharmas set up their businesses by taking a molecule through clinical trials and finally outsourcing it to a bigger pharma on a royalty basis. Eventually, the most competent biopharmas, went after the traditional pharmaceutical business model, that is building a fully integrated pharmaceutical company (FIPCO) that would commercialize new biopharmaceuticals, manufacture, promote, distribute, and sell them, and so on. In the three decades that ensued since the commercialization of the very first biopharmaceutical, a lot has changed in biotechnology business models, hence the present chapter. In summary, thousands of healthcare biotechnology companies are now involved with only a small corner of the biotech value chain, as we will discuss in the present chapter. Figure 13.1 details several service- or product-based biotechnology business models, while Table 13.1 shows the contribution of either protein or vaccine manufacturers within the global biopharmaceutical market during 2008, as well as the respective market projections for 2013.

Source: Granstrand, O. and Sjölander, S., *Res. Policy*, 19, 35, 1990.

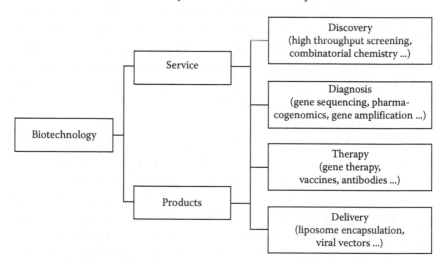

FIGURE 13.1   Biotechnology business models. (Reprinted from Granstrand, O. and Sjölander, S., *Res. Policy*, 19, 35, 1990. With permission from Elsevier.)

TABLE 13.1   Global Biopharmaceutical Market Size
Projections to 2013 (in $ Billion)

	2008	2013
Total pharmaceutical market	625	698
Small molecule	512	533
Proteins	94	138
Vaccines	17	25

Source: Courtesy of Johnson & Johnson, Global biopharmaceutical market size projections to 2013
(in USD billion), in Corporate Presentation,
Pharm Day, 2009, Posted at: http://www.jnj.com.

BLOCKBUSTER MODEL

In studying the biopharmaceutical business models in existence today, one cannot escape analyzing the omnipotent blockbuster model, which was originally implemented by big pharma, until the most prominent biopharmaceuticals reached the same status after years of their own commercial availability. A blockbuster biopharmaceutical product is defined as a product with annual sales of at least $1 billion, or $5 billions in 5 years postlaunch. Furthermore, the mega blockbuster status (annual sales of at least $10 billion) awaits the most successful biopharmaceutical brands, trying to catch up with their pharmaceutical equivalents, such as the likes of Prozac, Zyprexa, or Lipitor before them.

It has been estimated that approximately 80% of growth of the pharma industry came from almost 8 drugs in the last 10 years. Some of the most critical factors behind blockbuster success are: (1) therapeutic areas with large patient population; (2) significant unmet medical needs; (3) chronic and severe diseases; (4) significant competitive advantages versus the previous "gold standard" in either efficacy, safety, or added value; (5) premium pricing; (6) global regulatory submissions; and (7) global promotional campaigns. In addition, (8) healthcare education and information globalization; (9) increasing penetration of the Internet; (10) large marketing budgets; (11) increasing influence of patent protection treaties; (12) significant patient pull toward stronger biopharmaceutical brands; (13) strong life cycle management by the manufacturers of blockbusters; and (14) frequent collaboration of two mega organizations in copromoting a single blockbuster.

By the way, how does a blockbuster reach high profitability even in the face of promotional mega campaigns? Let us hypothesize that a single blockbuster is being promoted in the U.S. market alone. It has probably cost $800 million to develop, and $300 million to launch. It has a 10%

cost of goods, and is being promoted by a $200 million campaign and 5000 sales reps costing their employer (including healthcare, mileage, and meal expenses) $200,000 each. The annual blockbuster profit and loss (P&L) statement would look like this:

Annual sales	$3,000,000,000
COGS	$300,000,000
Marketing	$200,000,000
Sales	$1,000,000,000
Gross profit	$1,500,000,000

or easily surpassing its complete R&D budget and still leaving a hefty profit.

Nevertheless, as we have previously discussed in Chapter 6 and will further analyze in the final chapter, significant risks await even the most successful blockbuster, due to previously unforeseen side effects or manufacturing and other mishappenings, that make the predicament of sustaining an entire biopharma organization on a single blockbuster, a disaster waiting to happen. In addition to the risks involved, the blockbuster model has been associated with these disadvantages: (1) severe loss of market share and volume and value sales due to generic competition, upon patent expiration; (2) organizational inability to easily produce successful successor products to blockbusters with expiring patents; (3) organizational resistance in shifting R&D focus away from the blockbuster therapeutic area; (4) significant dependence of the biopharma's share price on the fate of its blockbuster sales; and (5) inability of national healthcare systems to support more than one blockbusters' products in any single therapeutic area at the same time.

The consequences of these blockbuster-associated risks are easily observed in the strategies undertaken by several major biopharma organizations. For example, one can observe: (1) choosing an alternative business model (see below), (2) focusing research on various therapeutic areas at a time, (3) supplementing existing blockbusters with smaller in-licensing opportunities, (4) further developing each blockbuster into additional therapeutic areas postlaunch, and (5) staying competitive and agile, unlike the severely hierarchical and bureaucratic big pharma organizations.

According to IMS Health (http://www.imshealth.com), in 2007, there were a total of 106 global pharmaceutical blockbusters, of which 22 were biotechnology blockbusters. The top-selling biologics are listed in the order of decreasing annual sales in Table 13.2. Furthermore, as Table 13.3

TABLE 13.2   Which Were the Top-Selling Biologics in 2007–2008?

Product Name	Type	First FDA Approval	First Full-Year Sales (in $) (M) (Year)	2008 Sales (in $) (M)	2007 Sales (in $) (M)
Enbrel	Recombinant fusion protein; soluble TNF receptor linked to IgG1	11/98	367 (1999)	6191	5275
Remicade	Chimeric monoclonal antibody; anti-TNF-alpha	8/98	124 (1999)	5866	4975
Rituxan/ MabThera	Chimeric monoclonal antibody; anti-CD20	11/97	163 (1998)	5536	4869
Avastin	Humanized antibody to vascular endothelial growth factor (VEGF)	2/04	1264 (2005)	4866	3624
Herceptin	Humanized monoclonal antibody; anti-HER-2	9/98	188 (1999)	4759	4282
Humira	Fully human monoclonal antibody to TNF-alpha	12/02	280 (2003)	4521	3064
Gleevec	Small molecule signal transduction inhibitor	5/01	615 (2002)	3670	3050
Neulasta	Pegylated version of Neupogen	01/02	1300 (2003)	3318	3000
Aranesp	Novel erythropoiesis-stimulating protein (second-generation EPO)	9/01	416 (2002)	3137	3614
Procrit	Recombinant erythropoietin	12/90	N/A	2460	2885

Source: Courtesy of IMS Health, Norwalk, CT, http://www.imshealth.com

TABLE 13.3   Billion Dollar Club (in U.S.$)

# of Companies	2001	2002	2003	2004	2005	2006	2007	2008
<99 million	112	162	82	92	104	91	91	184
100–249 million	90	66	85	100	104	101	103	59
250–499 million	60	46	68	70	54	65	66	38
500–999 million	36	19	32	47	46	44	45	26
>1 billion	58	36	48	51	55	49	60	49

Source: Burrill, G.S., Biochemistry 241y, Winter 2010, January 4 to March 15, Mondays, 4:00–6:00 pm, Genentech Hall, N 106, Mission Bay Campus, UCSF, 2010, Posted at: cbe.ucsf.edu/cbe/9212-DSY/version/default/part/AttachmentData/data. With permission.

indicates, in 2008, there were 49 biopharmaceutical companies reaching more than $1 billion in annual sales (Burrill & Company, 2009).

ORPHAN DRUG MODEL

Orphan Drugs in the United States

We have just discussed the frequent predisposition of both big pharma and biopharma organizations with the development and marketing of the next blockbuster product, one enjoying a large patient base and global campaigns. What happens, though, with the tens of thousands of other diseases that would not enjoy such epidemiological characteristics? The answer is simple: lack of investment, lack of research, no new commercial product launches, huge unmet needs, and poor quality of life for all their sufferers and their families.

In order to combat the significant research absence in rare diseases, the U.S. Orphan Drug Act (ODA) was designed to offer incentives to those organizations investing into the field in the form of financial incentives for research, and also a market exclusivity (monopoly) for a set period of time, significant enough for the organizations to recuperate their initial investments. First, orphan diseases had to be defined as those that affect less than 200,000 Americans at any given time (prevalence). The prevalence ceiling led to the identification of approximately 7000 rare diseases in the United States and more than 25 million sufferers from them.

The basic incentives offered by ODA were (1) research grants from various state sources, such as those coming from the National Institutes of Health (NIH); (2) tax incentives on R&D-related expenses; (3) eligibility for expedited regulatory approval; and, most importantly, (4) a 7 year market exclusivity period following the commercial launch of a new product. The U.S. FDA is quoting on its Web site a Tufts Center for the Study of Drug Development (CSDD) study (2010), according to which since the ODA of 1983 was signed into law in the United States, more than 2000 products in development have been designated as orphan drugs, while FDA has granted market approval to 350 drugs and biologicals.

Orphan Drugs in the European Union

The rare diseases regulatory framework in the European Union is similar in nature to that in the United States. According to the European Medicines Evaluation Agency, rare diseases are life-threatening or chronically debilitating conditions affecting no more than five in 10,000 EU citizens, which translates to approximately 246,000 sufferers from a single rare disease in the EU 27 Member States. It is estimated that between 5000 and 8000 distinct rare diseases exist today, affecting between 6% and 8% of the population in total—in other words, between 27 million and 36 million people in the European Union (EMEA, 2007).

The European regulatory authorities inform interested parties that the EU orphan-drug designation criteria are the following:

- RARITY (prevalence)/RETURN ON INVESTMENT: Medical condition affecting not more than 5 in 10,000 persons in the community. Without incentives, it is unlikely that the marketing of the product would generate sufficient return to justify the necessary investment.

- SERIOUSNESS: Life threatening or chronically debilitating.

- ALTERNATIVE TREATMENTS AUTHORIZED: If satisfactory method exists, the sponsor should establish that the product will be of significant benefit.

The incentives for orphan drug research in the EU include the following: Economic/marketing: Fee reduction/exemption, extended incentives for SMEs (post authorization), and market exclusivity; product development: protocol assistance; community marketing authorization; and national incentives (EC inventory). Table 13.4 lists some of the EMEA-authorized orphan-designated medicines per therapeutic area, approved by November 2008.

As far as medicinal products for human use are concerned, the procedure is free of charge, it can be requested at any stage of development, the sponsor can be either company or individual—established in the community (EU, Iceland, Liechnestein, Norway), and a European Commission Decision gives access to incentives. The ways to obtain orphan designation are the following: (1) application submitted either by companies or individuals (sponsors); (2) established in the EU; (3) application form; (4) description of the condition; (5) description of the medicinal product, prevalence calculation of the condition, justification of severity; and (6) justification of "significant benefit" (when applicable), and description of product development (current and future).

TABLE 13.4   List of EMEA-Authorized Orphan-Designated Medicines per Therapeutic Area

Year	Oncology	Endocrinology/ Metabolism	Hematology	Cardiovascular and Respiratory	Nervous System	Other
2008	Ceplene		Thalidomide	Volibris		Firazyr
2007	Atriance, Gliolan, Yondelis, Torisel	Elaprase Cystadane	Revlimid Soliris		Diacomit Inovelon	
2006	Evoltra, Sutent, Nexavar, Sprycel	Naglazyme Myozyme	Exjade	Thelin		Savene
2005		Orfadin		Revatio	Prialt Xyrem	
2004	Photobarr, Litak, Lysodren	Wilzin	Xagrid	Pedea		
2003	Onsenal	Carbaglu Aldurazyme	Busilvex	Ventavis		

Source: European Medicines Agency's (EMEA), Committee for Orphan Medicinal Products (COMP). Orphan medicines in numbers—The Success of ten years of orphan legislation, Press Release, 3 May 2010. Posted at: http://www.ema.europa.eu/docs/en_GB/document_library/Report/2010/05/WC500090812.pdf

Orphan Drug Example: Yondelis (PHARMA MAR)

Yondelis® (trabectedin) is an antitumor agent of marine origin discovered in the colonial tunicate Ecteinascidia turbinata. It is currently produced by chemical synthesis. Yondelis® has a unique action mechanism. It binds to the minor groove of the DNA and interferes with cell division and the gene transcription processes and repair machinery of the DNA. In September 2007, it received marketing authorisation from the European Commission for the treatment of advanced or metastatic soft tissue sarcoma. In 2008, it was announced the submission of a registration dossier to the European Medicines Agency (EMEA) and Federal Drugs Administration (FDA) for Yondelis® when administered in combination with DOXIL®/Caelyx® (pegylated liposomal doxorubicin) for the treatment of women with relapsed ovarian cancer (ROC). Yondelis® has been designated an orphan drug by the European Commission (EC) and the U.S. Food and

Drug Administration (FDA) for soft tissue sarcoma and ovarian cancer. PharmaMar markets Yondelis® in Europe and Japan and Ortho Biotech Products, L.P. does so in the United States and the rest of the world. Phase II trials with Yondelis® are also being carried out for breast cancer, lung cancer and prostate cancer and for paediatric tumours.

Source: Courtesy of PHARMA MAR, Madrid, Spain, http:// www.pharmamar.com/company.aspx

Orphan Drugs in Japan

Orphan drugs in Japan were first approved in 1993, and until the writing of this book, there have been close to 200 product approvals. The orphan designation criteria are along the lines of the U.S. and EU framework, (1) disease sufferers must be less than 50,000 Japanese citizens: (2) there should not be an identical product approved in the marketplace, otherwise the new product should be a significant improvement over the existing treatment; and (3) the biopharma developer should have a sound clinical development program based on a peer-reviewed scientific and medical rationale.

The incentives offered by the Japanese authorities to the orphan drug developers are (1) removal of the applicable regulatory fees, (2) access to financial aid for the clinical trials conducted, and above all, (3) a significant market exclusivity period spanning 10 years. Table 13.5 summarizes some of the national orphan drug regulations existing in various pharmaceutical markets.

TABLE 13.5   National Orphan Drug Regulations

	EU	United States	Japan
Year	2000	1983	1993
Prevalence per 10,000	<5	<7.5	<4.2
Protocol assistance	80% reduction	Yes	Yes
Fees waiver	50% reduction	Yes	C35% reduction
Market exclusivity	10	7	10
Research grant	No	Yes	Max 50% p.a.
Tax credit	Up to member state	50%	% varies

VIRTUALLY INTEGRATED MODEL

As the healthcare biotechnology environment turned 30-something, and countless entrepreneurs left the safety of academic research on the way to biopharmaceutical success, fame, and fortune, so the industry providers grew in sophistication, size, and services offered to cover the entrepreneurial needs. Simultaneously, the collective experience of healthcare biotechnology executives grew significantly; new scientific tools have offered the uncontested benefits of R&D automation, while previously skeptic investors went on an all-out war of identifying, investing in, and securing the rights to the next best things emerging from the industry. These powerful winds of change have brought about the advent of the first healthcare biotechnology virtual firms, a term originally belonging to Internet dotcoms that rose and fell by the thousands.

In summary, a biotechnology virtual firm has compartmentalized the entire value chain of biotechnology research, development and commercialization, allocating responsibility on these multiple compartments to different provider firms with respective expertise. Above all these external collaborators, a core team of experienced industry executives has maintained ultimate supervisory and coordinating responsibility, mimicking the art of puppeteers in directing their creations into fully blown lively characters in the minds and hearts of their young audiences.

In other words, preclinical research has been outsourced to a research organization, clinical research has been assigned to an experienced contract research organization, manufacturing is being provided by a contract biomanufacturer, regulatory submissions are being submitted by external experts, while sales and marketing is done by a contract sales organization. What remains is a board of directors who, together with a lean team of experts, directs the different dominoes into a coherent, value-adding healthcare biotechnology organization. Progressively, as the first outcomes of this virtual strategy are being validated, approved, and commercialized, the virtual biopharma may decide to start internalizing select segments of the value chain, on the way to a full-fledged FIPCO we have discussed earlier in this chapter. Table 13.6 summarizes the advantages and disadvantages of virtual companies.

For a virtually integrated company example see: BioGenerix, Company profile, BIOGENERIX, Mannheim, Germany, 2010, Posted at: http://www.biogenerix.com/index1.html

TABLE 13.6   What Are the Advantages and Disadvantages of Virtual Companies?

Advantages	Disadvantages
Management focuses on business development	Management overload
Flexibility and speed	Pressure on decision making
Outsource best quality specialist support	High cost of contractors and need good support
Lower fixed costs	Ownership of IP
Builds strong small team with ownership with sense of mission	Possible confidentiality issues
Perceived as "small"	Less scope to develop new IP

DRUG DEVELOPMENT COMPANY MODEL

We have now briefly studied the two extremes of the healthcare biotechnology business model continuum, namely, the FIPCO focusing on blockbuster development, versus the leanest virtual organization possible. In between these two extremes, however, there are thousands of biotechnology organizations that are focusing on distinct components of the value chain, with varying degrees of integration, and even more varying degrees of commercial success and long-term sustainability. The organizations found in the middle of the continuum are collectively called drug development companies, or DEVCOs for short. Numerous attempts have been made in categorizing these widely diverse business models into distinct categories. For example, Reponen (2002) has identified three new major business models: (1) platform or tool business model, (2) product business model, and (3) hybrid business model.

DEVCOs are specializing in upstream early discovery and research around structural genomics to proteomics; most of them never taking their discoveries past the first-in-man clinical trial milestone. According to Sabatier et al. (2009), DEVCOs tend to be specialists in various processes along the "gene-to-drug (g-2-d) pathway," ranging from experts in structural genomics applications (content providers) and companies that determine gene function, genetic variability single nucleic polymorphisms (SNPs) and epigenomics, to companies that specialize in validation, lead generation, and final clinical product development.

For a DEVCO example see: deCODEs Corporate Profile, Reykjavik, Iceland, http://www.decodecom/

TECPROs

Among the DEVCOs we have just mentioned, countless healthcare organizations specialize on any given preclinical research technological platform, and offer their invaluable services to either FIPCOs or virtual organizations who are lacking this specific field of ultrasophisticated technological expertise. These specialized providers are said to be focusing on specific platform technologies, thus called TECPROs. For example, these organizations may be focusing on gene sequencing, high-throughput screening, informatics, microassays, or reagents. Taken together, they have added a significant new level of sophistication, expertise, speed, and know-how to the know-how available in-house by larger biopharma organizations, and have assisted many of the latter in closing critical freedom-to-operate gaps, resource and facility constraints, or just time limitations on their way to successful biopharmaceutical commercializations. The modern healthcare biotechnology industry would not have been the same without the voluminous assistance of specialized TECPROs along the R&D pathway. But let us study some of these game-changing, revolutionary platform technologies that have changed biotech forever.

Platform Technologies

The access to platform technologies is of paramount importance to any healthcare biotechnology today. In fact, the number of different technologies existing in-house is one of the most important benchmarks determining the degree of R&D know-how that a biopharma possesses in-house. Let us name a few: rational drug design, where a genetically synthesized antibody is designed to fit a biological receptor; automated peptide and nucleic acid analysis (introduced by B. Merrifield in 1964); combinatorial chemistry (introduced by R. Houghten in 1985), where millions of peptides are synthesized to be tested for biologic activity; polymerase chain reaction (introduced by K. Mullis in 1983), where minute samples of DNA can be multiplied millions of times making their characterization easier; gene sequencing, where millions of bases can be identified within a short period of time; and computer automation, where laboratory functions are being monitored and analyzed by sophisticated hardware and software.

Bioinformatics Companies

The word bioinformatics describes the application of information technology into molecular biology. Imagine, comparing the billions of nucleic acid bases existing within specific species with each other for identifying evolutional coherence. Or imagine comparing DNA samples taken from thousands of rare disease sufferers for locating SNPs. Finally, imagine combing through the medical archives of millions of patients suffering from a single disease and comparing their long-term therapy outcomes to various modalities of treatments. These examples underscore the power of bioinformatics and the increasing role they may be playing in health and disease in the near future.

Subscription Companies and Other Models

Subscription companies create genomic databases of millions of patients suffering from the same diseases or a single remote geographic location, and then making these results available to interested biopharmaceutical organizations looking for R&D clues in their battle with chronic and severe diseases, for a subscription fee. Examples include Human Genome Sciences and Millenium Pharmaceuticals. Chemistry services companies are involved in made-to-order chemical synthesis, for example, a biopharma asking for their expertise in building a better monoclonal antibody, or an enzyme-resistant biomolecule, or a long-acting molecular side chain. Examples include Tripos and Synexis Chemistry and Automation.

In addition, smart screening companies develop proprietary animal models to biopharmas. Imagine, for example, a biopharma acquiring exclusive patent rights to a biomolecule originating from an academic technology transfer office (TTO) and with potential effects on Parkinson's disease, for which both a small and a large animal Parkinson's disease model are needed. Examples include EnVivo. Other companies may be selling tools as product, instead of proprietary services, for example, producing and selling DNA chips such as Affymetrix. And the list of specialized providers keeps growing, such as specialized clinical supply biomanufacturers, formulation companies, injection device companies, skin patch designers, and more.

PHARMACOGENOMICS (PGX) MODEL

We have just described the importance of studying genomic polymorphisms in attempting to identify the molecular basis of a disease. A similar approach would be to collect vast amounts of patient genomic data and then attempt to correlate those, not with their predisposition to a disease, but to their response to specific therapeutic modalities. Let us think of a colorful example. Before selling a brand new automotive, car companies design them with computer-aided design and then construct life-sized models that are purposedly smashed on walls in a detailed study of their safety standard. Now how about doing the same with patients (without the smashing part), that is, how about studying the pharmacokinetic (PK) and pharmacodynamic (PD) reactions of millions of patients to a given therapy, and later picking and choosing the right medication, route of administration, dosage, and formulation for patients exhibiting the optimally responding genotype?

According to Ahn (2007), such an approach could potentially have a revolutionary effect on therapeutics. For example, it would optimize the drug used, it would decrease disease relapses and hospitalizations, it would increase patient compliance and quality of life, it would minimize side effects and drug interactions, and so on. The combined study of patient genomics and their reactions to therapy has thus been called pharmacogenomics, and is meant to have a tremendous rise in R&D in the near future. Table 13.7 lists some of the main functions of proteins in the body.

FDA's Critical Path Initiative

In 2004, the U.S. FDA launched the Critical Path Initiative with the release of report *Innovation/Stagnation: Challenge and Opportunity on the Critical Path to New Medical Products* (http://www.fda.gov/oc/initiatives/criticalpath/whitepaper.pdf). According to the Personalized Medicine Coalition (Ahn, 2007), the report indicated concern on the rising difficulty and unpredictability of drug development and called for a concerted effort to modernize the scientific tools and exploit the potential of bioinformatics for the evaluation and prediction of safety, effectiveness, and manufacturability of candidate drugs.

TABLE 13.7   Protein Functions (Potential Products and Targets)

Structure	Muscle, bone, epithelium, endothelium, nerves, hair, cells
Communication/ mediation—intercellular	Hormones, stimulating factors, interleukins, interferons, receptors
Functional	Catalysis (enzymes), blood clotting glucose processing
Immune defense/reactions	Identification, recognition, tagging, adhesion
Cell function	Signaling, chaperones, degradation, differentiation, reproduction, energy production, death

PGx Example:

> Roche AmpliChip Cytochrome P450 Genotyping test and Affymetrix GeneChip Microarray Instrumentation System—K042259
>
> Product Name: Roche AmpliChip Cytochrome P450 Genotyping test and Affymetrix GeneChip Microarray Instrumentation System
>
> Manufacturer: Roche Molecular Systems, Inc. and Affymetrix, Inc.
>
> Address: 4300 Hacienda Dr., Pleasanton, CA 94588 and 3380 Central Expy., Santa Clara, CA 95051
>
> Clearance Date: December 23, 2004
>
> Clearance Letter: http://www.accessdata.fda.gov/cdrh_docs/pdf4/k042259.pdf
>
> What is it? The Roche AmpliChip Cytochrome P450 Genotyping test for use on the Affymetrix GeneChip Microarray Instrumentation System is a new laboratory test system that will help doctors personalize treatment options for their patients. Doctors can use a patient's genetic information to help them determine appropriate drugs and doses to prescribe. This will help minimize harmful drug reactions and prevent patients from being improperly treated with sub-optimal doses.
>
> This system uses DNA extracted from a patient's blood to detect certain common genetic mutations that alter the body's ability to break down (metabolize) specific types of drugs. The enzyme produced from the gene that is tested, called cytochrome P4502D6 (CYP4502D6), is active in metabolizing many types of drugs including antidepressants, antipsychotics, beta-blockers, and some chemotherapy drugs. Variations in this gene can cause a patient to metabolize these drugs abnormally fast, abnormally slow, or not at all. For example, the same dose that is safe for a patient with one variation might be too high (and therefore toxic) to a patient with a different variation who cannot metabolize the drug.
>
> With genetic information for this gene, many harmful reactions resulting from inappropriate dosing and treatment may be significantly reduced as clinicians can adjust the patient's regimen accordingly.
>
> How does it work? A doctor orders the genetic test in patients to gather information on the predicted metabolic activity of their enzyme encoded by CYP4502D6.
>
> A sample of blood is collected and taken to the lab.

The lab extracts DNA from the blood sample.

The lab processes and applies the DNA to the Cytochrome P450 Genotyping test.

The GeneChip Microarray Instrumentation System reads the test.

The genetic result for the Cytochrome P450 Genotyping test is sent to the doctor.

The doctor uses the Cytochrome P450 genetic test results, clinical evaluation and other lab tests as an aid in individualizing patient treatment options.

Sources: U.S. Food and Drug Administration (FDA), Silver Spring, MD, Posted at: http://www.fda.gov/MedicalDevices/Productsand MedicalProcedures/DeviceApprovalsandClearances/Recently-ApprovedDevices/ucm078879.htm (accessed on July 19, 2010).

Ahn, C., *Genomics Inform.*, 5(2), 41, June 2007. With permission.

MOLECULAR DIAGNOSTICS IN NUMBERS

According to a report by DATAMONITOR (Ref. DMHC 2430, November 2008) the global molecular diagnostics market was valued at over USD 2.6 billion, comprising about 7% of the total in vitro diagnostics (IVD) market, and predicted to grow by an estimated CAGR of 14% by 2013. Furthermore, CLINICAL DATA reported in their 2009 Annual Report (CLINICAL DATA INC FORM 10-K, Filed 06/15/09 for the Period Ending 03/31/09) that there were more than 900 labs worldwide performing laboratory-developed assays, with more than 90% of them located in the US, Europe, and Japan. Figure 13.2 describes the in vitro diagnostics market.

Source: Courtesy of William Blair & Company, Chicago, IL, in Burrill & Company, *Biotech 2009—Life Sciences: Navigating the Sea of Change*, Burrill & Co, San Francisco, CA, 2009.

PERSONALIZED MEDICINE MODEL

As discussed above, pharmacogenomics promises to eventually develop more effective and safer medicines by administering the right biopharmaceutical, to the right patient, at the right dosage, with the right route

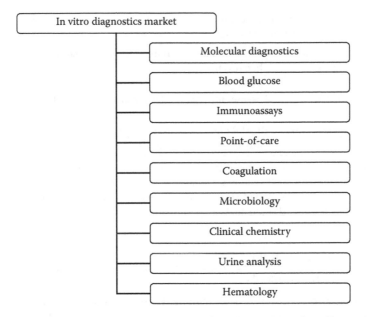

FIGURE 13.2 The in vitro diagnostics market. (Courtesy of William Blair & Company, Chicago, IL, in Burrill & Company, *Biotech 2009—Life Sciences: Navigating the Sea of Change*, Burrill & Co, San Francisco, CA, 2009. With permission.)

of administration, and for the right duration of treatment. According to Hu (2005), pharmacogenomic technologies could deliver additional value by enhancing biopharma R&D productivity by (1) producing higher quality targets, (2) providing early target screening and validation approaches, (3) enabling faster lead validation and preclinical studies, (4) filtering out nonoptimal candidates early via toxicology screening, and (5) resulting in more efficient clinical development programs. Some of the best known targeted treatments include Gleevec (Novartis)—pH + CML kinase inhibitor, Iressa (AstraZeneca)—EGFR tyrosine kinase inhibitor, Tarceva (Genentech/OSI)—HER1/EGFR inhibitor, and Favrille—and Genitope—MyVax for non-Hodgkin's lymphoma.

Some of the potential benefits of pharmacogenomics and personalized medicine often cited include more powerful, safer drugs and vaccines, improvement of drug discovery and approval, and decrease in overall healthcare cost. Table 13.8 presents an analysis of the molecular profiles of body functions in health and disease.

TABLE 13.8   Analyzing the Molecular Profiles (Biosignatures) of Body Functions in Health and Disease

The molecular basis of biological processes	The molecular heterogeneity of disease	Individual genetic variation	
Alterations in disease	Disease subtypes	Pharmacogenetics	Disease predisposition
New targets for Dx, Rx, Vx	Right Rx for disease	New targets for Dx, Rx, V	PDx PRx

Source: Burrill, G.S., Biochemistry 241y, Winter 2010, January 4 to March 15, Mondays, 4:00–6:00 pm, Genentech Hall, N 106, Mission Bay Campus, UCSF, 2010, Posted at: cbe.ucsf.edu/cbe/9212-DSY/version/default/part/AttachmentData/data. With permission.

BIOSIMILARS MODEL
Generic Pharmaceuticals

As discussed in Chapter 2, a pharmaceutical patent confers upon its holders the legal monopoly to manufacture, promote, sell, and distribute their product for a given period of time, usually 20 years from filing that patent. During this period, the pharmaceutical manufacturer enjoys a period of commercial monopoly and is free to price and sell its product at such a price that is sufficient to cover all its fixed and variable costs during its commercial phase, as well as the total costs incurred during its long R&D phase (that take an average of 10 years out of the 20 years under patent protection). In fact, due to the lack of similar competition, the price can come at a premium that the manufacturer expects to bring its forecasted profitability.

Later, upon patent expiration, additional manufacturers are free to manufacture the same molecule, by using the same manufacturing methods, and soon launch their own commercial versions of the molecule at a fraction of the R&D and regulatory costs the originator company had to incur. The limited costs incurred by the so-called generic manufacturers of pharmaceuticals are due to the available legislation (see Chapter 12) that gives them the right to avoid the costly preclinical and clinical trials needed for the original, provided that they can only prove a bio-equivalence of their own version with the original medicine.

Based on the fact that the vast R&D and regulatory costs have been already avoided, and that a cheap manufacturing method exists that leads to a fairly negligible cost-of-goods (less than 5% for a chemical drug, and around 10% for a mainstay biopharmaceutical), the generic manufacturers can in turn offer really competitive product prices that quickly capture significant market shares from the original product, especially in price-sensitive, partially reimbursed therapeutic area markets. But generic strategies do not stop there. By avoiding investing in significant innovative therapies, that is, instead of becoming an innovation leader, they opt to become the therapeutic area price leaders, by limiting their expenses across every single component of the pharmaceutical value chain, for example, development, manufacturing, distribution, and marketing. The final outcome is a large plethora of generic alternatives with significantly lower prices compared with the previously patented original, leading to a newly competitive, off-patent and freemarket competitive landscape.

Biogenerics, Biosimilars, or Follow-On Biologics

Although generic equivalents of chemical medicines have been around for decades, the situation has not been the same for commercially available generic copies of biopharmaceuticals. This is historically due to the fact that the first biopharmaceutical was launched back in 1982, and given the long patent protection, the additional patents that might have prevented generic competition immediately following its patent expiration, as well as the lack of a previously existing common regulatory path for the approval of generic equivalents of biopharmaceutical medicines have not allowed the availability of such generics in various markets until today.

As we will further discuss below, this situation is soon about to change. The drivers behind such a change are the following: (1) a significant number of patented biopharmaceuticals will soon lose their patent protection in the next 5 years, (2) the EU and Japan have already approved regulatory pathways for generic alternatives of off-patent biopharmaceuticals, while the United States is slowly following in their footsteps, and (3) healthcare systems around the world are focusing on significant cost reductions under the burden of rising costs and median life expectancies, and (4) the annual treatment costs of many patented biopharmaceuticals are significant, showing the way for their generic equivalents as soon as this becomes a regulatory possibility.

Before we embark on the study of the emerging field of generic alternatives of biopharmaceuticals, we should raise our attention to the fact that exact bioequivalent products of biopharmaceuticals (completely down to stereochemical molecular structure, PK, and PD effects) are difficult to produce, leading to a contested nomenclature for these products around

TABLE 13.9   Small Molecule Generics versus Biosimilars

	Small Molecule Generics	Biosimilars
Product characteristics	Small molecules	Large, complex molecules
	Often very stable	Stability requires special handling
	Mostly without a device	
		Device is often a key differentiator
Production	Produced by chemical synthesis	Produced in living organisms
		Highly sensitive to manufacturing changes
		Often comparatively high costs
Development	Very limited clinical trials (often only Phase I PK/PD studies)	Significant R&D (i.e., cell lines)
		Extensive clinical trials, including Phase I and Phase III studies
Regulation	Abbreviated registration procedures in Europe and the United States	Regulatory pathway now defined by EMEA
	Usually enjoy "substitutability" status	"Comparability" status
		No pathway yet in the United States under BLA
Marketing	No or limited detailing to physicians	Detailing to (specialist) physicians required
	Key role of wholesalers and payers	Pharmacists may not substitute
	Market substitution in pharmacies	
	High price discounts	Price discounts smaller; price sensitivity is product specific

Source: Courtesy of (SANDOZ), Small molecule generics versus biosimilars, Holzkirchen, Germany, Posted at: http://www.sandoz.com/site/en/product_range/more_about_biosimilars/index.shtml, 2010.

the world, where they have been called biogenerics, biosimilars, or "follow-on" biologicals. Overall, there are significant differences observed between traditional small molecule generics and biosimilars, as summarized in Table 13.9.

For a biosimilar product example see: EPO-ZETA (STADA), STADA Corporate Presentation, Bad Vilbel, Germany, October 2009, http://www.stada.de/english/investorrelations/presentations/

THE GENERIC DRUG APPROVAL PROCESS

The Drug Price Competition and Patent Term Restoration Act in the United States

We will start our analysis of the generics and biogenerics regulation from the U.S. market. It would be an understatement to declare that it has been an epic battle between the interests of originator (commonly called "ethical research" manufacturers) and their generic manufacturer opponents over the years. On the one hand of the battleplace, ethical manufacturers used to argue that (1) generics could not use the original research findings in coming up with their copies bypassing R&D, (2) generics should start their full R&D efforts following the expiration of the original patent, (3) generics would inhibit original research and innovation from ethical manufacturers, (4) the usual patent-protection period was too short for ethical manufacturers to recuperate their R&D investment, and that (5) cheaper generic alternatives would not produce significant savings for healthcare systems and patients alike.

On the other hand of the spectrum, generic manufacturers argued that (1) generic pharmaceuticals are safe, effective, and significantly cheaper; (2) generic development should not have to repeat the exact clinical trial program taken by the innovators, due to an unnecessary waste of resources; (3) generic development should begin even before patent expiration of the original, while approval could happen immediately after the patent expiration; and (4) the ethical manufacturer's profits far surpassed the resources spent for drug development.

The defining moment for this fierce debate was the approval of the *The Drug Price Competition and Patent Term Restoration Act of 1984*, commonly known as the *Hatch–Waxman Act* (1984), which was enacted to facilitate faster introduction of generic drugs. The Act achieved the following: (1) it gave ethical manufacturers a longer patent life; (2) it gave generic manufacturers a right to initiate their development efforts before the patent expiration of the original, a shortened pathway for regulatory approval, protection from patent infringement suits from ethical manufacturers, and a pathway for challenging the original pharmaceutical's patent validity and enforceability; and (3) it gave the U.S. society generic pharmaceuticals at a reduced cost and, therefore, price, insurance providers cheaper therapeutic alternatives, and uninsured patients access to cheaper medicines.

Nevertheless, we still have not addressed the issue of launching a generic medicine only because it had a similar molecular structure to that of the patented medicine. This was addressed by making all generics undergo a standardized, short, and economical bioequivalence testing, for example studying the drug's PK profile in 30–40 healthy volunteers and comparing these findings with those provided by the original medicine (Bhat, 2005). One important point: the Act did not apply to antibiotics and biopharmaceuticals.

Abbreviated NDA (ANDA)

As discussed above, the Hatch–Waxman Act of 1984 provided to all generic medicines a new, shorter, more economical, and standardized method of applying for regulatory approval, as described in Figure 13.3. This new pathway avoided the repetition of phase I–III clinical trials by the generic manufacturer, only requiring short PK and PD studies proving equivalence to the original medicine. In exchange, it gave the originator companies a prolonged market exclusivity period, to take into account the long R&D phases that would previously consume a significant portion of the overall patent protection period of 20 years. Figure 13.3 describes the abridged new drug application (ANDA) in the United States.

The FDA's Orange Book

Since the Hatch–Waxman Act required the generic manufacturer to maintain its part in the abbreviated approval procedure, while respecting the rights of the ethical manufacturer, all sides of the regulatory divide (ethical and generic) were either required to list their proprietary patents in an FDA-regulated database—the so-called Orange Book—or to describe how they planned to challenge the original medicine's patent protection with a new generic. In other words, for a new generic to be approved, its

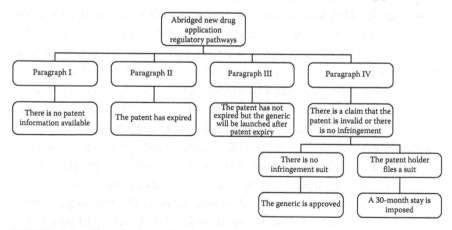

FIGURE 13.3 The ANDA in the United States.

manufacturer needed to describe one of the following four regulatory possibilities, respectively, called certifications or paragraphs:

I patent information on the drug has not been filed.

II the patent has already expired.

III the date on which the patent will expire.

IV the patent is invalid or use or sale of the drug will not infringe the patent.

Now let us review the respective procedures. Certifications I and II authorize the FDA to approve the submitted ANDA. Certification III authorizes the agency to wait until the applicable patents expire, and then approve the ANDA. Finally, Certification IV indicates that the generic manufacturer mounts a challenge to the originator company. This triggers an automatic notification to the originator company, who may wish to respond to the challenge by filling an infringement suit versus the generic applicant within 45 days of being notified. Following the suit, the owner of the patent gets a 30 month stay from the FDA from approving the generic. The matter is then up to the relevant Courts. They may decide one of the following three routes: (1) the patent had expired, so the ANDA proceeds, (2) the generic manufacturer was within the research exemption period and can proceed with their testing, and (3) nothing of the previous two applies, and the generic manufacturer has to honor the 30 month stay and then proceed with the generic application.

BIOSIMILAR DEVELOPMENT UNDER FDA

We have previously discussed how the Hatch–Waxman Act allowed the abbreviated regulatory approval of generic pharmaceuticals following the patent expiration of the original drugs. Unfortunately, the Act had a significant limitation at the time of its approval into law: it only applied to drugs regulated under the *Federal Food, Drug and Cosmetic Act* ("FD&C Act"). Most medicines sold in the United States are covered by the FD&C Act, including not only the hundreds of small molecule or chemical drugs, but also some biologic drugs (mainly hormone therapies). All other biologics, including most biotech medicines, are licensed under the *Public Health Service (PHS) Act*. While drugs already enjoy a generic approval process as well as a second-generation pathway, neither exists for PHS Act biologics.

According to Engel et al. (2009), the lack of an approval process for generic biologics means that, even when the patents expire on these products, there is no ability for generic biologics to be approved by FDA. This is significant given that PHS Act biologics have become an increasingly important treatment option across a range of medical conditions—many of which may be more common among older adults and the annual treatment costs can be quite substantial.

Hatch–Waxman and Biologics

When the Hatch–Waxman Act was effected into law, it defined as one of the basic prerequisites of generic pharmaceutical approvability the term "same," indicating the interchangeability between the original medicine and its generic equivalent. Although this simple four-letter definition can easily be argued effectively for most chemical copies of small molecule pharmaceuticals, this is not the case for large, complex, multidimensional, and multi-domain biopharmaceuticals, for which a minute change in their nucleic acid synthesis, or their stereochemical structure may result in a loss of its famous "lock-and-key" affinity to a biological target (e.g., cell surface receptor), resulting in reduced efficacy, lower safety, host antibody formation, and more.

Therefore, among the more than 200 biopharmaceuticals approved to date, a very small minority of biopharmaceutical molecular entities can be safely and dependably reproduced by a biomanufacturing method in such a way that identical "sameness" is maintained, and thus, both bioequivalence and pharmacological equivalence of the resulting biogeneric versus the original molecule can be guaranteed. In summary, the Act is not and cannot be safely used in assessing the sameness of generic biological medicines.

Section 505(b) (2) Drug Application

In the biogeneric industry's efforts to go head-to-head versus the original biopharmaceuticals and prove their full bioequivalence gaining an abbreviated regulatory pathway to approval, attempts have been made to utilize another existing regulatory pathway, namely, the mechanism described under section 505(b) (2) of the FD&C Act.

Let us review this possibility for a while. In essence, what every biogeneric manufacturer is looking for is a standardized and abbreviated regulatory pathway whereas a biogeneric copy of a biopharmaceutical can prove that (1) it is safe, (2) it is effective, and (3) it is similar or

identical to the original, giving it access to refer to previously conducted and published clinical trial results by the originator company.
Could this 505(b) (2) pathway of the FDCA be the solution? First it
calls for safety (check one prerequisite), second it calls for efficacy
(check two), third it calls for an abbreviated pathway (check three),
and fourth it calls for abbreviated clinical findings that are "relevant
and applicable" for the originator product being challenged. In other
words, it does not call for the ANDA's rigid "sameness" requirement,
but it does apply to generics drugs that can justify being exact copies of the original, anyway (easy for small molecules, but difficult for
biopharmaceuticals).

The Case of Sandoz's Omnitrope

The approval of SANDOZ's Omnitrope®, a follow-on version of recombinant human growth hormone (somatropin) by the U.S. FDA is a case
in point for the 505(b) (2) procedure. Following a long regulatory scrutiny, and a monumental persistence by the biogeneric manufacturer, the
FDA finally approved Omnitrope in 2006, although its original comparator, Pfizer's Genotropin, was originally approved following an NDA
under the FDCA.

Could this be the forgotten castle door that remained open for biogeneric challengers into the FDA's world of regulatory approval heaven?
The answer is no. This is because the FDA closed the door for biogeneric
copies of biopharmaceuticals originally approved under the PHSA (the
vast majority of them). At the same time, FDA explained its decision on
Omnitrope by arguing that human growth hormone was well characterized physicochemically, structurally, pharmacologically, toxicologically,
and, above all, it had a molecule lacking glycosylation, the make-or-break
tertiary structural element that is hard to immitate by using a different
biomanufacturing method.

BIOSIMILAR DEVELOPMENT UNDER EMEA

European Regulatory Guidance

Years before the FDA could decide on an abbreviated regulatory approval
pathway for biogenerics, the EMEA (see Chapter 6) developed a guidance
for how a manufacturer can submit an application for approval of a follow-
on biologic in the EU. EMEA's system depends on the following principles:
(1) every biogeneric under scrutiny needs to be compared with a "reference" biopharmaceutical already approved in the EU; (2) every biogeneric

must be compared with the same reference product as far as its efficacy, safety, and quality are concerned; and (3) all biogenerics are divided into four different "reference classes": (i) biological products that contain biotechnology-derived proteins as the active substance, (ii) immunologicals such as vaccines and allergens, (iii) blood- or plasma-derived products and their recombinant alternatives, and (iv) other biological medicinal products.

As far as biotechnology-derived proteins are concerned, EMEA requires three different nonclinical investigations to be performed: (1) physicochemical properties (e.g., molecular weight, melting point, primary, secondary, tertiary structure); (2) assessments of biological activity (e.g., efficacy in biological assays); and (3) determinations of purity and impurities (amino acid sequence, molecular weight, etc.) (MacNeil and Douglas, 2007).

In assessing the biological activity of protein therapeutics, EMEA's guidelines are fairly general: (1) biological assays using different approaches to measure the biological activity should be considered as appropriate; (2) the biologic should be examined to identify the impurities in the product and compare them with those found in the reference product; (3) manufacturers should test the purity of the product under stress conditions that induce selective degradation; (4) manufacturers should perform studies in a species "known to be relevant"; and (5) manufacturers should attempt to develop animal studies that investigate PD endpoints, and measure nonclinical toxicity via at least one repeat dose toxicity study.

On the other hand, the guidelines stipulate that (1) there are some routine toxicology studies that will not be required of follow-on biologics, such as safety pharmacology, reproduction toxicology, and mutagenicity and carcinogenicity studies—unless the repeat dose toxicity studies raise issues in these areas, and (2) as for clinical studies, the manufacturer should perform PK and PD studies followed by clinical efficacy and safety trials.

European Biosimilar Approvals to Date

In 2006, biosimilars received regulatory approval for the first time in Europe. Two recombinant human growth hormones, Holzkirchen, Germany-based Sandoz's Omnitrope and Valtropin, offered by Biopartners of Baar, Switzerland, were approved in the EU. Table 13.10 lists the European biosimilar approvals by December 2009.

TABLE 13.10   European Biosimilar Approvals to Date

#	Trade Name	Generic Name	Manufacturer	Approval Date
1	Omnitrope	Somatropin	Sandoz	April 12, 2006
2	Valtropin	Somatropin	Biopartners	April 24, 2006
3	Binocrit	Epoetin Alfa	Sandoz	August 28, 2007
4	Epoetin Alfa Hexal	Epoetin alfa	Hexal	August 28, 2007
5	Abseamed	Epoetin alfa	Medice	August 28, 2007
6	Retacrit	Epoetin zeta	Hospira	December 18, 2007
7	Silapo	Epoetin zeta	Stada	December 18, 2007
8	Ratiograstim	Filgrastim	Ratiopharm	September 16, 2008
9	Biograstim	Filgrastim	CT Arzneimittel	September 16, 2008
10	Tevagrastim	Filgrastim	Teva Generics	September 16, 2008
11	Filgrastim Ratiopharm	Filgrastim	Ratiopharm	September 16, 2008
12	Filgrastim Hexal	Filgrastim	Hexal	February 13, 2009
13	Zarzio	Filgrastim	Sandoz	February 13, 2009
14	Ratioepo	Epoetin theta	Ratiopharm	Positive CHMP opinion: July 23, 2009
15	Eporatio	Epoetin theta	Ratiopharm	Positive CHMP opinion: July 23, 2009
16	Biopoin	Epoetin theta	CT Arzneimittel	Positive CHMP opinion: July 23, 2009

Source: European Medicines Evaluation Agency (EMEA), European biosimilar approvals to-date, EMEA, Brussels, Belgium, last updated: February 2010, Posted at: http://www.emea.europe.eu/htms/human/epar/a.htm

BIOSIMILAR DEVELOPMENT UNDER THE JMHW AND IN THE ROW

Biosimilar Development in Japan

Following Europe, Japan has put forward during 2009 the biosimilar guidance to give a clear instruction on the definition of this group of drugs, and requests for development and registration. As per the guidelines, "biosimilars are drugs which are equivalent and homogeneous to original biopharmaceuticals in terms of quality, efficacy and safety and which are developed by manufacturers different from those of the original biopharmaceuticals."

IHS Global Insight (*Source:* IHS Global Insight, MHLW issues guidelines on biosimilars development and regulatory applications, March 26, 2009, http://www.ihsglobalinsight.com/SDA/SDADetail16336.htm. With permission.) has previously summarized the biosimilar approval framework in Japan as described below:

Development: Biosimilars should be developed to be equivalent and homogeneous to original drugs. However, biosimilars are also requested to be developed with updated technologies and knowledge, therefore only need to demonstrate enough similarity to guarantee the safety and efficacy instead of absolute identity.

Application filing: Biosimilars' regulatory approval applications will be categorized separately from conventional generic drugs. In general, the applications should be submitted, as in new drug applications, with data on clinical trials, manufacturing methods, long-term stability and information on overseas use. The MHLW will assess the data on absorption, distribution, metabolism, and excretion (ADME) on a case-by-case basis. The applicants do not need to provide data on accessory pharmacology, safety pharmacology, and genotoxicity.

Naming: Biosimilars are requested to use brand names and nonproprietary names of the original biopharmaceuticals less the genetic recombination description. The nonproprietary names should also be followed by kozoku-1, meaning follow-on-1 and so on. In November 2009, the MHLW received Japan's first biosimilar marketing approval application from Japan Chemical Research (JCR) and Japanese pharma company Kissei Pharmaceuticals for JR-013, a treatment for renal anemia in dialysis patients based on recombinant human erythropoietin.

For a biosimilar with JMHW approval example see: Somatropin (SANDOZ), Sandoz has received marketing authorization for the first-ever Japanese biosimilar, recombinant human growth hormone somatropin, SANDOZ Press Release, Holzkirchen, Germany, June 25, 2009, http://www.sandoz.com.

Other ROW Countries' Biosimilar Guidelines

Following EMEA's leadership, several other countries, except Japan, have issued their own guidance on the regulatory approval pathways for follow-on biologicals. Table 13.11 summarizes the biosimilar guidelines issued to date in other ROW countries.

DATA EXCLUSIVITY, APPROVAL EXCLUSIVITY, AND MARKETING EXCLUSIVITY

FDA Market Exclusivity Rules

As previously mentioned, the Hatch–Waxman Act created provisions that provided protections for both pharmaceutical patent holders as well as their generic challengers by imposing compromises on either side's demands.

TABLE 13.11   Other ROW Countries' Biosimilar Guidelines to Date

Country	Final Guidelines on Abbreviated Licensing Pathways for Biosimilars Released
Argentina	Draft guideline issued July 2008 by ANMAT Title: "Registration and registry modification of biological medicinal products"
Australia	EU guidelines have been adopted in August 2008
Brazil	Final guideline was issued on October 26, 2005 Title: "Technical rules for registration of biological products"
Canada	2nd Draft guideline on SEBs issued in March 2009, open for comments for 60 days (May 26, 2009) Reference product: "…in appropriate circumstances, a biologic product that is not authorized for sale in Canada may be used as a reference product…"
Colombia	Issue date not known, Draft guideline Title: "License for manufacturing facilities of biological products"
India	Final guideline was issued on July 11, 2008 Title: "Preparation of the quality information for drug submission for new drug approval: Biotechnological/biological products"
Malaysia	Final guidance: July 30, 2008 issued by the Ministry of Health Malaysia Title: "Guidance document for registration of biosimilars in Malaysia"
Mexico	Draft guideline was issued on October 9, 2008 Title: "Ley generalde medicamentos biotecnológicos"
Middle East	The consensus group recommended the implementation of the EMEA guidelines as the basis of Regional guidelines for the registration of biosimilar in the Near and Middle East. Saudi Arabia: Draft guidance issued August 2008 Title: "Drug master file requirements for the registration of biosimilars"
Taiwan	Final guideline issued on November 21, 2008 by Department of Health Title: "Review criteria for registration and market approval of pharmaceuticals—Registration and market approval of biological products"
Turkey	Final Guideline issued August 2008 by General Directorate of Pharmaceuticals and Pharmacy Title: "Instruction Manual on Biosimilar Medical Products"
Venezuela	Final guideline was issued on August 3, 2000 Title: "SRPB-R guidelines: Application for Health Registry of DNA recombinant products, monoclonal and therapeutic antibodies, subclassification for active substances already on the market"

Source: Schwarzenberger, I., Global development, the way forward the EGA's perspective, in *European Biopharmaceutical Group 7th EGA Annual Symposium on Biosimilars*, London, April 23/24, 2009, PowerPoint presentation posted at: http://www.egagenerics.com/doc/ega_biosimilars_Schwarzenberger_090424.pdf. With permission.

For example, it has created a data exclusivity period, preventing generic challengers from using publicly available clinical trial and related data to substantiate the safety of their medically equivalent/ similar medicines. Generic drug suppliers may not be able to contest the patents of a brand provider unless the generic supplier has filed with the FDA. The Act has also created approval exclusivity, sometimes referred to as market exclusivity, a period of time during which a generic drug supplier can file for FDA approval, but cannot receive approval (Kotlikoff, 2008).

Every time a new patent is added in the Orange Book, the brand manufacturer gets a 30 month stay from approving the ANDA. However, the 30 month stay obtained for each patent runs concurrently. Currently, the brand manufacturer can only get one 30 month extension. The first generic manufacturer who files ANDA with paragraph IV certification is rewarded with 180 day market exclusivity, if its generic drug is approved.

EMEA Data and Marketing Exclusivity Rules

The provisions described on data and marketing exclusivity apply to applications filed in the framework of the centralized procedure as well as to applications filed in the framework of national authorizations procedures. Rules on data exclusivity have been further harmonized at the EU level in 2004. However, the new periods of protection do not apply to reference medicinal products for which the initial application for authorization was submitted before the implementation of the new legislation (November 20, 2005 for centrally authorized products and October 30, 2005 for nationally authorized products).

According to the European Commission's Pharmaceutical Sector Inquiry Final Report (2009), data and marketing exclusivity rules for marketing authorization applications submitted after November 20, 2005/ October 30, 2005 are as follows: The 6 or 10 years of protection under the previous rules are replaced by a period of 10 years broken down into the so-called 8 + 2 formula. As they apply to marketing authorization applications for original products submitted after November 20, 2005/October 30, 2005, the 8 year protection period for such applications will expire at the earliest in 2013. For a generic product of a reference medicinal product for which the initial application was made after the mentioned dates, an abridged application is possible after 8 years from the initial marketing authorization (data exclusivity period).

THE GLOBAL GENERIC INDUSTRY IN NUMBERS

Generic Medicine Policies

The regulatory approval procedures implemented by various regulatory agencies for biogenerics comprise only a small component of their market regulation. An additional critical component is the implementation of varying national policies dictating the use of these medications, as well as incentives or disincentives set up by national governments in order to enhance (or inhibit) the further penetration of cheaper generic therapeutic alternatives, that may be nationally produced or imported. Table 13.12 presents representative generic medicine policies of European governments.

Global Generics Market

According to IMS data, the 2008 global generics sales amounted to USD 78 billion. Growth was down to 3.6% from 11.4% in 2007. The top eight global markets—the U.S., Germany, France, the U.K., Canada, Italy, Spain and Japan—accounted for 84 percent of total generics sales. The top 10 generics companies had a 47 percent share of the generics market worldwide. The three leading generics manufacturers were Teva (11% market share), Sandoz (9%) and Mylan (8%). Furthermore, IMS predicted that generics companies would benefit as products generating $139 billion in branded sales

TABLE 13.12   Generic Medicine Policies of European Governments

I. Countries with a coherent generic medicines policy	Sweden, United Kingdom, Denmark, France
II. Generic medicines competition within existing regulatory frameworks	Poland, Netherlands, Denmark, Germany, United Kingdom, Sweden
III. Countries with incentives for physicians to prescribe generic medicines	Germany, France, United Kingdom, Sweden
IV. Countries with incentives for pharmacists to dispense generic medicines	Netherlands, Denmark, United Kingdom, Italy, France, Poland, Sweden
V. Countries with incentives for patients to demand generic medicines	Italy, Denmark, Germany, Sweden, France, Poland

Source: Bongers, F. and Carradinha, H., How to increase patient access to generic medicines in European healthcare systems—A report by the EGA Health Economics Committee. European Generic Medicines Association, Brussels, June 2009—Revised and updated with additional country data (July 2009), Posted at: http://www.egagenerics.com/doc/ega_increase-patient-access_update_072009.pdf. With permission.

in the top eight world markets would lose their patent protection through 2012.

Source: IMS Health, IMS Health Reports Annual Global Generics Prescription Sales Growth of 3.6 Percent to $78 Billion, Norwalk, CT, Press Release, December 10, 2008.

Global Biogenerics Market

According to a Markets and Markets' (2009) report, Biosimilars (2009–2014), the biogenerics sector is currently highly fragmented and this, coupled to the shift in regulations, means there are opportunities for growth. In particular, the opening up of the U.S. market will drive growth in the sector. Currently, Asia is the primary market for biosimilars, accounting for 34.1% of sales, but the U.S. market is predicted to rise to the top spot once legislation is passed. Compound annual growth rate (CAGR) is predicted to be 89.1% from 2009 to 2014, in part because of the expected establishment of a regulatory pathway in the United States. The other aspect is that biologics with sales totaling $25 billion will be off patent by 2016, and recombinant non-glycosylated protein products account for a sizeable proportion of this.

Table 13.13 provides an overview of biogeneric companies, their products and timescales.

BIOSIMILAR DEVELOPMENT COSTS

DiMasi and Grabowski (2007) found the cost of development of a new innovative biotechnology drug approximated $1.2 billion (including unsuccessful or failed drugs), comprised of $615 million of preclinical expenses and $626 million of clinical expenses. This compares to an estimated $0.5 billion–$0.8 billion for traditional new chemical drugs (Reiffen and Ward, 2007).

According to Fuhr and Blackstone (2008), biopharmaceuticals take 97.7 months to get through the regulation process compared to 90.3 months for traditional chemical drugs. The cost of developing a simple biosimilar ranges between $14.5 million and $17 million compared to between $0.9 million and $2.6 million for a chemical generic. The development period for a biosimilar is estimated to be 7 years. They have also published that the production costs of the biosimilar are 60% higher relative to active price than chemical generics. The profit margin is much less for a biosimilar than a chemical drug. Especially significant are the expenditures required for clinical trials. Clinical trials for biosimilars in Europe have been estimated to require expenditures of $26.5 million–$53 million.

TABLE 13.13 Biogeneric Companies, Products, and Timescales

Company	Country	rh GH	rh EPO	Rh G-CSF	rh GM-CSF	rh IFN Alpha	Rh IFN Beta	rh Insulin
						Developing Product/Filling for EU Approval		
BioGeneriX	Germany		Yes	Yes	Yes		Yes (rh IFN beta-1a)	
BioPartners	Switzerland	Yes	Yes	Yes	Yes	Yes	Yes	
Dr. Reddy's Laboratories	India		Yes	Yes		Yes		
GeneMedix	United Kingdom	Yes earliest launch 2007	Yes	Yes launch in 2007	Yes	Yes	Yes	Yes
Novartis/Sandoz	Switzerland	Yes						
Pliva	Croatia		Yes	Yes				
Prolong Pharmaceuticals	United States		Yes	Yes		Yes	Yes	
Ranbaxy	India		Yes	Yes		Yes		
Rhein Biotech	Germany							
Savient	Israel	Yes	Yes					Yes on market
Stada	Germany		Yes	Yes			Yes	
Teva (now acquired Sicor)	Israel	Yes marketed				Yes		
Transkaryotic Therapies	United States		Yes					
Wockhardt	India	Yes	Yes					Yes

BIOSIMILAR PRICING

Biologic Therapy Costs

According to Christopher (2006), the high cost of biologics has intensified battles over the U.S. government's right to control drug pricing and access to lower-cost generics. For example, several months' dose of a biologic such as Genentech's bevacizumab (Avastin; used to treat colorectal cancer and also to help prolong life for non-small-cell lung cancer patients) can cost from $55,000 to more than $100,000, including very high co-pays. In response to outcries about the medicine's price, in October, Genentech announced a $55,000/year per patient price tag for people with lower incomes. The *Access to Life-Saving Medicine Act* is designed to help resolve the ongoing debate by defining a biogenerics approval process for the FDA.

Biosimilar Market Penetration

The production, testing, and distribution costs for biologics are expected by many experts to be higher than the costs of bringing small molecule generics to market, and therefore FOB discounts will be less than those experienced in the small molecule generic market. Brand biologics manufacturers will increase the price of their product in the first year FOB competitors enter the market and then produce a gradual lowering by 30% in pricing of the brand biologic.

> The pricing strategy for each biosimilar needs to balance two competing forces. On the one hand, the price will have to reflect the high investment in development and manufacturing and marketing, as well as pharmacovigilance commitments. These high barriers mean the competitive intensity will be weak, which translates into more pricing leverage. Therefore, price differentials between originator product and biosimilar can be much less than for traditional generics. On the other hand, a small price differential reduces the incentive to switch. The consensus seems to be that a 20–25% discount is optimum.

> *Source:* Ahlstrom, A., King, R.(G.), Brown, R., Glaudemans, J., and Mendelson, D., 2007. Modeling federal cost savings from follow-on biologics. AVALERE HEALTH LLC, Washington, DC. Posted at: http://www.avalerehealth.net/research/docs/Modeling_Budgetary_Impact_of_FOBS.pdf

Factors reducing FOB market penetration are (1) clinical development and marketing costs, (2) biosimilar NOT substitutable for reference product at retail pharmacy level, (3) state generic substitution laws may not provide for biosimilar or biogeneric substitutability, (4) introduction of second-generation product threatens to limit potential of biosimilars to save money by retaining reference product market share and price premium, and (5) 64% of biotech drugs are used in a physician's office, which limits effectiveness of retail pharmacy substitution (if it is even possible). Medicare Part B payment system provides incentive for doctors to use the more expensive drug.

On the other hand, a factor increasing FOB market penetration is the following: Payers and pharmacy benefits managers (PBMs) have clearly indicated their intention to move quickly and aggressively to encourage the utilization of FOBs as they have done with small molecule generics.

Omnitrope was launched in Germany and Austria at a price 20% below Genotropin and has been able to gain less than 1% of the European market. It was also launched at a 20% discount compared to Eli Lilly's Humatrope in Germany. However, the discount is likely to increase when Biopartners' Valtropin is launched. Biosimilar human growth hormone in Australia costs 25% less than the brand. Originator products' pricing strategies will have a huge influence on the uptake of biosimilars. Many brands have raised the price of first-generation products to encourage switching to their second-generation products. The introduction of biosimilars may increase the cost differential and increase the switch back to first-generation products (Pisani and Bonduelle, 2007).

Heldman (2008) has reported that ESA brand-name competitors reduce prices before and after introduction of biosimilars in Germany and the United Kingdom. Amgen reduces price 13%–16% in early 2008 in Germany. However, Amgen says it maintains a 15%–30% price premium to first generation ESAs in Europe. Other data suggest price premium is narrower in Germany. ESA biosimilars priced at about 25% discount to innovator product.

BIOSIMILAR MARKETING

According to Fuhr and Blackstone (2008), an important factor distinguishing chemical generics from biosimilars is the greater reliance on marketing and detailing of biosimilars. Unlike chemical generic drugs, substitution will not be automatic. Brand loyalty will be especially difficult to overcome. The first successful drug may enjoy a strong first-mover advantage, making entry quite difficult. Biosimilars companies will have to assure physicians (and hospital purchasing authorities) that their biosimilar will be safe and perform as well as the brand name drug. This will be difficult and require substantial expenditures of time and money, adding to the risk of entry. Direct advertising to consumers is unlikely to be successful. These factors mean high costs for marketing since direct contact with physicians may be required.

For a biosimilar marketing example see: OMNITROPE, SANDOZ, Holzkirchen, Germany, http://www.sandoz.com.

QUESTIONS

1. What is defined as a business model? Provide different business model examples from various industries.
2. Which are the main biopharmaceutical business models in existence today? Provide actual examples.
3. What are the pros and cons of the biopharmaceutical blockbuster model?
4. What are the prerequisites for an orphan drug designation in the U.S., EU, and Japanese markets?
5. Which are the alternative orphan drug company scenarios? Provide an actual company example for each scenario.
6. What does it take to build a virtual biopharmaceutical company? Where would you start?
7. What is the importance of pharmacogenomics in biopharmaceutical drug development?
8. Which are the main benefits offered by molecular diagnostics?
9. Which are the main factors increasing or reducing biosimilar market penetration?
10. What is the importance of biosimilar marketing?

EXERCISES

1. Take the top 10 biopharmaceuticals by global sales during the last year data is available for. Then, by visiting the USPTO and FDA pages, describe their patent and market exclusivity status in the United States.
2. Describe the case study of Sandoz's Omnitrope approval by the FDA.
3. By the time this book hits the bookshelves, biosimilar development in the United States may have dramatically changed. What is the current regulatory framework and how does it compare to Europe's?

4. You are an experienced regulatory professional hired by a start-up biopharma early in its life cycle. What are the USPTO and FDA filling processes you are recommending to your board of directors?

5. Describe the U.K. policy versus generic pharmaceuticals. Would you consider it supportive, inhibiting, or neutral toward their further market penetration and usage?

6. Taking into account the various national policies versus the use of generic pharmaceuticals around the world, which countries would you select as the most positive and which as the most negative toward their further market penetration?

7. There are various biosimilar molecules commercially launched in the EU market to date. What is their pricing strategy versus their respective branded biopharmaceuticals? What was the pricing response of the originator companies?

8. You are the marketing executive of a biogeneric coming into the marketplace soon. What kind of marketing activities do you undertake in support of your molecule?

9. Study the Web sites of three subscription companies, and provide examples of how major biopharmas are capitalizing on their technology offerings.

10. What is the standing of personalized medicine today, and where can it take us in the next 10 years? Name actual biomolecules currently under development that can make another step toward individualized medicine.

REFERENCES

Ahlstrom, A., King, R.(G.), Brown, R., Glaudemans, J., and Mendelson, D., 2007. Modeling federal cost savings from follow-on biologics. AVALERE HEALTH LLC, Washington, DC. Posted at: http://www.avalerehealth.net/research/docs/Modeling_Budgetary_Impact_of_FOBS.pdf

Ahn, C., 2007. Pharmacogenomics in drug discovery and development. *Genomics Inform* 5(2): 41–45, June.

Bhat, V.N., 2005. Patent term extension strategies in the pharmaceutical industry. *Journal Pharmaceuticals Policy and Law* 6: 109–122.

BioGenerix, 2010. Company profile, BioGenerix, Mannheim, Germany. Posted at: http://www.biogenerix.com/index1.html

Bongers, F. and Carradinha, H., 2009. How to increase patient access to generic medicines in European healthcare systems—a report by the EGA Health Economics Committee. European Generic Medicines Association, Brussels, June 2009—Revised and updated with additional country data (July 2009). Posted at: http://www.egagenerics.com/doc/ega_increase-patient-access_update_072009.pdf

Burrill, G.S., 2010. Biochemistry 241y, Winter 2010, January 4 to March 15, Mondays, 4:00–6:00 pm, Genentech Hall, N 106, Mission Bay Campus, UCSF. Posted at: http://cbe.ucsf.edu/cbe/9212-DSY/version/default/part/AttachmentData/data

Burrill & Company, 2009. *Biotech 2009—Life Sciences: Navigating the Sea of Change*. San Francisco, CA: Burrill and Co.

Christopher, A., 2006. Biogenerics and drug pricing: A battle royal. *Pharmacy Times*, Published Online: December 1, 2006. Posted at: http://pharmacytimes.com/issue/pharmacy/http://2006/2006-12/2006-12-6122.

deCODE, Reykjavik, Iceland, http://www.decode

DiMasi, J.A. and Grabowski, H.G., 2007. The cost of biopharmaceutical R&D: Is biotech different? *Managerial and Decision Economics* 28: 469–479.

Engel, J.M., Hughes, E.C., and Woollett, G.R., 2009. *AARP Issue Paper: The EU Biosimilars Pathway*. AARP Office of International Affairs, Washington, DC. Posted at: http://www.aarpinternational.org/usr_attach/AARPIssuePaper_Biosimilars_May2009_footnotes.pdf

European Commission—Commission of the European Communities, 2009. *Pharmaceutical Sector Inquiry Final Report*. Brussels, Germany: EC. SEC(2009) 952, July 8, 2009. Posted at: http://ec.europa.eu/competition/sectors/pharmaceuticals/inquiry/communication_en.pdf

European Medicines Evaluation Agency (EMEA), 2007. Orphan drugs and rare diseases at a glance. EMEA, Brussels, Belgium, July EC, 2007. Posted at: http://www.emea.europa.eu/pdfs/human/comp/29007207en.pdf

European Medicines Agency's (EMEA), Committee for Orphan Medicinal Products (COMP), 2010. Orphan medicines in numbers—The Success of ten years of orphan legislation, Press Release, 3 May 2010. Posted at: http://www.ema.europa.eu/docs/en_GB/document_library/Report/2010/05/WC500090812.pdf

European Medicines Evaluation Agency (EMEA), 2010. European biosimilar approvals to-date. EMEA. Last updated: February 2010. Posted at: http://www.emea.europe.eu/htms/human/epar/a.htm

Food and Drug Agency (FDA), 2004. *Innovation/Stagnation: Challenge and Opportunity on the Critical Path to New Medical Products*. FDA, Washington, DC, March 2004. Posted at: http://www.fda.gov/oc/initiatives/criticalpath/whitepaper.pdf

Fuhr, J.P. Jr. and Blackstone, E.A., 2008. Why biosimilars will have a smaller competitive edge than generics. PowerPoint presentation posted at: http://www.consumerinstitute.org/Biosimilarspowerpointrevised%203-16.pdf

Granstrand, O. and Sjölander, S., 1990. Managing innovation in multi-technology corporations. *Research Policy* 19: 35–60.

Hatch-Waxman Act, 1984. Drug Price Competition and Patent Term Restoration Act of 1984, Pub. L. No. 98-417, 98 Stat. 1585—codified at 21 U.S.C. 355(b), (j), (l); 35 U.S.C. 156, 271, 282.

Heldman, P., 2008. Follow-on biologic market: initial lessons and challenges ahead. Potomac Research Group, Friday, November 21, 2008. Posted at: http://www.ftc.gov/bc/workshops/hcbio/docs/fob/pheldman.pdf

IHS Global Insight, 2009. MHLW issues guidelines on biosimilars development and regulatory applications, March 26, 2009. Posted at: http://www.ihsglobalinsight.com/SDA/SDADetail16336.htm

IMS Health, 2008. *IMS Health Reports Annual Global Generics Prescription Sales Growth of 3.6 Percent, to $78 Billion.* IMS Health, Norwalk, CT, Press Release, December 10, 2008.

Johnson & Johnson, 2009. Global biopharmaceutical market size projections to 2013 (in USD billion). In: Corporate Presentation, Pharm Day 2009. Posted at: http://www.jnj.com

Kotlikoff, L.J., 2008. Stimulating innovation in the biologics industry: A balanced approach to marketing exclusivity. Teva USA Government Affairs, Washington, DC, September 2008. Posted at: http://people.bu.edu/kotlikoff/New%20Kotlikoff%20Web%20Page/Kotlikoff_Innovation_in_Biologics21.pdf

MacNeil, J.S. and Douglas, F., 2007. *Challenges to Establishing a Regulatory Framework for Approving Follow-On Biologics: A Background Paper.* Massachusetts Institute of Technology, Cambridge, MA. Posted at: http://web.mit.edu/cbi/publications/FOB_macneil.pdf

Markets and Markets, 2009. *Biosimilars (2009–2014) Report.* Markets and Markets, Dallas, TX, September 2009.

PHARMA MAR, Madrid, Spain, http://www.pharmamar.com/company.aspse

Pisani, J. and Bonduelle, Y., 2007. *Opportunities and Barriers in the Biosimilar Market: Evolution or Revolution for Generics Companies?* PricewaterhouseCoopers LLP, London. Posted at: http://www.pipelinereview.com/joomla/content/view/10955/286/

Reiffen, D. and Ward, M., 2005. 'Branded generics' as a strategy to limit cannibalization of pharmaceutical markets. *Managerial and Decision Economics* 28(4–5): 251–265.

Reponen, T. (ed.), 2002. *Information Technology Enabled Customer Service.* IGI Global, Herschey, PA, November.

Sabatier, V., Mangernatin, V., and Rousselle, T., 2009. From business model to business model portfolio in the European biopharmaceutical industry. hal-00430782, version 1–November 12, 2009. Posted at: http://hal.grenoble-em.com/docs/00/43/07/82/PDF/Business_Model_Portfolio_V7_2_.pdf

SANDOZ, 2009. Sandoz has received marketing authorization for the first-ever Japanese biosimilar, recombinant human growth hormone somatropin. SANDOZ Press Release, Holzkirchen, Germany, June 25, 2009. Posted at: http://www.sandoz.com

SANDOZ, 2010. Small molecule generics versus biosimilars. SANDOZ, Holzkirchen, Germany. Posted at: http://www.sandoz.com/site/en/product_range/more_about_biosimilars/index.shtml

Schwarzenberger, I., 2009. Global development, the way forward the EGA's perspective. In: *European Biopharmaceutical Group 7th EGA Annual Symposium on Biosimilars,* London, April 23/24, 2009. PowerPoint presentation posted at: http://www.egagenerics.com/doc/ega_biosimilars_Schwarzenberger_090424.pdf

STADA Corporate Presentation, October 2009, Bad Vilbel, Germany, http://www.stada.de/english/investorrelations/presentations/

Tufts Center for the Study of Drug Development, 2010. U.S. orphan product designations more than doubled from 2000–2002 to 2006–2008. Impact Report 12(1) January/February 2010.

U.S. Food and Drug Administration (FDA), Silver Spring, MD. Posted at: http://www.fda.gov/MedicalDevices/ProductsandMedicalProcedures/DeviceApprovalsandClearances/Recently-ApprovedDevices/ucm078879.htm (accessed on July 19, 2010).

Venkatadri, B., 2007. Follow on protein products: Opportunity or overblown? In: *VENTUREAST Conference*, November 2, 2007. PowerPoint presentation posted at: http://www.ableindia.org/bobba.ppt

## CHAPTER 14

Biocompany Life Cycle

The market turmoil led to significant declines in funding in 2008. Overall, capital raised by biotech companies fell by 46%, from US$30 billion in 2007 to US$16 billion in 2008. Not surprisingly, the most dramatic fall-off was in funds raised from public investors. The amount of capital raised in IPOs fell by a dramatic 95%, from US$2.3 billion in 2007 to US$116 million in 2008.

Source: Ernst & Young, *Beyond Borders: 2009 Global Biotechnology Report*, E&Y, Boston, MA, 2009.

WE HAD LEFT OUR friendly Advanced Therapies start-up back in Chapter 10, struggling to come up with a proper pricing for its first biopharmaceuticals still under clinical investigation. In this chapter, we review our courageous start-up's entire company life cycle, starting from its own incorporation, discussing some of the challenges it has faced along the way, reviewing the major risks it has faced, and also the founders' ongoing debate about taking the company forward. By the way, for those of you who are still wandering, Advanced Therapies has successfully launched its first biopharmaceutical through its own subsidiary within the U.S. market, while it has out-licensed its global non-U.S. product rights to a big pharma organization. Luckily, the company's founders had managed to see their diluted share holdings reach maturity and are now dividing their time at homes in Santa Monica, Lake Tahoe, and Lake Geneva.

We had started our Advanced Therapies' review while it was an aspiring, yet struggling, healthcare biotechnology start-up. These companies are defined as small organizations, in their early research and development years, still years away before their first products enter human clinical trials, trying to secure financing from a variety of sources in order to take their product forward. Start-ups became a household word back in the early dotcom era in the late 1990s, where thousands of Internet-based start-ups rose to fame and some of them flourished, as the world was entering a new technology paradigm. Coming back to biotechs, they have initially emerged back in the late 1970s, launched their first products with the assistance of big pharma in the early 1980s, and later became fully integrated in the early 1990s. Their meteoric rise gave the impetus needed for thousands more to be set up in the early 1990s across the world, although very few have managed to commercialize their biopharmaceuticals yet, and even fewer have reached profitability to date.

In general, a high-technology based start-up (such as Advanced Therapies) is characterized by the following signs: (1) a limited operating age, (2) a small, entrepreneurial, and highly skilled work force, (3) usually no commercial income, necessitating the need for successive rounds of external financing, (4) one or more products in early research and development, and (5) a strong intellectual property base, that if financed and developed properly, may give rise to significant commercial opportunities and financial returns in the future.

Biotech start-ups, in particular, have their own unique characteristics: (1) a biotechnology patent, eventually conferring the freedom to operate for a start-up to develop a new biopharmaceutical, vaccine, or diagnostic, (2) a large unmet clinical need for which a challenging target product profile has been created, (3) a long, arduous, and risky preclinical and clinical research road, (4) a prolonged regulatory approval period, and (5) a profoundly competitive, yet potentially financially rewarding, pharmaceutical marketplace. These are the very characteristics upon which industry pioneers such as Genentech and Amgen were created, and yet the same obstacles that led hundreds of other biotechnology start-ups to fade away before ever reaching regulatory approval.

ORGANIZATIONAL LIFE CYCLE

In Chapter 12, we reviewed the biopharmaceutical product's life cycle. A similar distinct life cycle also defines all healthcare biotechnology companies in existence today. Let us review their most defining moments.

Modern Healthcare Biotechnology Era

Millions of prescribers and patients today take biosynthetic biopharmaceuticals for granted. However, in the not-so-distant past human therapeutics included the use of urinary gonadotrophins extracted from the urine of postmenopausal women, or cadaver insulin. The defining moment for this new, exciting, and life-saving industry to come into existence is considered by many to be the U.S. Supreme Court (1980) decision of June 16, 1980 in the case of *Diamond vs. Chakrabarty* (see Chapter 2) that a genetically modified microorganism could be patented. Ever since, countless biotechs utilized the same molecular tools to come up with genetically modified hosts that could produce human biotherapeutics in commercial quantities. And so the life of modern healthcare biotechnology had just begun.

Conception and Gestation

Armed with thorough knowledge of these genetic engineering techniques, mostly academic but also corporate researchers come across (1) a new method of synthesizing a biological protein, (2) a new protein able to bind and alter the function of a biological disease-related target, or (3) a wholly new biological target, that if therapeutically manipulated, may result in satisfying an unmet clinical need. These scientists, usually with the assistance of an academic TTO, then secure the rights to their invention by obtaining a patent. A newly acquired IP right often gives the impetus for an academia-to-industry leap, leading to a new biotech start-up incorporated, which then attracts its first rounds of financing.

Infancy

Funded by their first meager financing rounds, healthcare biotechnology entrepreneurs establish their first laboratory space, attract the research and development talent needed to take their planned molecules further, and set up the preclinical assays, including in vitro or in vivo models, that will allow the thorough investigation of the first molecules in cellular or whole animal models related to the disease being investigated. After several rounds of testing, and progressively moving from the smallest assay to small animals, and later larger animal models resembling progressively more the human physiology and pathology, investigators are hopefully able to sort their long list of molecules into their primary candidates for entering clinical trials called "leads."

Adolescence

Following the successful completion of the preclinical research phase, biotechnology start-ups secure the approval of the relevant regulatory agency to enter human clinical trials by obtaining an investigational new drug (IND) approval and later attract the significant additional financing needed for them to enter this arduous pathway. Upon the IND's approval, the lead molecules enter their first-in-man trials, leading to initial pharmacokinetic and dose-ranging findings.

Company Maturity and Investor Exit

Having progressed through the Phase I clinical trials in healthy human volunteers, the biotechnology start-ups are then faced with an entirely different ball game. That is the need to expand their small-scale, dose-finding studies into multicenter, multinational, large Phase II and later Phase III trials that will eventually prove the lead molecule's efficacy, safety, and superiority over the existing commercially available medicines. It is common at this stage that the start-ups decide to "go public" thus listing their company shares on a public stock exchange, through the IPO process we have reviewed back in Chapter 4. This is a defining moment for the entire biotech start-up organization, since the initial investors (VC and others) are exiting the company by selling their share portfolio, the company's founders see their own share holdings significantly reducing but giving them a significant capitalization, while the organization acquires a capitalization which will hopefully allow its progression through the entire clinical trial program and up to regulatory submission.

Regulatory Approval and Commercial Product Launch

Having completed a long, expensive, and risky clinical trial program, the biotech organization reaches the golden gate of make-or-break regulatory approval. By submitting a voluminous new drug application (NDA) or a biologics license application (BLA) to the U.S. FDA, for example, the biotech enters its final defining months before its regulatory approval and launch. A series of meetings and potential responses by company executives or external experts hopefully leads to the full resolution of all outstanding issues, upon which FDA confers the NDA license for commercial availability to the biotech organization.

Immediately after, the company may launch its product within the U.S. market, either on its own or through biopharma or big pharma collaborators. Soon after, similar NDA applications to European, Japanese, or RoW regulatory authorities produce additional regulatory approvals and subsequent product launches around the world.

Company Growth, Diversification, or Exit

The final period in a biopharma's life cycle is its eventual progression into a rapid growth phase, including additional biopharmaceuticals being commercially launched, several foreign subsidiaries being created, growing product sales, and more products entering and going through R&D. Following years of successful commercial presence, the biopharma may reach its peak sales, complete with strong R&D and commercial portfolios, several foreign subsidiaries and a large global workforce, which in the case of industry leaders has surpassed the 10,000 strong organizations.

On the other end of the spectrum, successive failures in the commercial arena, a potential product withdrawal due to unforeseen product side effects, or a stagnating R&D portfolio may bring a biopharma to its knees. At this point, all options are considered, and the company liquidation may not be excluded, ending an exhilarating, yet unsustained life cycle and eventual closure through liquidation.

As reviewed above, a biopharma life cycle is full of struggles, exhilarating moments of discovery, rewarding moments of regulatory approvals, and stressing moments of commercial launches. In the final pages of this book, we review some of the trials and tribulations of a young biopharma start-up on its way to financial success, and long-term sustainability and growth.

START-UP CHALLENGES IN RESEARCH AND DEVELOPMENT

In Chapter 6, we have reviewed the long and arduous road through the preclinical and clinical trials required by biopharmaceuticals for approval. Along the way, currently approved biopharmaceuticals have faced serious challenges and have managed to overcome most of them. Let us review some of these R&D-related challenges below, constituting one of the most critical risks a biopharma is faced with along its life cycle.

Lack of Efficacy or Safety

It is not uncommon for a biopharmaceutical product candidate to fail during its clinical trial phase. There can be many potential reasons for such a failure. For example, the product is (1) failing to meet its primary efficacy and/or safety endpoints, (2) proving effective only in combination with previously existing therapies, (3) proving effective only as a second- or third-line option, meaning that more effective therapeutic alternatives have to be applied first, and after the patient exhibits a disease relapse then the new trial medicine may be useful, (4) showing a very narrow therapeutic index (i.e., a very small differential between its effective and toxic doses), (5) exhibiting frequent drug interactions with concomitant disease medications, (6) having a very short half-life, requiring frequent administrations, (7) causing a low patient compliance due to administration or tolerability issues, or (8) requiring constant medical monitoring of the patient making its out-hospital administration impractical.

Development Shortcomings

These research-associated challenges discussed above may be corroborated by additional development challenges, having to do with either the product itself, or the entire biopharma start-up. For example, development problems may be related to: (1) inability to come up with stable formulations, (2) very short shelf life, (3) intravenous administration only, making its out-hospital usage impossible, (4) existence in a cumbersome lyophilized plus diluent form, making its reconstitution difficult and time consuming, (5) difficult to titrate in its final concentration due to narrow therapeutic index, or (6) only available in formulations containing inactive substances or excipients that are facing mounting regulatory obstacles, e.g., albumin or gelatin.

Organizational Shortcomings

A biopharma having its primary product candidate through clinical trials may face previously unforeseen challenges forcing to it either scale back its R&D program, temporarily withdraw its product from the clinical trial program, or even decide to abandon its program all together. But let us see how some of these problems may come about.

Frequent R&D problems facing a biopharma organization are (1) a potential challenge to their IP base, leaving them open to litigation and eventual punitive damages paid for patent infringement, (2) shortage of financing for moving their product through the very expensive clinical trial phase, (3) differences in strategy among the founders leading to a contested battle for company control, or (4) insurance and reimbursement changes bringing an abrupt challenge to their planned product development and eventual pricing model.

And the organizational challenges do not end there. It has been a frequent occurrence in the world of biopharmaceutical R&D that the biopharma's licensing agreements (either in-licensing or out-licensing) upon which an entire biopharmaceutical R&D program is based to face insurmountable challenges that may eventually necessitate the abandonment of the entire program all together, and the change of the company's direction into alternative product candidates or even new therapeutic areas. For example, (1) an in-licensing partner (e.g., an academic TTO) may decide to renegotiate the financial terms of its out-licensing to the biopharma, or (2) issue additional technology licenses to formidable big pharma competitors that may outrun the small biopharma to the finish line, or (3) even decide to withdraw its license all together arguing that the biopharma has utilized it in a previously unauthorized way or in a different therapeutic field.

As far as the biopharma's out-licensing agreements are concerned, a big pharma organization receiving the rights to further development and commercialization may either: (1) decide that the biopharmaceutical product candidate is less effective or safe than their initial due diligence had indicated, thus returning the rights to the biopharma, or (2) get acquired by a larger organization possessing competing molecular candidates, or (3) develop it in additional therapeutic areas or usages, thus turning the agreement terms unfavorable for the out-licensing biopharma.

Having mentioned all the pessimistic biopharma R&D scenarios above, we may have inadvertently labeled biopharmaceutical R&D overly unfavorable and risky to start with. However, the modern healthcare biotechnology industry is replete with stories of biopharmaceutical product candidates which initially failed in their R&D efforts, or were returned to their developers, and were later either fully developed in new indications, or managed to surpass their R&D obstacles and eventually triumphed in the marketplace even reaching blockbuster status.

START-UP CHALLENGES IN SALES AND MARKETING

Through the course of this book, we have talked about the defining differences between modern healthcare biotechnology and the traditional pharmaceutical industry. In the process, we have argued for biopharmaceutical industry's superiority in innovation, entrepreneurial spirit, cutting-edge research and development, as well as its propensity to take on challenging therapeutic problems.

Whatever those advantages may be, however, the biopharmaceutical industry is still faced with the same healthcare stakeholders, identical unmet medical needs, and the very same competitive battleground faced by big pharma themselves over their longer and equally challenging industry evolution. In other words, on the day of FDA approval, biopharma and big pharma become fierce competitors in the same pharmaceutical market, facing the same prescriber hesitations, patient demands, reimbursement authority doubts, and PBM threats that the new commercial biopharmaceutical may not live up to everyone's expectations and demands.

It is exactly this defining moment in a biopharmaceutical organization's life cycle that the function of marketing rises above all other functions, and is required to take over the company's efforts in identifying the product's unique selling points, segmenting, positioning, and targeting it versus the optimal segments, and finally communicating its unique product value versus that of competitive products. In addition, some of the previously approved products may be the therapeutic area "gold standards" at a fraction of the biopharmaceutical's cost, while the insurance providers may have severe financial constraints to face, or patients may be unwilling to pay their contributions for the yet untested new commercial alternative. Faced with these sales and marketing challenges, every biopharma organization must face head-on its new realities, and both quickly and effectively switch from a research-oriented organization to a more commercial, fast-paced, sales target–oriented, competitive, and "glossy" enterprise. Let us briefly take a look at what this paradigm-changing switch entails for the biopharma organization.

Disease Prevalence and Unmet Medical Need

Before the entire R&D plan was even conceived, the biopharma should have targeted a therapeutic area with a large incidence and prevalence base, as well as significant unmet medical needs. A large patient base, coupled with the majority of patients experiencing significant unmet needs leading to a poor quality of life, is giving impetus to the emerging commercial biopharma to quickly capture market share from less effective or safe therapeutic competitors, and later expand the market by either (1) educating undiagnosed patients to seek the advice of a physician, (2) providing diagnostic tools to prescribers in order to improve the disease diagnosis rate, (3) maintaining an active role in asking the global medical opinion leaders to create and cascade globally acceptable therapeutic guidelines, (4) improving the product's intrinsic value by offering improved formulations, friendlier administration routes and frequencies, or patient-friendly administration devices, and also (5) continuing the product's R&D development into additional disease phases (e.g., earlier or later stages), or even new therapeutic indications.

Product Portfolio

Having succeeded with their first commercial biopharmaceutical product introduction, most biopharmas quickly embark on supplementing this portfolio with additional pipeline or even in-licensed commercial products. The reasons are multiple, for example: (1) additional pipeline products confer increased company valuation, financing, stability, and sustainability, (2) a therapeutic area product franchise is critically important in providing prescribers, nurses, patients, and their carers with complete therapeutic solutions, (3) multiple products within the same therapeutic area create the branding and bundled-product opportunities for sales teams, while (4) additional products in different therapeutic areas attract more talent while also giving a signal to prescribers, patients, and investors that the organization is successful and sustainable and thus merits their preference and even championship.

Intellectual Property

A successful commercial biopharmaceutical introduction produces a growing revenue stream, a stable cash flow, a rising product profitability, as well as company valuation and capitalization over the long run. Armed with a newly discovered financial chest, biopharmas should quickly and efficiently move toward attracting additional intellectual property in-house, for example, through in-licensing acquisitions of pipeline or commercial products. Furthermore, for R&D obstacles still remaining in-house, significant investments need to be made in order to ensure the missing freedom to operate on the way to additional product approvals and commercial introductions.

Technology Platform

In addition to new IP brought in-house, the aspiring biopharma that has just launched its first commercial biopharmaceutical needs to strengthen its technology platform, by enhancing its existing capabilities (additional laboratory space, more lab devices, and more test animals) with additional research and development platforms. We have previously discussed the paramount importance of platform technologies in our discussion of various business models, where entire biopharmaceutical providers were based on specific technology platforms. In the case of our Advanced Therapies' poster-biopharma, its founders and present owners need to quickly identify missing gaps in their technology platform capabilities and fill them with investments that will give them a new boost in R&D capabilities and achievements.

Early Marketing (Premarketing)

Throughout this book, we have taken the reader through every single phase of a biopharmaceutical company's life cycle and analyzed the prerequisites and challenges along the way. However, although it may have appeared that a biopharma company's life cycle is a rigid sequential process, where financing follows licensing, and regulatory approval follows clinical trials, a single overarching company function remains of paramount importance over the company's entire life cycle.

This function is no other than marketing that has to be thoroughly planned, initiated, and followed early into the company's evolution, and later implemented continuously and forcefully throughout the company's life cycle. The reasons behind the absolute necessity for early marketing are the very fact that each biopharma faces numerous stakeholders along its life cycle. Therefore, even though in the absence of regulatory approval patients and prescribers are not the primary marketing target, still a large effort needs to be directed toward other "earlier" stakeholders, both external and internal. For example, new employees need to be enticed, potential investors need to be convinced, important opinion leaders and clinical investigators need to be recruited, and regulatory officials need to be informed of every aspect of the company's efforts. The entire company's existence thus depends on the introduction of early marketing, and the often young, science oriented, and untested company's founders remain to be convinced and become champions of marketing early on.

Stronger Marketing

As the biopharma start-up achieves its first product regulatory approval, sales and marketing organizations need to be already in place, specially selected, trained, and motivated, and following exact marketing plans detailing every single step of a huge marketing and branding effort, often on a global basis. Such marketing efforts of the early biopharmas were very science focused and limited in their extent in their earlier life cycle years. For example, (1) small marketing budgets were planned due to resource constraints, (2) small campaigns were planned only to prescribing specialists, (3) there were no direct-to-consumer promotion since all early biopharmaceuticals were seen as very "experimental," "complex," and hard to communicate, and (4) the public opinion was left uninformed or "unbiased" in an effort to avoid initial public doubts over the safety of a then-untested new technology.

The situation just described could not be further from the truth today! For example, (1) steady revenue streams have given rise to massive, global biopharmaceutical campaigns, (2) medical promotion is targeted not only to specialists but also to general pathologists (family doctors) who may be the "gatekeepers" to specialist referrals, (3) there is a significant DTC promotion of biopharmaceuticals, in an attempt to capture large patient populations, for example, in diabetes, and (4) the biopharma marketing efforts targeting the public opinion are now strong, focused, and coming from the vantage point of "experience," "proven superiority," and "life-saving efficacy."

START-UP CHALLENGES IN HUMAN RESOURCES

We have just discussed the most common challenges start-up biopharmas face in research, development, sales, and marketing. In addition to these, there is an overarching, and common denominator to all the previous key success factors (KSFs): the start-up's human resources. Countless reviews and benchmarking analyses have been issued on the essential traits a healthcare biotechnology company's human resources team needs to possess on the way to success and long-term sustainability. In addition, further analyses have focused on the paradigm-switching, critical changes a start-up biopharma is going through during its life cycle, resulting in a different set of capabilities and skills required by its workforce as the company matures.

The evolutionary steps of a start-up biopharma have been described earlier in this chapter. As far as the changes affecting its human resources over the company's life cycle are concerned, let us briefly focus on the bio-pharmaceutical start-up culture, as indicated in Table 14.1.

These characteristics, however, are soon to be tested, as the biopharma start-up progresses through the initial research and development phases and enters its first human clinical trials. Suddenly, the skills required by the company human resources enter a more competitive, fast-paced, and marketing-oriented stage. That is the time when the initially existing research and development talents are not enough to take the company forward on their own. As a consequence, new talent needs to attracted, possessing the following characteristics: (1) commercial marketing expertise

TABLE 14.1   What Is the Usual Biopharmaceutical Start-Up Culture?

University style—academic (origin)	Cutting edge science
Research predominates	Small companies
Scientists predominate	Team concepts for decision making
CEO and Board scientists	Best ideas predominate
Dress casual	Naiveté' in marketing and product needs
Communications very open and challenging	

Source: Evens, D.P., Biotechnology and Industry Research and Practice: Part 1—The Exploding Science, the Expanding Products, the Usage Challenges and Opportunities. University of Florida, College of Pharmacy Course PHA 5172, 2005, PowerPoint presentation posted at: http://www.cop.ufl.edu/safezone/pat/pha5172/evens-powerpoint-05.htm. With permission.

in the therapeutic area being developed, (2) medical affairs experience, (3) marketing planning and corporate strategy skills, (4) financial experience, especially in taking biopharmas through all rounds of financing and even initial public offerings (IPOs), (5) regulatory experience, (6) public relations and investor relations, (7) supply chain and biomanufacturing expertise, and (8) pricing, reimbursement, and managed markets experience.

It thus becomes apparent that a monumental change in prior experience and skills is taking place over the biopharma's precommercial evolution. As far as the minimum required capabilities and traits from all its human resources are concerned, the following are some of the most frequently mentioned prerequisites: (1) initial skills: scientific background, seed fund financing, business development, flexibility, resourcefulness, entrepreneurism, open-mindness, focus, and ownership, (2) later skills: venture capital financing, project management, marketing, sales, medical affairs, financial, IPO expertise, regulatory, PR, supply chain, manufacturing, pricing, and reimbursement, (3) essential traits: commitment, entrepreneurism, teamworking, and multitasking management.

Commitment

We have previously mentioned the defining differences between biopharma and big pharma. One of the most prominent differences is the lean and flat organizational graphs found within the more entrepreneurial biopharmas. Obviously, the lack of several hierarchical levels and skills commonly found in big pharma would require a higher degree of commitment from the much fewer, and more stressed biopharma employees. In general, such a commitment within the biopharma ranks is warranted by a higher exposure into exciting new areas of science, multiple organizational functions at the same time, as well as the increased potential for higher rewards, for example, a higher advancement through the various ranks, increased visibility within the industry and in the media, and also a significant potential for significant financial rewards in the form of company stock options.

Entrepreneurism

According to Iversen et al. (2008), the word entrepreneur was initially coined by Jean-Baptiste Say, a French economist, in about 1800, who proclaimed that an entrepreneur is "one who undertakes an enterprise, especially a contractor, acting as intermediatory between capital and labour." In the modern world of healthcare biotechnology, his definition still holds true after more than two centuries. In summary, a biotechnology entrepreneur is somebody who, armed with a strong scientific rationale and a resulting IP protection is willing to enter into an entirely new scientific domain, adapt within uncharted environments, withstand significant opposition and scepticism, and be persevering, target-oriented, focused, adaptive, pragmatic, and visionary.

Teamworking Skills

Academic biological science professionals are highly educated, extremely focused, introverted, and superspecialized on a single biological target or process. In fact, the author of this book as a holder of two successive postdoctorals in pharmacology can only verify the superspecialization that comes with the profession. There comes a time, however, when an invention idea strikes. The boldest and most entrepreneurial biological scientists will quickly transform their idea into a tangible commercial application, and seek for a patent. Depending on the patentability and other conditions, they may eventually decide to leave the relatively safe academic confines of research and set up a biotechnology start-up where teamworking and sharing everything with a core team of trusted colleagues is of paramount importance.

Multitasking Management

As previously mentioned, the core team of entrepreneurs initially manning a biopharma start-up is asked to fully embrace their start-up idea, to work very long hours with minimum or no pay, to endure countless disappointments and challenges, and find quick and efficient answers to a vast number of obstacles along the way. As their common background is often only biological sciences and they cannot afford the specialized services of experienced colleagues in additional company functions, they are forced to rise above the occasion, teamwork, compromise, adapt, and manage multiple tasks at the same time. Their efficiency in multitasking management is thus a prerequisite for the entire company's early viability and long-term sustainability.

COMPANY NETWORKING

In addition to the critical success factors for any biopharma we have reviewed above, there is still a plethora of other factors that may play an important role in the company's success and sustainability. Such additional factors include the degree and efficiency of the company's networking, its effectiveness in dealing with uncertainties, as well as its capability to successfully identify a future growth strategy and implement it. Let us start by focusing on the networking prerequisite.

Networking is essential for any healthcare biotechnology start-up around the world. This is due to the fact that the very nature of biopharmaceutical regulatory approval and commercial availability requires the networking and collaboration of countless specialists, found both internally or externally, and even professionals who can be active on the opposite side of the planet but still possess a critical skill needed for further biopharmaceutical development. In other words, how the company utilizes its internal personnel, and how efficiently and successfully it manages to interact with all its external stakeholders will dictate its future viability and success.

Focusing on external stakeholders, a biopharma is principally interacting with (1) academic institutions, (2) medical and other experts (regulatory, manufacturing, legal, etc.), (3) foreign partners (e.g., importers, distributors, PR companies, etc.), (4) other biopharma or big pharma corporations, and most importantly with (5) several government officials across the healthcare regulation spectrum, dispersed across the major national pharmaceutical markets the biopharma intends to enter. We start our analysis by focusing on networking with the first three groups (Rautiainen, 2001).

Networking

Networking of biopharma start-ups with academic investigators, medical opinion experts, other external experts critical for the company's multiple functions, and foreign partners is essential for the following reasons: (1) access to new ideas, (2) expert advice saving time and effort and avoiding risks, (3) strategic direction, and (4) preservation of the company's minute resources. Networking at this level can be achieved through (1) prior personal acquaintances of the company's founders, (2) direct contact and inclusion of external experts in company's advisory boards, (3) consulting arrangements, (4) company's attendance of important scientific, medical, or business development congresses, (5) through the company's Web site, and also (6) anonymously, through the company's involvement in innovation-centered, web-based think-tanks or innovation networks.

Clustering

The interaction of a biopharma start-up with the previous three groups of stakeholders, as well as with fellow biopharmaceutical or even big pharma companies can also be enhanced by the biopharma's location within a biotechnology cluster. Some of the most well-known global biotechnology cluster's include the San Francisco Bay area, Boston Houston, London, Cambridge, Medicon Valley, Biovalley BioAlps, and Shanghai. The common characteristics of such a cluster are (1) proximity of high-technology-focused academic institutions, (2) availability of free or subsidized research, development, IT, web, and library facilities, (3) availability of a specialized labor pool, (4) availability of research incentives, and (5) availability of angel or venture capital investors who are critical for the biopharma's evolution. The obvious advantages of a biotechnology cluster are shared facilities, informational exchange, employee mobility, and financing availability.

General Infrastructure

In the same way with clustering, general infrastructure interacts with the geographic location of a company. Endersby (1999) listed some critical factors in the infrastructure: transportation, telecommunications, energy, and education thereby maintaining prosperity and high quality of life.

National Policies

Gilmartin (1998) brought up national policies as an external success factor in a biopharmaceutical company. Some enabling activities that nations often provide include national, or federal, support of basic biomedical research, support for start-up companies, and tax reductions.

Company Climate

Small corporations possess a quality that cannot easily be transferred into a larger, well-established company: the small corporate environment. A small firm can offer the employees an entrepreneurial environment, technology enthusiasm, innovative climate, and culture. Lester (1998) emphasized the importance of entrepreneurial cross-functional teams, or venture teams, when developing a new product even in a larger company.

MATURITY CHALLENGES IN DEALING WITH UNCERTAINTY

Throughout the course of this book, we have overemphasized the tremendously arduous, long, capital-intensive, and risky road leading to healthcare biotechnology commercialization. Our own Advanced Therapies' brainchild has had its own ups and downs, which are still keeping the original founders awake at nights. In fact, the significant risks facing a biopharma do not stop by its first biopharmaceutical commercial launch, not even with its 10th consecutive launch for that. This is due to the fact that each and every biopharmaceutical remains susceptible to the occasional manufacturing mishaps, previously unforeseen side effect, or a potential financial crisis within the biopharma. For all these reasons, biopharmaceutical companies need to identify their potential sources of risk, study them in detail, and create a robust and effective lifelong plan to limit their occurrence or manage their consequences. In the next few paragraphs, we attempt to identify some of these biopharma life-threatening risks.

Sources of Uncertainty

The art of risk analysis is fundamentally about first identifying potential failures (categorizing events into "risk types"), then estimating the frequency of occurrence of these failures, and, finally determining the magnitude of the consequences. Risk can be divided into financial and nonfinancial risks.

Financial Risk

This is the risk of loss from holding investments that are subject to change in value with changing market conditions. This risk includes all changes in market conditions, such as prices, volatility, liquidity and credit risk, and the ability and willingness of counterparties to honor their contractual obligations.

Nonfinancial Risk

Market risk: This is the risk that investments can lose value due to changing market conditions including prices, volatility, and market liquidity.

Operational risks: This is the risk of loss arising due to the procedure errors, omissions, or failure of internal control systems. These risks are due to actions on or by people, processes, infrastructure, or technology or similar which have an operational impact, including fraudulent activities.

Regulatory risk: The risks of noncompliance with legal or regulatory requirements. There are two types of regulatory risk: one is compliance risk (incorporating approval process risk) and the other unregulated goods/services approval risk.

Legal risk: Intellectual property risk transforms could lead into "a new form of investment risk when rivals are unequally matched according to financial and human resources." Legal challenges of small biotech firms from larger more established and more resourced biotech firms may bankrupt the smaller firm or provide significant setbacks to product and market development.

Business risk: The risk of failing to achieve business targets due to inappropriate strategies, inadequate resources, or changes in the economic or competitive environment. Table 14.2 summarizes some well-known pharmaceutical product withdrawals from the marketplace after their commercial launch.

TABLE 14.2   Selected Pharmaceutical Product Withdrawals from the Marketplace after Their Commercial Launch

Date Approved	Drug Name	Use	Risks	Date Withdrawn
2004	Tysabri	Multiple sclerosis	Rare, frequently fatal demyelinating disease of CNS	2005
2001	Bextra	Pain reliever	Heart attack/stroke; fatal skin reactions	2005
1999	Vioxx	Pain reliever	Heart attack/stroke	2004
1997	Baycol	Cholesterol	Severe damage to muscle that is sometimes fatal	2001
1999	Raplon	Anesthesia	An inability to breathe normally	2001
1993	Propulsid	Heartburn	Fatal heart rhythm abnormalities	2000

Political risk: It is the risk that includes tax, trade, regulation, education, and social policies.

Industry risk: The risk associated with operating in a particular industry.

Environmental risks: The risk that an organization may suffer loss as a result of environmental damage caused by themselves or others which impacts on their business.

Risk Management by Biopharmas

According to Deloitte (2006), life sciences companies respond to these pressures and risks by taking steps that

- Feed product development pipelines with the help of alliances, joint ventures, in-licensing, and other strategies
- Meet production requirements through outsourcing, contract manufacturing, and alliances, which heighten concerns about quality, security, privacy, and control
- Work against lengthening development times
- Address increasing demand for lower priced products as well as a desire for higher returns
- Deal with a rising call from consumers for safer or risk-free breakthrough therapies
- Cope with heightened media scrutiny and escalating litigation

Source: Deloitte, The risk intelligent life sciences company, Deloitte Risk Intelligence Series, 4, 2006, Posted at: http://www.deloitte.com/assets/Dcom-Shared%20Assets/Documents/us_risk_intell_lifesci_180407.pdf

MATURITY CHALLENGES IN CHOOSING A GROWTH STRATEGY

According to Chatigny et al. (2003), the product life cycle of a drug is characterized by highly variable cash flows. Rather than the four main phases of a typical product life cycle (introduction, growth, maturity, and decline), prescription drugs have three distinct phases: discovery and approval, patent protection, and post-patent expiration. Based on this product life cycle, drug companies need to time the release of their products to protect their areas of competence and guard against periods of negative cash flow. As a result, smaller companies (e.g., biotechs) are at a strategic disadvantage over the long term.

Growth Options

Make, Buy, or License: For example, Johnson & Johnson has employed three vehicles, make, buy, and license to grow its product line. Of the company's top six revenue-producing drugs two were developed by J&J scientists, two were obtained by acquisition, and two were licensed in from other firms. The pros and cons of various business models for biopharmaceutical growth are shown in Table 14.3.

TABLE 14.3   What Are the Pros and Cons of Various Business Models for Biopharmaceutical Growth?

	Description	Pros	Cons
Outsourcing	Outsource art of R&D chain activities to a Chinese local vendor (or government research institution)	Time to test the water Broadened experience Cost savings Exit flexibility	The possibility that cost savings and vendor choices may be smaller than in other regions (e.g., India for chemistry) Limitation of lower complexity work because of IP concerns Risk of lower quality when using new vendors
Partnership or alliance	Provide scientific training and management oversight to a local vendor	Control over quality with management oversight Better communication and trust owing to the longer term relationship	The possibility of a partner taking capability elsewhere as a service provider and of the management-training effort being leverage by competitors
Captive investment	Build an R&D center from scratch Hire employees, or scientific staff	Larger commercial benefits Control over assets, skills, knowledge, and culture Quicker advancement into more complex work Fewer IP concerns	Lower cost savings Potential political risks (asset ownership) Potential regulatory risks

Source: Boston Consulting Group, 2005. A Game Plan for China: Rising to the Productivity Challenge in Biopharma R&D, Boston, MA, 2005, Posted at: http://www.bcg.com/documents/file14715.pdf. With permission.

The various healthcare biotechnology growth strategies used to date include

- Sustainable independent growth (bench to bedside)
- Traditional pharma-biotech relationship (at start of Phase IIb)
- Collaborative development (as early as at start of Phase I)
- Pharma's preferred relationship (at start of Phase III)
- Intra-biotech collaborative growth (bench to bedside)
- High-risk independent growth (bench to bedside)

Mergers

Since the late 1980s, the pharmaceutical industry has witnessed significant industry consolidation, most of which has occurred as a result of a spree of mergers between large commensurately sized industry players. These mergers can offer

- Broadening and/or specializing therapeutic focus
- Curtailing competition by building a dominant position in specific therapeutic areas
- Combining therapy area synergies to save costs and drive sales

For companies having similar therapeutic area focus, current revenues for products under patent are combined, while concurrently containing costs through the elimination of redundant support organizations (sales and marketing). There are similar effects on the pipeline of drugs still in development.

Organic Growth

A second alternative is organic growth. Pharmaceutical companies traditionally invested in R&D to grow their product pipelines. Historical performance has demonstrated that allocating more resources to internal R&D projects does not sustain long-term growth. As a result of the power of institutional buyers, the industry has trended toward a focus on volume growth as opposed to price-driven growth. Firms choosing not to merge cannot keep pace with the R&D potential of merging firms. Moreover, increased R&D activity tends to raise unit costs and reduce the return on capital demands.

According to Chatigny et al. (2003), large firms resisting major mergers have increasingly pursued alternative means to cooperate and compete with merging firms. Companies can build a "virtual mass" by forming a network of alliances with various industry players to achieve growth. Codevelopment and copromotion agreements permit firms to boost their late-stage pipelines, while allowing the participants to maintain long-term strategic and operational flexibility.

QUESTIONS

1. Which are the main steps in the biopharmaceutical organizational life cycle?
2. What are some of the most common challenges in R&D faced by healthcare biotechnology start-ups?
3. How early in a biopharma's organizational life cycle is marketing needed?
4. How does a start-up biopharma prepare its product reimbursement plan?
5. What are the main employee skills a biopharma start-up should be looking for in all its new hires across functions?
6. How important is networking and what are the main potential partners of a start-up biopharma?
7. Which are the main sources of uncertainty for a start-up biopharma?
8. What are the main risk minimization strategies that a start-up biopharma should employ?
9. What are the pros and cons of various business models for biopharmaceutical growth?
10. What is meant by "organic growth" of biopharmaceutical companies? Can you provide recent actual examples?

EXERCISES

1. You are a start-up biopharma entrepreneur with a promising product portfolio in preclinical development. What are the potential commercialization scenarios for your early product candidates? What are their respective pros and cons?
2. You are an American biopharma entrepreneur in close liaison with your U.S. (doctoral) and your U.K. (postdoctoral) alma mater. You are now at the crossroads of company incorporation. Which location would you choose, and what is the rationale behind each?

3. You are the CEO of a start-up biopharma making the transition from preclinical to clinical research for its main product, requiring a significant new financing effort. What additional skills and functions does your company need at this point?

4. You are an experienced business development executive hired by a biopharmaceutical start-up. What activities and organizations do you suggest to your board of directors for the better networking of your organization with academia, big pharma, and foreign partners?

5. Which are the main biotechnology clusters in the United Kingdom and Germany? How do you compare the two sides as far a new biopharma start-up is concerned?

6. Describe in brief the efforts of three major bionations in support of their national biotechnology initiatives.

7. Your company's biopharmaceutical pipeline is exposed to various regulatory risks. What are the main sources of these risks and how do you tackle them?

8. You are the head of a biopharma's R&D department developing a new psoriasis biopharmaceutical, until your business development colleagues come up with an important in-licensing opportunity for the same indication. How do you evaluate the pros and cons of either approach?

9. Pick one of the top biopharmaceutical companies in the world. Then, by studying its web pages, describe one example each for (a) an internally developed product, (b) an in-licensed product, (c) an out-licensed product, and (d) a discontinued one.

10. As CEO of a young biopharma you are about to set up your first foreign subsidiaries. What countries do you select, how do you proceed, and what budgets do you foresee for each subsidiary?

REFERENCES

Boston Consulting Group, 2005. A game plan for China: Rising to the productivity challenge in biopharma R&D, Boston, MA. Posted at: http://www.bcg.com/documents/file14715.pdf

Business Insights, 2008. *Biotech M&A Strategies: Deal Assessments, Trends and Future Prospects*. Business Insights Ltd: London, October 2008.

Chatigny, N., Higginbotham, K., Walsh, J., and Williams, K., 2003. Growth strategies in the pharmaceutical industry: Strategic acquisition. April 29, 2003. Posted at: http://www.mcafee.cc/Classes/BEM106/Papers/UTexas/2003/JandJ.pdf

Deloitte, 2006. The risk intelligent life sciences company. Deloitte Risk Intelligence Series, 4, 2006. Posted at: http://www.deloitte.com/assets/Dcom-Shared%20Assets/Documents/us_risk_intell_lifesci_180407.pdf

Endersby, J.M., 1999. Kick-starting biotechnology in Ontario. *Nature Biotechnology* 17: 444–446.

Ernst & Young, 2009. *Beyond Borders: The Global Biotechnology Report 2009.* E&Y: Boston, MA.

Evens, D.P., 2005. Biotechnology and industry research and practice: Part 1—The exploding science, the expanding products, the usage challenges and opportunities. University of Florida, College of Pharmacy Course PHA 5172. PowerPoint presentation posted at: http://www.cop.ufl.edu/safezone/pat/pha5172/evens-powerpoint-05.htm

Gilmartin, R.V., 1998. Winning in pharmaceutical research. *Research Technology Management* 41(4): 9–12.

Iversen, J., Jorgensen, R., and Malchow-Moller, N. 2008. Foundations and Trends in Entrepreneurship, 4(1), January 2008.

Lester, D.H., 1998. Critical success factors for new product development. *Research Technology Management* 41(1): 36–43.

Rautiainen, T., 2001. *Critical Success Factors in Biopharmaceutical Business a Comparison Between Finnish and Californian Businesses.* TEKES: Helsinki, Finland, Technology Review, p. 113.

U.S. Supreme Court *Diamond vs. Chakrabarty*, 1980. 447 U.S. 303 (1980)–447 U.S. 303–No. 79–136. Argued March 17, 1980. Decided June 16, 1980.

Appendices

APPENDIX A: LIST OF ABBREVIATIONS

ANDA	Abbreviated New Drug Application
ATC	Anatomical therapeutic chemical
BD	Business development
BDI	Brand-driven innovation
Biotechs	Biotechnology companies
BLA	Biologics license application
CBER	Center for Biologics Evaluation and Research
CDER	Center for Drugs Evaluation and Research
CGMP	Current good manufacturing practice
CMS	Centers for Medicare and Medicaid Services
CNS	Central nervous system—neurology
CRM	Customer relationship manager
CRO	Clinical Research Organization
CTA	Clinical trial application
CTM	Clinical trial material
DMF	Drug master file
DOE	Department of Energy (United States)
EC	Environment Canada
EMEA	European Agency for the Evaluation of Medicinal Products
EPO	Erythropoietin
FD&C	Food, Drug and Cosmetic Act
FDA	Food and Drug Administration
FDAMA	Food and Drug Administration Modernization Act
FIPCO	Fully Integrated Pharmaceutical Company
FTO	Freedom to operate
GMP	Good manufacturing practices
HC	Health Canada

IND	Investigational new drug
IP	Intellectual property
IRB	Institutional Review Board
MHRA	Medicines and Healthcare Products Regulatory Agency
NCE	New chemical entity
NDA	New drug application
NICE	National Institute for Health and Clinical Excellence (United Kingdom)
NME	New molecular entities
NPD	New product development
ODA	Orphan Drug Act
OECD	Organization for Economic Cooperation and Development
OTC	Over-the-counter
PDUFA	Prescription Drug User Fee Act
Pharma	Pharmaceutical companies
PhRMA	Pharmaceutical Research and Manufacturers of America
PHS	Act Public Health Service Act
PM	Project manager
PMA	Premarket approval
R&D	Research and development
RCT	Randomized controlled (clinical) trial
RFP	Request for proposal
ROI	Return on investment
SOP	Standard operating procedure
TRIPS	Agreement on trade-related aspects of intellectual property rights
VC	Venture capitalist
WHO	World Health Organization
WIPO	World Intellectual Property Organization
WTO	World Trade Organization

APPENDIX B: BIOPHARMACEUTICAL MARKETING PLAN OUTLINE

1 Executive Summary
2 Core Analysis
   2.1 Company Resources
   2.2 Product Strengths and Weaknesses

APPENDIX C: LIST OF NAMES

454 Life Sciences
AAH Pharmaceuticals
Abbott Laboratories
Abingworth Management
Abseamed
Academy of Managed Care Pharmacy (AMCP)
Acceleron
Accordant
Accredo Health, Inc.
Aclara
Actavis
Actemra
Activase
AD_THER_51
ADTHER57
Advanced Cell Technology, Inc.
Advanced Therapies
AdvancePCS
Advate
Affymetrix
Afinitor
Africa
African Regional Industrial Property Organization (ARIPO)
Agennix, Inc.
Agreement on Trade Related Aspects of Intellectual Property Rights (TRIPS)

Albany Molecular Research
Albuferon (albinterferon alfa-2b)
Albumin
Alcimed
Aldurazyme
Alere
All India Biotechnology Association
AllianceBernstein
Alloy Ventures
Allston Landing
Alnylam
Alpheon
Altana Pharma
Alteplase
Ambien CR
American Association for the Accreditation of Laboratory Animal Care
    International (AAALAC International)
American College of Rheumatology
American Express (AMEX)
American Lung Association
American Marketing Association
American Medical Association (AMA)
American Neurological Association
American Society for Microbiology
American Society of Health System Pharmacists (ASHP)
Amerisource
Amevive
Amgen
Amgen Ventures
Amicore
Amitiza
AmpliChip
Angel Capital Association (ACA)
Ann Arbor, MI
Annenberg School of Communication, University of Southern California
Antithrombin
APP Pharma
Applied Biosystems
Aprotinin

China
Cialis
Ciba-Geigy
Cimzia
Cincinnati, OH
Cinryze
Cipla
Citigroup
City of Hope National Medical Center
Claritin
Coartem
Cohen, Stanley
Coley
Columbia University
Committee for Orphan Medicinal Products (COMP)
Copaxone
Copegus
Copenhagen
Cora Biomanufacturing
Cornell University
Coumadin
Crédit Agricole Private Equity
Crick, Francis
Crixivan
Croatia
Crucell N.V.
CT Arzneimittel
Cuba
Cumberland Pharmaceuticals
CuraScript Pharmacy, Inc.
CVS/Caremark Rx, Inc.
Cyanokit
Cyclacel
Cyprus
Cystadane
Czech Republic
DAG Ventures
Datamonitor
Decision Resources

Synagis
Synexis Chemistry & Automation
Syngenta Biotechnology
Synta
Synvisc
T. Rowe Price
Taiho Pharmaceutical Co., Ltd.
Takeda
Talactoferrin
Tamoxifen
Tanox
Tarceva
Tarumi, Yuzo
Tasigna
Taxol
TCA Cellular Therapy
Teachers' Private Capital
Tegretol
Temodar
Tenecteplase
Teradata magazine
Teva (now acquired Sicor)
Teva Generics
Teva Pharma United States
Teva Pharmaceuticals
Teva/Barr
Tevagrastim
Thalidomide
Thalomid
The Wellcome Trust
Thelin
Therapies
Thomson Financial
Thomson Medical Economics
Thousand Oaks, CA
ThromboGenics
Thymoglobulin
Thyrogen
Tissue Plasminogen Activator

Xolair
Xyntha
Xyrem
Yahoo
Yale University
Yondelis
YouTube
Zactima
Zantac
Zarzio
Zavesca
Zenapax
Zentiva
zeta
Ziagen
Zocor
Zolinza
Zometa
Zurich
Zymogenetics

Index

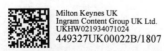